POCKET GUIDE TO UROLOGY

Sixth Edition

Volume 1: Oncology

Jeff A. Wieder, M.D.

IMPORTANT NOTICE

- This book is intended for use by health care professionals.
- During our rigorous attempts to make *Pocket Guide to Urology* accurate, we have depended on references that are presumed to be true and correct. Typographical errors, printing errors, omissions, and inaccuracies may be present despite our meticulous efforts to make the contents of this book error-free. The information in this book may be inaccurate, incomplete, and out of date. Health care professionals should verify the information contained within this text before applying it to any circumstance.
- This book provides methods of working up, diagnosing, and treating various medical conditions. There may be alternatives that are not listed. This book is not meant to serve as a strict guideline, but rather to provide suggestions to consider when making *your* decision regarding the work up and treatment of a patient. Appropriate work up and treatment must be determined by the health care professional based on each patient's unique circumstance.
- This book is not a substitute for appropriate medical training and education.
- Some medications and medical devices listed in this book are not approved by the Food and Drug Administration (FDA) for the indication given herein. Furthermore, this book does not provide complete or current prescribing information. Before prescribing any medication or medical device (including the ones listed within this book), the health care provider should completely read a product's label, package insert, instructions, and prescribing information and should be aware of a product's appropriate use, including (but not limited to) its FDA status, its FDA approved indications, contraindications, dose, route of administration, adverse reactions, drug interactions, and duration of therapy.
- The information in this book is subject to change at any time.
- This book comes without warranties and guarantees expressed or implied. The author, publisher, editors, and sponsors disclaim any and all liability, injury, loss, damage, expense, and any other consequences caused by the use, misuse, or application of the information in *Pocket Guide to Urology.*
- If you do not want to be bound by the conditions, stipulations, and warnings listed above, other reference books are available for your use.

ISBN # 978-0-9672845-7-6
Printed in the United States of America

Produced by J. Wieder Medical
www.pocketguidetourology.com

POCKET GUIDE TO UROLOGY

Sixth Edition

_____

"If I have been able to see farther than others, it was because I stood on the shoulders of giants."
—Sir Isaac Newton

In the references, consensus statements, guidelines, and best practice policies are in bold print. I encourage you to read these publications on your own. With your support, I hope to continue improving and updating the *Pocket Guide to Urology*. Thanks to all the professors, residents and co-workers who contributed to my education and helped make this book a reality.

Jeff A. Wieder, M.D.

To order additional copies of this book and for more information, please visit my website:

www.pocketguidetourology.com

CONTENTS

Volume 1: Oncology

Volume 2: Non-oncology

Voiding & Incontinence

Hematuria, Urolithiasis, Strictures, & Imaging

Pregnancy, Development, & Pediatric

CONTENTS

RENAL TUMORS

Presentation
1. Many tumors are found incidentally during the evaluation of unrelated medical issues; therefore, renal tumors are often asymptomatic.
2. Symptoms include flank pain, hematuria, weight loss, fever, and sweats.
3. Signs include flank mass, hypertension, new varicocele (especially rapid onset), and paraneoplastic syndromes (see page 12).
4. The classic triad (flank mass, hematuria, and flank pain) is now rare because tumors are often detected incidentally at a low stage. The presence of the classic triad signifies advanced disease.

Work Up

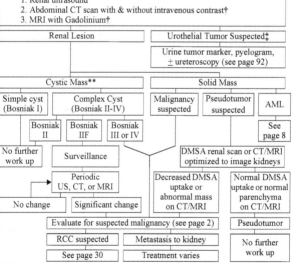

AML = angiomyolipoma, RCC = renal cell carcinoma, US = ultrasound,
CT = computerized tomography, MRI = magnetic resonance imaging
* Complex cysts and solid renal masses should be evaluated with CT and/or MRI.
† Inspect tumor size and location (is it amenable to nephron sparing surgery?), renal vein and vena cava (is tumor thrombus present?), contralateral kidney (is it normal?), adrenal glands, lymph nodes, and other organs (are metastases present?)
** See Imaging of Renal Cysts on page 469 and Bosniak Classification on page 469.
‡ Centrally located tumors, especially those that appear to fill the collecting system, are suspicious for urothelial carcinoma.

1

Evaluation of Suspected Renal Malignancy

1. Physical exam—including blood pressure, skin exam, and lymph node exam. Hypertension may be caused by a paraneoplastic syndrome from RCC (see page 12) or by a juxtaglomerular tumor. Skin lesions that are associated with genetic renal tumor syndromes are shown below.

Skin Lesion	Description	Syndrome
Adenoma sebaceum	Pink or red colored papules, usually overlying the cheek bones or the nasolabial folds.	Tuberous Sclerosis
Ash-leaf spots	Hypopigmented macules on the trunk or buttock.	
Shagreen patches	Orange-peel textured plaques on the lower back.	
Periungual fibromas	Flesh-colored papules near the nail bed.	
Fibrofolliculomas	Small white or flesh-colored papules on the face, neck, back, or upper trunk.	BHD
Cutaneous Leiomyoma	Small pink-purple papules in the same location as hair follicles. The papules are often painful.	HL RCC
Papillomas	Hard smooth flesh colored papules, usually on the face, lips, mouth, hands, and feet.	PTEN Hamartoma (Cowden) Syndrome
Trichilemmomas	Wart-like flesh colored papules, typically on the face or dorsum of the hands and feet.	
Keratosis	Skin thickening on the palms of the hands and/or on the soles of the feet.	
Glans Macules	Macular pigmentation of the glans penis.	

BHD = Birt-Hogg-Dubé Syndrome
HL RCC = Hereditary Leiomyomatosis Renal Cell Carcinoma.

2. Obtain imaging until the mass is adequately characterized (see page 1). If vena cava invasion is suspected, obtain an abdominal and chest MRI.
3. Obtain lab tests—BUN, creatinine, alkaline phosphatase, liver function tests, LDH, serum calcium, complete blood count, and urinalysis. If urinalysis shows proteinuria, obtain a quantitative measure of urine protein (such as spot urine protein/creatinine ratio, spot urine albumin/creatinine ratio, or 24 hour urine for protein).
4. Assign a chronic kidney disease (CKD) stage using proteinuria level and calculated glomerular filtration rate (GFR).
5. For patients with renal dysfunction, consider pre-treatment referral to a nephrologist, especially in patients with pre-treatment GFR < 45 ml/min, proteinuria, medical diseases that could worsen renal function (such as diabetes mellitus, hypertension, etc.), or when their post-treatment GFR is expected to be less than 30 ml/min.
6. Measurement of differential renal function by renal scan may help guide therapy, especially when the contralateral kidney is small or appears to have decreased function based on the CT or MRI nephrogram.
7. Obtain a chest x-ray or chest CT—obtain a chest CT if the patient has an abnormal chest x-ray, pulmonary symptoms, or higher risk for metastasis.
8. If the patient has bone pain, hypercalcemia, elevated alkaline phosphatase, bone fracture, or suspicious bone lesions on other imaging, then obtain a bone scan. Hypercalcemia and elevated alkaline phosphatase may be caused by bone metastases or by a paraneoplastic syndrome (see page 12)
9. If neurologic exam is abnormal or neurologic symptoms are present, obtain a brain MRI to look for metastasis and for lesions associated with von Hippel Lindau and tuberous sclerosis. Spine imaging should be performed if symptoms or exam suggest the spinal cord is affected.
10. In women at risk for breast cancer, consider performing a breast exam and a mammogram (breast cancer may metastasize to the kidney).
11. Biopsy of the renal lesion may be indicated in some cases.

Biopsy of Renal Masses

1. In general, *biopsy of a solid or complex cystic renal mass is not necessary before excision because most of these lesions are malignant.* The AUA 2021 guideline states that biopsy of a suspicious renal mass is "not required" for young healthy patients who are unwilling to accept the uncertainties associated with biopsy or for older or frail patients who will be managed conservatively regardless of the biopsy results. Although biopsy is not part of the standard evaluation, it should be considered when:
   a. There is suspicion that the renal lesion may be infectious, inflammatory, angiomyolipoma, lymphoma, or a tumor metastatic to the kidney.
   b. A candidate for nephrectomy that chooses to undergo surveillance, ablation, or embolization.
   c. To confirm the diagnosis of RCC before systemic therapy in a patient with metastases who is not a candidate for cytoreductive or palliative nephrectomy. In this case, the renal lesion or a metastatic lesion may be biopsied.
2. Renal mass biopsy technique—biopsy is performed percutaneously under CT or ultrasound guidance using a 16 or 18 gauge needle. *The biopsy needle is advanced coaxially through a sheath to minimize the risk of tumor seeding along the biopsy tract. At least 2 to 3 cores should be taken from each mass. Core biopsy is preferred over fine needle aspiration (FNA) because core biopsy has a higher diagnostic yield.*
3. Diagnostic yield
   a. Renal mass biopsy is nondiagnostic in approximately 14% of cases; however, a repeat biopsy will be usually be diagnostic. When the initial biopsy is nondiagnostic, cancer is usually discovered on subsequent biopsies.
   b. The negative predictive value of a benign biopsy is approximately 63-80% (which means that 20-37% of patients with a benign biopsy will actually have a cancer). For example, in the rare situation when RCC coexists with oncocytoma, a false negative biopsy can arise when the needle samples only the benign oncocytoma.
   c. The positive predictive value of a malignant biopsy is 99.8% (which means that only 0.2% of patients with a malignant biopsy will actually have a benign lesion).
   d. The concordance of biopsy pathology and surgical pathology is approximately 50-75% for tumor grade and > 75% for RCC type. Grade can vary within a tumor and biopsies may miss the area of maximum grade. In one study, the risk of underestimating tumor grade was 16% (in patients with low grade cancer on preoperative biopsy, 16% had high grade tumor in the nephrectomy specimen).
4. Side effects
   a. Serious side effects occur in 1% of cases, and include bleeding requiring transfusion, severe pain, pneumothorax, and severe infection.
   b. Tumor seeding along the biopsy tract—tumor seeding is rare (estimated to be < 0.01% of cases, with less than 30 cases reported since 1977, but several cases reported after 2010). Tumor seeding is more likely when the biopsy is done with a needle ≥ 20 gauge and without a coaxial sheath. Thus, *biopsy of a renal mass should use a needle < 20 gauge and a coaxial sheath to minimize the risk of tumor seeding along the biopsy tract.* Biopsy of a cystic mass may have a higher risk of tumor spillage.
5. Metastatic melanoma and renal angiomyolipoma (AML) stain positive for HMB-45. If a biopsy of a renal tumor stains positive for HMB-45, then it is usually either AML or melanoma.

General Information About Renal Masses

Primary Renal Masses
1. Benign examples
   a. Simple renal cyst—the most common benign renal mass.
   b. Papillary adenoma—the most common benign *solid* renal mass.
   c. Other examples include pseudotumors, angiomyolipoma (AML), oncocytoma, juxtaglomerular tumor, multilocular cystic nephroma, and mesoblastic nephroma.
2. Malignant examples
   a. Renal cell carcinoma (RCC)—the most common primary renal cancer in adults.
   b. Wilms' tumor—the most common primary renal cancer in children.
   c. Other examples include clear cell sarcoma and rhabdoid tumor.

Secondary Renal Masses (Metastases to Kidney)
Metastases to kidney (listed most common to least common):
1. Lymphoma/leukemia
2. Lung
3. Breast
4. Other less common sites include stomach, colon, cervix, and melanoma.

Pseudotumors
1. These appear to be solid renal masses on some imaging studies, but are actually *normal* renal parenchyma. Examples include column of Bertin, fetal lobation, dromedary hump, hilar lip or uncus, and nodular compensatory hypertrophy.
2. The following imaging studies can help differentiate pseudotumors from true tumors: CT optimized to examine the kidneys, MRI optimized to examine the kidneys, and DMSA renal scan. On DMSA renal scan, pseudotumors have normal isotope uptake, whereas true tumors have decreased isotope uptake.
3. Dromedary hump—a focal bulge at mid-lateral kidney thought to be from downward pressure from the spleen or liver during development. It is more common on the left.

Relative Frequency of Renal Neoplasms
1. Small solid renal masses are more likely to be benign than large renal masses (20% of solid masses $\leq$ 4 cm are benign, whereas only 8% of masses > 4 cm are benign).
2. Solid masses are usually malignant. The most common solid renal mass in adults is renal cell carcinoma (RCC).

Solid Primary Renal Tumor	Relative Frequency*
Clear cell RCC	65%
Papillary RCC	10-15%
Chromophobe RCC	5-10%
Unclassified RCC	1-4%
Collecting duct carcinoma	< 1%
Oncocytoma	7%
Angiomyolipoma	1-2%

* When lesions of all sizes are included.

Bosniak Classification of Cystic Renal Masses
See page 469 for details. Bosniak I and II masses are usually benign; thus no treatment or follow up are required. IIF lesions are monitored. Bosniak III and IV lesions are usually malignant and are treated with surgical excision.

Hereditary Syndromes & Genetic Testing

Compared to sporadic RCC, RCC caused by a genetic syndrome is more likely to occur at an earlier age and is more likely to be multifocal.

Germline Genetic Testing and Genetic Counseling
1. Genetic counseling (with possible germline genetic testing) is recommended for patients with any of the following characteristics.
   a. Diagnosed with renal cancer at ≤ 46 years of age.
   b. Multifocal or bilateral renal masses (synchronous or metachronous).
   c. The tumor pathology suggests a genetic syndrome (e.g. a mixture of RCC and oncocytoma suggests Birt-Hogg Dubé syndrome).
   d. Personal history that suggests a genetic syndrome (e.g. a female with a prior breast cancer who develops RCC may have a CHEK2 mutation).
   e. Family history suggests a genetic syndrome.

Examples of Hereditary Syndromes Associated with Renal Tumors

Hereditary Syndrome	Gene	Renal Tumor Type(s)
von Hippel Lindau	VHL	Clear Cell RCC
BAP1 Syndrome	BAP1	Clear Cell RCC
CHEK2 Syndrome	CHEK2	Clear Cell RCC
Chromosome 3 Translocation Syndrome	Chromosome 3	Clear Cell RCC
PTEN Hamartoma (Cowden) Syndrome	PTEN	Clear Cell RCC
Hereditary Papillary RCC Type 1	MET	Papillary RCC type 1
Hereditary Leiomyomatosis RCC†	FH	Papillary RCC type 2†
Birt-Hogg Dubé (BHD)	FLCN	*RCC mixed with oncocytoma,* Oncocytoma alone, and Chromophobe RCC alone*
Succinate Dehydrogenase (SDH) Deficiency RCC†	SDH (subunits B, C, & D)	RCC (various types)†
Tuberous Sclerosis	TSC1, TSC2	RCC (various types), AML

RCC = renal cell carcinoma; AML = angiomyolipoma
* These patients also rarely develop clear cell RCC.
† RCC in these genetic syndromes tends to behave aggressively; thus, surveillance for these tumors is not recommended (even if the tumors are small).

Birt-Hogg-Dubé Syndrome (BHD)
1. BHD may cause skin fibrofolliculomas, air filled pulmonary cysts, spontaneous pneumothorax, and renal tumors.
2. Fibrofolliculomas are benign small white or flesh-colored papules on the face, neck, back, or upper trunk and usually appear after age 20.
3. Approximately 25% of people with BHD develop renal tumors. Most develop bilateral renal tumors and multiple tumors per kidney. Renal tumors that develop include clear cell RCC, chromophobe RCC, oncocytoma, and *mixture of oncocytoma and RCC. Any patient who presents with oncocytoma and RCC should be evaluated for BHD.*
4. BHD is autosomal dominant. BHD arises from mutations in the FLCN gene on chromosome 17.

PTEN Hamartoma (Cowden) Syndrome
1. This disorder results from a mutation in the PTEN gene.
2. RCC develops in up to 35% of cases (usually clear cell RCC).
3. This syndrome is associated with RCC, breast cancer, endometrial cancer, thyroid cancer, macular pigmentation of the glans penis, skin lesions (papillomas, trichilemmomas, keratosis), macrocephaly, and autism.

Hereditary Leiomyomatosis Renal Cell Carcinoma

1. This rare disorder results from a mutation in the fumarate hydratase gene (FH).
2. RCC develops in 15% of cases (usually type 2 papillary RCC).
3. *RCC in these patients usually behaves very aggressively; thus surveillance for these tumors is not recommended.*
4. Patients typically have cutaneous leiomyomas. Females may have uterine leiomyomas (fibroids).

Tuberous Sclerosis

1. The classic triad of tuberous sclerosis (*mental retardation, seizures, and adenoma sebaceum*) is seen in only 30% of cases.
2. Tuberous sclerosis is an autosomal dominant disease caused by a mutation of the TSC1 gene (chromosome 9) or the TSC2 gene (chromosome 16).
3. Tuberous sclerosis causes hamartomas, which usually occur in the retina, brain (cerebral cortex tubers, subependymal nodules, subependymal giant cell astrocytomas), skin (adenoma sebaceum), kidney (angiomyolipoma), lung (lymphangioleiomyomatosis), and heart (cardiac rhabdomyomas).
4. Urologic manifestations—renal cysts, angiomyolipoma (AML), or RCC may develop.
   a. Renal cysts usually develop in childhood.
   b. 60% of adults with tuberous sclerosis develop AML, with most patients having multiple and/or bilateral AML.
   c. There is an increased risk for renal cell carcinoma (2% develop RCC). RCC can be of any type.
5. Adenoma sebaceum are pink or red colored papules usually on the skin overlying the nasolabial folds or the cheek bones. They appear between age 4 and puberty and may be mistaken for acne. Other skin manifestations include hypopigmented macules on the trunk or buttocks (ash-leaf spots), orange-peel textured plaques on the lower back (shagreen patches), and flesh-colored papules near the nail bed (ungual or periungual fibromas).

von Hippel Lindau (VHL)

1. VHL is an autosomal dominant disorder caused by mutation of the VHL gene on chromosome 3p, with manifestations that may include
   a. Non-urologic—cerebellar hemangioblastomas, spinal hemangioblastomas, and retinal angiomas.
   b. Urologic—renal cysts (75%), clear cell RCC (50%), pheochromocytomas (15%), epididymal cystadenomas (10%), and epididymal cysts (7%).
2. Renal cell carcinoma
   a. Clear cell RCC occurs in 50% of patients with VHL.
   b. VHL is associated with mutation of chromosome 3p; therefore, *clear cell RCC is the most common renal cancer in VHL.*
   c. RCC is often multi-focal and bilateral.
   d. RCC develops at an earlier age in VHL (usual age < 40 years) than in sporadic RCC (usual age > 40 years).
   e. In patients with VHL, all renal cysts (including simple cysts) have malignant potential.
3. In patients with VHL and a renal neoplasm, surveillance of renal masses < 3 cm is reasonable because these masses have a low metastatic potential. When intervention is indicated, renal sparing therapy is the treatment of choice. If extensive bilateral RCC is present and renal sparing surgery is not possible, treatment usually consists of bilateral nephrectomy and dialysis.

Benign Renal Tumors

Papillary Adenoma

1. Papillary adenoma are usually found incidentally during autopsy.
2. An adenoma is a lesion < 5 mm in size whose microscopic appearance is similar to low grade papillary renal cell carcinoma. Microscopically, papillary adenoma and papillary RCC are indistinguishable. However, the benign behavior of lesions < 5 mm is inferred based on the frequency of adenomas and the rarity of metastases.
3. Adenomas arise from the proximal tubule and have similar cytogenetic abnormalities as papillary RCC.

Oncocytoma

1. Oncocytoma is a benign renal tumor that arises from the collecting duct and is composed of oncocytes (oncocytes are cells with an *eosinophilic* granular cytoplasm). "Malignant" oncocytomas have been reported, but these were probably chromophobe RCC or oncocytoma mixed with RCC that were misdiagnosed as pure oncocytoma.
2. Presentation—most common in males age 40-60 years. They may be asymptomatic or symptomatic.
3. Imaging
   a. Oncocytoma cannot be distinguished from RCC using imaging studies; therefore, it is often treated as RCC.
   b. Arteriogram may show a *"spoke wheel"* pattern of tumor arterioles with a lucent rim around the tumor (from the avascular capsule). However, these findings are not specific for oncocytoma and can occur with RCC.
4. Pathology
   a. Gross—mahogany or tan mass with a fibrous capsule and *often with a central scar.* Necrosis and hemorrhage are rare.
   b. Microscopic—*nests* of polygonal cells with a granular *eosinophilic* cytoplasm. Mitoses and necrosis are rare.
   c. Electron microscopy—*the cytoplasm is packed with mitochondria.*
   d. It may be difficult to distinguish between chromophobe RCC and oncocytoma (see Chromophobe RCC, page 9).
   e. Approximately 10% of oncocytomas will also contain RCC, although the range reported in the literature is 2-32%.
5. Treatment—surgical excision is the treatment of choice because
   a. Imaging cannot distinguish between RCC and oncocytoma.
   b. RCC may coexist with oncocytoma.
   c. Renal biopsy cannot rule out coexisting malignant elements.

Juxtaglomerular Tumor

1. A rare benign renin-secreting tumor that arises from the juxtaglomerular apparatus. They are usually < 3 cm in diameter.
2. Presentation—young (average age is 25 years old), diastolic hypertension, headaches, elevated renin, and hyperaldosteronism with hypokalemia.
3. Treatment—nephron sparing excision is the treatment of choice.

Mesoblastic Nephroma—see page 46.

Multilocular Cystic Nephroma—see page 46.

Metanephric Adenoma/Metanephric Adenofibroma

1. Metanephric tumors are benign, and very rare.
2. They consist of small uniform tubules lined with cuboidal epithelium.

Angiomyolipoma (AML)
1. AML is a benign renal mass composed of blood vessels (angio), smooth muscle (myo), and fat (lipo).
2. Presentation
   a. AML occurs most often in the following populations.
      i. Females age 40-60 years.
      ii. Tuberous sclerosis—up to 60% of patients with tuberous sclerosis develop AML, usually multiple and bilateral. However, most patients with AML do not have tuberous sclerosis. See page 6.
   b. AML is often asymptomatic. If symptoms develop, they may include flank pain, hematuria, and hemorrhage with hypotension.
   c. AML ≥ 4 cm are more likely to be symptomatic and to hemorrhage.
3. Imaging and diagnosis

	AML Size	
	< 4 cm	≥ 4 cm
Symptomatic	0-24%	46-82%
Hemorrhage	0-13%	33-51%

   a. AML is rarely calcified. A calcified solid renal mass is probably RCC.
   b. CT scan—AML enhances (indicating vascularity) and *Hounsfield units (HU) are usually -20 to -80 on noncontrast CT* (indicating fat content). AML can be diagnosed by CT scan if its classic features are present (enhancing, HU = -20 to -80, homogenous, not calcified, and not cystic).
   c. Ultrasound—AML is hyperechoic. AML cannot be diagnosed using ultrasound because AML and RCC may look similar on ultrasound.
   d. *Among renal masses, HMB-45 expression usually occurs only in AML and metastatic melanoma. If a primary renal mass stains positive for HMB-45, then it is an AML and not an RCC.*
   e. If CT scan cannot confirm AML, options include surgical removal or percutaneous biopsy. If the biopsy does not confirm AML (especially if it is HMB-45 negative), suspect malignancy and excise the mass.
4. Treatment
   a. Stable patients with hemorrhage may undergo arterial embolization. If embolization fails, perform surgery. Unstable patients with life threatening hemorrhage should undergo immediate surgical exploration
   b. For asymptomatic AML that is < 4 cm, observation is recommended. Follow up includes a yearly renal ultrasound (check for growth > 4 cm).
   c. For asymptomatic AML that is ≥ 4 cm, options include surveillance or treatment. Surveillance may be problematic because the risk of hemorrhage is higher when AML is ≥ 4 cm and growth of the AML may make nephron sparing treatment impossible in the future.
   d. Patients with persistent symptoms should be treated.
   e. Elective treatment options include arterial embolization, ablation, or excision. For excision, nephron sparing surgery is preferred, but a large or centrally located AML may require total nephrectomy.
   f. Everolimus (see page 28) is FDA approved to shrink AML in patients with tuberous sclerosis whose AML does not require surgery.

Treatment of Angiomyolipoma (AML)

Significant active bleeding		No significant bleeding	
Life threatening hemorrhage	Not life threatening	AML < 4 cm & asymptomatic	AML ≥ 4 cm or symptomatic
Surgical Excision‡	Embolization → Bleeding persists	Surveillance* preferred	Consider Treatment†

*Surveillance involves imaging every 6-12 months (usually using ultrasound). Consider treatment if AML grows to size > 4 cm or becomes symptomatic.
†Treatment options include embolization, ablation, and excision‡.
‡ Nephron sparing surgery is preferred when possible.

Renal Cell Carcinoma (RCC)

Risk Factors for RCC
1. Tobacco smoking
2. Obesity—obese patients are more likely to develop RCC, but their tumors tend to be low grade and low stage.
3. Hypertension
4. Chronic renal failure treated with dialysis—1-3% develop RCC.
5. Adult polycystic kidney disease—less than 1% develop RCC.
6. Family history
7. Genetic risk factors—see page 5. Genetic syndromes such as von Hippel Lindau (VHL), tuberous sclerosis, Birt-Hogg-Dubé, and CHEK2 mutation (particularly I157T) can increase the risk of RCC.
8. Exposure to chlorinated solvents, especially trichloroethylene.
Note: The incidence of RCC in the general population is 0.04%.

Prevention
1. Avoiding obesity, smoking, and hypertension may decrease the risk of developing RCC.
2. Data are conflicting, but some studies suggest that consumption of fruits, vegetables, and fatty fish can reduce the risk of RCC.

Presentation
1. The most common age of presentation for RCC is 60 to 70 years.
2. Most RCCs are found incidentally during the evaluation of unrelated medical issues; therefore, RCC is often asymptomatic.
3. Symptoms include flank pain, hematuria, weight loss, fever, and sweats.
4. Signs include flank mass, hypertension, new varicocele (especially rapid onset), and paraneoplastic syndromes (see page 12).
5. The classic triad (flank mass, hematuria, and pain) is now rare because tumors are often detected incidentally at a low stage. The presence of the classic triad signifies advanced disease.

Classification of RCC
1. Sarcomatoid elements may be present in any RCC; therefore, sarcomatoid is not a unique type of RCC. The presence of sarcomatoid elements indicates a high grade tumor and a worse prognosis.
2. Clear cell (conventional) RCC—*clear cell RCC is the most common primary renal malignancy in adults.* Microscopically, it has a *clear cytoplasm* and a low nuclear/cytoplasmic ratio. The cytoplasm is filled with glycogen and lipids (which dissolve during tissue processing, resulting in a clear cytoplasm). Clear cell RCC arises from the *proximal tubule* and is associated with the *loss of 3p (short arm of chromosome 3).* Clear cell RCC is the most common type of RCC in patients with VHL.
3. Chromophobe RCC—this tumor has abundant cytoplasm and distinct cell borders. It usually has two cells types based on the appearance of the cytoplasm: granular eosinophilic cells (often with a perinuclear halo) and pale, almost transparent cells. It arises from the *collecting duct* and is associated with multiple chromosomal losses. Chromophobe RCC and oncocytoma may have a similar microscopic appearance. In oncocytoma, Hale's colloidal iron stains the cell border blue, but *not* the cytoplasm (negative stain). In chromophobe RCC, it stains the entire cytoplasm blue (positive stain). Under electron microscopy, the cytoplasm of oncocytoma is filled with mitochondria (microvesicles are rare), while the cytoplasm of chromophobe RCC is filled mainly with *microvesicles* (although some mitochondria are seen).

Feature	Oncocytoma	Chromophobe RCC
Cell Cytoplasm Types	One (granular eosinophilic)	Two (granular eosinophilic or pale)
Electron microscopy of cytoplasm shows	Rare microvesicles, *Many mitochondria*	*Many microvesicles*, Some mitochondria
Hale's colloidal iron stain	Negative	Positive
Binucleate	Rare	Common
Nucleus outline	Smooth	Irregular
Cell origin	Collecting duct	Collecting duct

4. Chromophil (papillary) RCC—the characteristic pathologic feature is *papillary architecture*. There are 2 histologic subtypes: Type I tumors have a basophilic cytoplasm and are usually low grade. Type II tumors have an eosinophilic cytoplasm are usually high grade. Type II papillary RCC has a worse prognosis. Papillary RCC arises from the *proximal tubule* and is associated with polysomy (especially of chromosome 7 and 17), MET gene mutations, or loss of the Y chromosome. *Papillary RCC is the most common renal cancer in patients with chronic renal failure on dialysis.*

5. Collecting duct carcinoma (Bellini duct carcinoma)—this rare, highly malignant cancer derives from the collecting duct (of Bellini) and is usually located in the renal medulla or papilla. Approximately 40% of these tumors present with metastases. Microscopic appearance often demonstrates hobnail cells lining tubular spaces. 5-year survival is rare.

6. Renal medullary carcinoma—this rare tumor is a form of collecting duct carcinoma. It occurs primarily in young adults of African ancestry with *sickle cell trait* (typical age is 10-39). These tumors are rarely confined to the kidney, rarely respond to chemotherapy or radiation, and have a poor prognosis (mean survival after nephrectomy is approximately 15 weeks). This is the only renal tumor with a racial predilection.

7. Unclassified RCC—the histology of these tumors does not match any of the other types. They usually have a poor prognosis because they are more likely to present with high grade and lymph node metastases.

8. Clear cell RCC appears to have a worse prognosis than papillary RCC and chromophobe RCC.

Feature	Clear Cell	Papillary	Chromophobe	Collecting duct
Characteristic pathologic features	Clear cytoplasm	Papillary architecture	Distinct cell borders, Perinuclear halo	Hobnail cells, Tumor located in medulla
Common cytogenetics	Loss of 3p	Polysomy 7 & 17, Loss of Y, or MET mutation	Multiple chromosomal deletions	?
Cell origin	Proximal tubule	Proximal tubule	Collecting duct	Collecting duct
Disease association	VHL, TC3, BAP1, Cowden, CHEK2	Chronic renal failure, HL RCC, HP RCC	BHD	Sickle cell**
Malignant potential	Moderate	Type I: Low Type II: High	Low	High

VHL = von Hippel Lindau; BHD = Birt-Hogg-Dubé; BAP1 = BAP1 syndrome;
TC3 = Translocation of chromosome 3; HL = Hereditary Leiomyomatosis;
HP = Hereditary papillary type 1 syndrome
* Abundant cytoplasmic microvesicles seen by electron microscopy
** Sickle cell trait is associated with renal medullary carcinoma, which is a variant of collecting duct carcinoma.

Comparison of Renal Masses

	Clear Cell RCC	AML	Oncocytoma
Potential	Malignant	Benign	Benign*
Origin	Proximal tubule	?	Collecting duct
Gender §	Male > Female	Female > Male	Male > Female
Average Age §	60	40-60	40-60
Side §	Left = Right	Right > Left	Left = Right
Gross Color	Golden yellow	Yellow or gray	Mahogany or tan
Common macroscopic features §	Solitary, Unilateral	Solitary, Unilateral	*Central scar,* Solitary, Unilateral
Common microscopic features	Clear cytoplasm	Fat, Smooth muscle, Blood vessels, HMB-45 positive	Nests of eosinophilic polygonal cells
Hypervascular	Most	Most	Few
Capsule	Pseudo-capsule	None	Fibrous capsule
Necrosis	Often	Rare	Rare
Mitosis	Common	Rare	Rare
Disease association**	VLH‡, TC3, BAP1, Cowden, CHEK2 Tuberous sclerosis‡	Tuberous sclerosis	BHD‡
Paraneoplastic	Up to 30%	No	No
Ultrasound	Hyperechoic	Hyperechoic	Hyperechoic
CT Scan	Enhances	Enhances, *HU -20 to -80*	Enhances
Arteriogram	Venous pooling, AV fistula, Neovascularity, Accentuation of capsular vessels	Hypervascular	*Spoke wheel* pattern of tumor arterioles, Lucent rim of tumor capsule†
Usual Treatment	Excision	Observe, excise, or embolize.	Excision
Diagnosis	Pathologic	Radiographic or pathologic	Pathologic

√HL = von Hippel Lindau, HU = Hounsfield Units, BHD = Birt-Hogg-Dubé
AML = angiomyolipoma, RCC = renal cell carcinoma; BAP1 = BAP1 syndrome;
TC3 = translocation of chromosome 3; CHEK2 = check 2 mutation syndrome.
§ Refers to sporadic tumors, not tumors associated with a genetic disease.
＊ Some reports of "malignant" oncocytomas have been published, but these were
    probably chromophobe RCC or oncocytoma mixed with RCC. Approximately
    10% of oncocytomas will also contain RCC.
* Tumors tend to be multiple and bilateral in these diseases.
† A spoke wheel pattern and a lucent rim of the capsule on arteriogram are not specific
    to oncocytoma and have been seen in RCC.
   Clear cell RCC occurs in 50% of patients with VHL and in 2% of patients with
   tuberous sclerosis. RCC occurs in 25% of patients with BHD, but it is usually
   chromophobe type.

Paraneoplastic Syndromes Associated with RCC

Approximately 10-20% of patients with RCC have a paraneoplastic syndrome. These syndromes are reversible with tumor resection. When paraneoplastic syndromes persist after tumor resection, metastatic disease is probably present and these patients have a poor prognosis. Paraneoplastic syndromes include

1. Elevated erythrocyte sedimentation rate (ESR)
2. Weight loss, cachexia
3. Fever
4. Anemia
5. Hypertension (from renin produced by the tumor)
6. Hypercalcemia (from a PTH-like substance produced by the tumor)
7. Stauffer's syndrome (hepatic dysfunction)—a reversible hepatitis associated with RCC that has *not* metastasized to the liver.
8. Elevated alkaline phosphatase
9. Polycythemia (from erythropoietin produced by the tumor)

Metastatic RCC

1. 20% of patients present with metastatic disease. Larger primary tumors have a higher risk of metastasis at presentation.
2. When metastatic disease is discovered, a solitary metastasis is present in only 1% of cases. Thus, metastases usually involve multiple sites rather than a single site.

Primary RCC Size	Risk of Metastasis at Presentation*
≤ 3 cm	< 4%
> 3 to 4 cm	7%
> 4 to 7 cm	16%
> 7 to 10 cm	30%
> 10 to 15 cm	41%
> 15 cm	51%

* Includes N1 and/or M1.
From J Urol, 181:1020, 2009.

3. Metastases occur by lymphatic spread and hematogenous spread with equal frequency.
4. Distant metastases are present in > 50% of patients with regional lymph node metastases.
5. Metastatic sites (most to least common): lung, bone, regional lymph nodes, liver, adrenal gland, contralateral kidney, brain. The most common site of bone metastasis is the spine.
6. Most metastases are symptomatic at the time of diagnosis.
7. Elevated alkaline phosphatase, calcium, or liver function tests (LFTs) may indicate a paraneoplastic syndrome or metastatic disease. Persistence of a paraneoplastic syndrome after nephrectomy indicates unrecognized or micrometastatic disease.
8. If metastases develop after nephrectomy for an M0 renal cancer, they usually occur within one year of surgery.

Integrated Staging for Renal Cancer

The UCLA Integrated Staging System (UISS) uses the TNM stage, Fuhrman grade, and the Eastern Cooperative Oncology Group performance status (ECOG PS) to stratify patients into categories that predict survival after treatment. For survival based on UISS, see page 31.

Grade

1. Higher grade implies a worse prognosis.
2. Chromophobe, collecting duct, renal medullary, and unclassified RCC are designated as high or low grade. Fuhrman grade is not appropriate.
3. Papillary RCC—Fuhrman may be used, but histologic subtype (type I or type II) should also be reported.
4. Clear cell RCC—Fuhrman grading should be utilized.

5. Fuhrman nuclear grading is used for clear cell and papillary RCC and is based on nuclear characteristics (size, contour, and nucleoli). Mitotic activity is *not* considered. The tumor is assigned the highest identified grade. If spindle shaped (sarcomatoid) cells are present, nuclear grade IV is assigned.

Fuhrman Nuclear Grade	Nuclear Size	Nuclear Contour	Prominent Nucleoli at x100†
I	Small (~10μ)	Round, smooth, uniform	No
II	Medium (~15μ)	Minor irregularities	No*
III	Large (~20μ)	Major irregularities	Yes
IV	Large (~20μ)	Major irregularities (often multi-lobulated, pleomorphic)	Yes

   † Low power magnification (x100).
   * Nucleoli may be seen with high power magnification (x400).

Stage (AJCC 2017)

The following TNM classification refers to both clinical and pathological staging. Higher stage implies a worse prognosis. This staging system applies only to renal cell carcinomas (and not to other renal tumors).

Primary Tumor (T)

Tx	Primary tumor cannot be assessed
T0	No evidence of primary tumor
T1	Tumor ≤ 7 cm in greatest dimension, limited to the kidney
T1a	Tumor ≤ 4 cm in greatest dimension, limited to the kidney
T1b	Tumor > 4 cm but ≤ 7 cm in greatest dimension, limited to the kidney
T2	Tumor > 7 cm in greatest dimension, limited to the kidney
T2a	Tumor > 7 cm but ≤ 10 cm in greatest dimension, limited to the kidney
T2b	Tumor > 10 cm, limited to the kidney
T3	Tumor extends into major veins or perinephric tissues, but not into the ipsilateral adrenal gland and not beyond Gerota's fascia
T3a	Tumor extends into the renal vein or its segmental branches, or invades the pelvicalyceal system, or invades perirenal and/or renal sinus fat but not beyond Gerota's fascia
T3b	Tumor extends into the vena cava below the diaphragm
T3c	Tumor extends into vena cava above the diaphragm or invades the wall of the vena cava
T4	Tumor invades beyond Gerota's fascia (including contiguous extension into the ipsilateral adrenal gland)

Regional Lymph Nodes* (N)

Nx	Regional lymph nodes cannot be assessed
N0	No regional lymph node metastasis
N1	Metastasis in regional lymph node(s)

Distant Metastasis (M)

M0	No distant metastasis
M1	Distant metastasis

* Regional lymph nodes include renal hilar, aortic, interaortocaval, and caval.

Treatment of Localized (Non-metastatic) RCC

General Information

1. Surgical excision is the most effective therapy for treating RCC. Thus, excision is usually the recommended primary treatment for localized RCC in surgical candidates.
2. Excision of a renal mass may not be necessary in the following situations.
   a. Small renal masses that will undergo active surveillance (see page 14).
   b. Some angiomyolipomas (see Angiomyolipoma, page 8).
   c. Bosniak category I, II, or IIF renal cysts (see page 469).
   d. Metastasis to the kidney (e.g. lymphoma)—treated with systemic therapy for the specific tumor type. Nephrectomy is seldom indicated.
   e. The patient cannot tolerate surgical extirpation.
   f. Unresectable tumor.
3. Radical nephrectomy is the gold standard for treating RCC. However, a nephron sparing procedure is recommended in the following scenarios.
   a. Renal masses < 7 cm that are amenable to nephron sparing therapy.
   b. There is an imperative indication for renal sparing (see page 16).
4. *A minimally invasive (laparoscopic or robotic) technique is preferred for excision of a renal mass when it does not compromise oncological control.*

Surveillance for Enhancing Renal Masses in the Absence of Metastases

1. The 2021 AUA guideline states that "When the oncologic risks are particularly low and the pathology of the lesion is uncertain (e.g. tumors < 2 cm), AS [active surveillance] with potential delayed intervention is an acceptable option for the initial management of all patients, not just those with limited life expectancy or poor performance status..." but "For patients...in whom the anticipated oncologic benefits of intervention outweigh the risks of treatment and competing risks of death, clinicians should recommend intervention." The EAU 2021 guideline states "offer active surveillance...to frail and/or comorbid patients with small renal masses." The NCCN 2021 guideline states "Active surveillance is an option for the initial management of patients with clinical stage T1...renal masses < 2 cm" or in patients with "clinical stage T1 masses and significant competing risks of death or morbidity from intervention."
2. *Tumors that arise from Hereditary Leiomyomatosis RCC or from Succinate Dehydrogenase Deficiency RCC behave aggressively even when they are small; therefore, tumors associated with these syndromes should not be managed by surveillance.*
3. The risk of surveillance is lowest when the renal mass is ≤ 3 cm.

   a. When enhancing renal masses ≤ 3 cm are initially discovered, 20% are benign, 13% are high grade, 6% extend locally outside the kidney (pT3), and < 4% have nodal or distant metastases. *The risk of malignancy, high grade tumor, local spread beyond the kidney, and metastasis rises as the size of the primary tumor increases.*

Primary RCC Size (cm)	Risk of Metastasis* at Presentation	Risk of High Grade Tumor
≤ 3	< 4%	13%
> 3 to 4	7%	16%
> 4 to 7	16%	21%
> 7 to 10	30%	27%
> 10 to 15	41%	33%
> 15	51%	38%

* Includes N1 and/or M1.
From J Urol, 181:1020, 2009 & J Urol 181: 29, 2009.

   b. *In untreated patients with an enhancing renal mass ≤ 3 cm in greatest dimension, the risk developing metastases within 2-3 years of diagnosis is 1%.* Larger tumors have a higher risk of developing metastases.

[handwritten: mean growth rate = .3cm/year]

4. Among patients undergoing surveillance for small renal masses, the mean tumor growth rate is approximately 0.3 cm per year. Tumor growth rate does not reliably distinguish between benign and malignant lesions. However, *metastases appear to be more likely in patients whose primary tumor demonstrates interval growth.*

5. *Surveillance for a renal mass ≤ 4 cm has a low risk of metastasis and local tumor growth in the short term. However, in the long term, surveillance of these masses may compromise survival.* In a retrospective study of patients with an enhancing renal mass ≤ 4 cm, Zini et al (2009) compared 9,858 patients who underwent partial or radical nephrectomy to 433 patients who underwent non-surgical management (no excision, no ablation). Excision improved cancer specific survival by as much as 9.4% at 5 years. ✓

6. Recommended baseline testing—before surveillance is begun, the following tests are recommended to obtain an accurate baseline assessment of the primary tumor and to check for metastasis.
   a. Abdominal cross sectional imaging (CT or MRI) with and without intravenous contrast (if there is no contraindication to contrast).
   b. Chest imaging (x-ray or CT)
   c. Lab tests—BUN, creatinine, estimated GFR, liver function tests, LDH, alkaline phosphatase, serum calcium, complete blood count, urinalysis.
   d. Additional metastatic evaluation should be done when symptoms, laboratory tests, or other imaging suggest metastatic disease.

7. Optional baseline testing—renal mass biopsy is optional. If the patient's medical condition would preclude treatment of the mass, then renal biopsy is not indicated. If the patient can tolerate treatment and would consider treatment based on biopsy results, then biopsy of the mass is reasonable. The intensity of follow up can be modified based on the tumor histology.

8. Assessing for growth of the renal mass
   a. The size of the mass on ultrasound appears to correlate well with the size of the mass on CT or MRI. Therefore, after the mass has been well characterized with a baseline CT or MRI, ultrasound may be used to monitor for changes in tumor size. If the ultrasound findings are of concern, then a CT or MRI can be obtained and compared to the baseline imaging to confirm tumor growth. *[handwritten: variability = 3mm]*
   b. Data suggests that inter-observer and intra-observer variability is < 3.1 mm when measuring tumor size. *Therefore, variations of < 3 mm in tumor size should not be interpreted as tumor growth unless there is a persistent increase in size over at least 2 imaging studies.*

9. Example follow up protocol—if a patient elects to undergo surveillance, the first follow up imaging should be conducted within 3-6 months after the initial diagnosis (even if a biopsy is benign) and should consist of abdominal cross sectional imaging (CT or MRI) with intravenous contrast. *This 3-6 month imaging is compared to the baseline imaging to determine growth rate.* Thereafter, follow up testing should include
   a. Renal imaging (with ultrasound, CT, or MRI) at least annually—imaging should be done even if a biopsy shows a benign tumor because benign tumors can grow over time and threaten the kidney's function.
   b. Chest imaging annually and as clinically indicated—chest x-ray is recommended in patients who had no renal mass biopsy or whose biopsy is nondiagnostic, oncocytoma, tumor with oncocytic features, or renal cell carcinoma. Although oncocytoma is considered benign, oncocytoma can coexist with RCC and it can be difficult to distinguish oncocytoma from an oncocytic cancer; thus, patients with oncocytoma are followed as if they have RCC. ✓
   c. Laboratory tests annually and as clinically indicated.

10. Treatment of the renal mass should be considered when any of the following criteria are present.
    a. The mass grows larger than 3 cm in greatest dimension.
    b. The mass demonstrates ongoing interval growth (especially more than 0.5 cm per year).
    c. The tumor develops an infiltrative appearance on imaging.
    d. The clinical stage increases.
    e. The patient develops symptoms attributable to the renal mass.
    f. Biopsy shows RCC with aggressive features.
11. During surveillance, symptoms may develop, a metastasis may develop, the tumor may grow (possibly eliminating the option of nephron sparing therapy), and the cure rate of subsequent treatment may decline. There is conflicting data about whether surveillance compromises cancer specific survival compared to treatment; however, close surveillance followed by delayed intervention appears to have acceptable oncologic outcomes for stage T1 renal tumors.

Radical Nephrectomy (RN)

1. RN is removal of Gerota's fascia and its contents (kidney and perirenal fat). In some cases, the adrenal gland (see page 22) and regional lymph nodes (see page 23) are removed. Tumor thrombus should be removed.
2. Open and laparoscopic RN achieve equivalent cancer control, survival, and quality of life, but laparoscopic RN results in less intraoperative blood loss, less postoperative pain, and shorter hospital stay.
3. Radical nephrectomy may be an option for renal cancer of any clinical stage. However, radical nephrectomy is best utilized in patients who meet all of the following criteria
    a. Partial nephrectomy would place the patient at high risk for positive surgical margin or would not preserve sufficient viable normal kidney to make the risk of partial nephrectomy worthwhile.
    b. No imperative indication for renal sparing.
    c. No preoperative renal insufficiency (e.g. GFR > 60 ml/min)
    d. No preoperative proteinuria
    e. Normal contralateral kidney
    f. Expected postoperative GFR > 45 ml/min.
4. *Partial nephrectomy is usually preferred for clinical stage T1 tumors (tumors ≤ 7 cm in greatest dimension confined to the kidney).*
5. *Radical nephrectomy is usually utilized for stage ≥ T2 tumors.*

Renal Sparing Treatment (Nephron Sparing Treatment)

1. Radical nephrectomy removes the entire kidney (including all normal and abnormal renal tissue), whereas renal sparing treatment attempts to spare as much of the normal ipsilateral kidney as possible. Nephron sparing treatment results in less reduction of the glomerular filtration rate (GFR) compared to radical nephrectomy.
2. Imperative indications for renal sparing treatment—renal sparing treatment may be indicated regardless of tumor characteristics when preservation of renal function is crucial. Imperative indications include
    a. Tumor in a solitary kidney
    b. Poor contralateral renal function
    c. Bilateral renal tumors
    d. Poor overall renal function
    e. Contralateral kidney is threatened by a disease that may worsen renal function (diabetes, hypertension, etc.).
    f. Contralateral kidney is threatened by a disease that can cause renal tumors (tuberous sclerosis, VHL, etc.).

3. The feasibility of renal sparing depends on the tumor size and its location within the kidney. Peripheral tumors ≤ 7 cm in size are more amenable to renal sparing treatment. When renal sparing would compromise complete excision of the malignancy or would not preserve sufficient normal kidney to make the risk worthwhile, then radical nephrectomy is preferred.

4. Renal sparing can be performed in situ or extracorporeal (nephrectomy with bench surgery and autotransplantation). In situ surgery is preferred.

5. Renal sparing surgery can be achieved by partial nephrectomy or by thermal ablation.

6. Partial nephrectomy (PN)—PN is excision of the tumor with a margin of normal tissue. *Partial nephrectomy is the preferred method of nephron sparing therapy because an abundance of long term data confirms its efficacy. Also, most population based analyses show that cancer specific mortality is lower after PN than after ablation.* ⅂ ✗

7. Thermal ablation—thermal ablation uses cold or heat to destroy the tumor in situ (i.e. without excision). *Thermal ablation appears to result in less decline in GFR than partial nephrectomy, but ablation has a higher local recurrence rate than partial or radical nephrectomy. Furthermore, retrospective data suggests that ablation results in a two fold higher risk of dying from kidney cancer compared to partial nephrectomy.*

8. Removal of renal tissue may decrease the glomerular filtration rate (GFR).
   a. Lower GFR after renal surgery corresponds to a higher risk of cardiovascular events, a higher risk of dying from cardiac events, and lower overall survival (especially when GFR is less than 60 ml/minute).
   b. Given the above findings, preserving as much renal function as possible may help reduce the risk of death.

Thermal Ablation

1. Thermal ablation is tumor destruction without excision, which is usually accomplished by freezing (cryoablation) or heating (radiofrequency ablation). Although no randomized trial has compared cryoablation and radiofrequency ablation, retrospective data shows that they have similar oncologic efficacy and similar complication rates.
   a. Cryoablation—the tumor is cooled to -20°C to -40°C (these temperatures induce cell necrosis). Two freeze-thaw cycles improve cell kill. A common regimen is 10 minutes of freezing, then 8 minutes of thawing, then another 10 minutes of freezing (the "10-8-10" protocol). Freezing is monitored by ultrasound. The necrosis zone is smaller than the frozen region revealed by ultrasound. In order to account for this, the hyperechoic edge of the ice ball on ultrasound must extend beyond edge of the tumor (by at least 5 mm). For details on cryoablation, including its mechanism of action and monitoring during freezing, see page 217.
   b. Radiofrequency ablation—the tumor is heated to between 50°C and 105°C (these temperatures induced cell necrosis). A probe delivers high frequency alternating current into the tumor (460-500 KHz). This current creates a electromagnetic field that agitates the molecules next to the probe. This agitation creates friction between molecules that heats the surrounding tissue (the source of the heat is not the probe; the heat arises from the agitated molecules around the probe). Heating the tissue to temperatures higher than 105°C can cause gas formation, which hinders the delivery of current. The goal is to ensure tumor necrosis by maintaining a temperature of 50°C to 105°C throughout the tumor, while not exceeding 105°C. Ablation can be monitored using ultrasound, CT, or MRI.

2. Ablation can be accomplished through an open, laparoscopic, or percutaneous approach. In most cases, *a percutaneous approach is preferred because it minimizes morbidity.*

3. *Biopsy of the renal mass is recommended before proceeding with tumor ablation.* The intensity of follow up can be modified depending on the tumor histology (benign tumors may require minimal follow up, whereas high grade or aggressive tumors may require more intense follow up).

4. *Thermal ablation is generally reserved for non-cystic clinical stage T1 tumors that are < 3 cm in size* because
   a. The risk of complications (such as tumor fracture and bleeding) are higher when tumor size is > 3 cm.
   b. The rate of recurrence is higher when tumor size is > 3 cm.
   c. Disease free survival is lower when tumor size is > 3 cm.
   d. Thermal ablation has not been well studied in cystic masses.

5. Tumors that are intrarenal, close to the renal hilum, or close to a renal sinus are more difficult to treat with thermal ablation. Peripheral exophytic tumors are easier to ablate.

6. When structures adjacent to the kidney are too close to allow for safe ablation of the tumor, the clinician can move these nearby structures away from the expected ablation zone to permit safe tumor ablation (using methods such as percutaneous hydro-dissection or spacer balloons).

7. Complications include hematoma, pain, and infection. Pneumothorax can occur when ablating upper pole renal masses. Rare serious complications include bleeding requiring transfusion, persistent urinary extravasation, complete loss of ipsilateral renal function, injury to nearby organs (such as the ureter or bowel), and tumor seeding along the probe tract.

8. *Thermal ablation appears to result in less decline in GFR than partial nephrectomy.*

9. *Local recurrence is more common after a single ablation (6%) than after partial nephrectomy (3%) or radical nephrectomy (1%). However, persistent tumor and local recurrence can be treated with repeat ablation. When repeat ablations are included, the risk of local recurrence is similar between ablation and PN.* Salvage excision of the tumor may be more difficult after ablation.

10. *Retrospective data suggests that ablation results in a two fold higher risk of dying from kidney cancer compared to partial nephrectomy.*

11. The EAU 2021 guideline states that ablation should be offered to "frail and/or comorbid patients with small renal masses..." and "inform patients about the higher risk of local recurrence and/or tumor progression." The AUA 2021 guideline states that physicians should consider thermal ablation as "an alternate approach for the management of cT1a solid renal masses < 3 cm in size..." and that patient counselling should include "an increased likelihood of tumor persistence or local recurrence...relative to surgical excision..."

12. Residual tumor after ablation and local recurrence—this is defined as any of the following
    a. *Imaging shows tumor in the same area of prior treatment that enhances with contrast more than 3-6 months after ablation, enlarges over time, or fails to regress over time.*
    b. Imaging shows new satellite tumors (tumors immediately surrounding the treated area).
    c. Biopsy shows tumor in the same area of prior treatment.
    d. Tumor detected along the tract where the probe was placed.

13. Renal biopsy for residual tumor or local recurrence
    a. If there is a suspicion of residual cancer or a local recurrence on imaging, then a renal mass biopsy should be performed.
    b. *The biopsy should sample the enhancing areas of the tumor.* Biopsies of non-enhancing areas are likely to show fibrosis (especially the center of the mass, where ablation is typically initiated).
14. For renal masses that have undergone successful ablation, immediate post-ablation imaging shows a slight enlargement of the tumor, and may show rim enhancement. Over the next few months, the tumor shrinks and no longer enhances (although with radiofrequency ablation, tumor shrinkage may be minimal).
15. Patients with no biopsy or patients whose biopsy is nondiagnostic, oncocytoma, or tumor with oncocytic features should probably be followed with the assumption that the tumor is renal cell carcinoma. Although oncocytoma is considered benign, oncocytoma can coexist with RCC, it can be difficult to distinguish oncocytoma from an oncocytic cancer, and it can grow enough over time to threaten the kidney's function.
16. Example follow up protocol—if a patient elects to undergo thermal ablation, *the first follow up imaging should be conducted at 3 months and 6 months after ablation and should consist of abdominal cross sectional imaging (CT or MRI) with and without intravenous contrast (unless contrast is contraindicated). These 3 and 6 month scans determine treatment success.* Thereafter, follow up testing should include
    a. For patients whose pre-ablation renal mass biopsy shows a benign tumor tumor that is not oncocytoma—if the 3 and 6 month scans show a treatment success and there are no ongoing treatment related complications, then further abdominal imaging and chest imaging is not necessary.
    b. For patients who did not have a renal mass biopsy or whose biopsy shows RCC, oncocytoma, tumor with oncocytic features, or nondiagnostic findings, use the follow up protocol described below.
        i. Renal imaging (with ultrasound, CT, or MRI) annually for 5 years and as clinically indicated. Renal imaging may be performed more often and using more detailed scans (CT or MRI rather than ultrasound) when there is concern about recurrence. Renal imaging after 5 years can be considered based on the patient's risk.
        ii. Chest imaging annually for 5 years and as clinically indicated. Chest imaging after 5 years can be considered based on the patient's risk.
        iii. Laboratory tests annually and as clinically indicated.

Partial Nephrectomy (PN)

1. PN removes the tumor with a margin of normal renal tissue. The method of removing the tumor can be classified into two categories.
    a. Incision—the normal kidney around the tumor is incised so the tumor can be removed with a modest macroscopic margin of normal kidney.
    b. Enucleation—the tumor is removed by blunt dissection between the tumor pseudocapsule and the normal kidney; therefore, there is a minimal (often microscopic) margin of normal renal tissue around the tumor. Some cancers do not have a pseudocapsule. If a pseudocapsule is absent, it may be more difficult to develop the correct tissue plane (which could cause dissection into the tumor). Also, tumor invades the pseudocapsule in up to one third of cases. Nonetheless. retrospective data suggests that incisional removal and enucleation have similar oncologic outcomes. For example, Minervini et al (2011) showed that enucleation and incisional partial nephrectomy achieved equivalent

10-year cancer specific survival, and that enucleation had a lower positive margin rate (3.4% vs. 1%). *The AUA 2021 guideline states "Until prospective evaluation is available for sporadic tumors, enucleation is best utilized on a selective basis..." and "should be considered in patients with familial RCC, multifocal disease, or severe CKD [chronic kidney disease]..."*

2. PN for stage T1 tumors—*when complete tumor excision can be achieved, partial nephrectomy is the treatment of choice for most clinical stage T1 tumors (tumors ≤ 7 cm in greatest dimension) because*
   a. PN results in a lower risk of chronic renal insufficiency than RN.
   b. PN and RN have equivalent oncologic efficacy in stage T1 tumors.
   c. Cancer specific mortality is lower with PN than with ablative therapies.

3. PN for stage T2—partial nephrectomy is an option for stage T2 tumors when PN will completely excise the cancer and will preserve a sufficient amount of normal kidney to make the risk worthwhile. In these cases, PN results in a higher blood loss and a higher risk of complications than RN. Also, large tumors have a higher likelihood of aggressive pathologic features (such as infiltration beyond the tumor capsule); therefore, it is crucial to only utilize PN when it can be done with minimal risk of leaving cancer behind. Radical nephrectomy is also an option for stage T2 cancer.

4. Stage T3 or T4—radical nephrectomy is generally performed for these stages of primary cancer unless there is an imperative indication for renal preservation.

5. Surgical margins—historically, a one centimeter margin of normal tissue was recommended. *However, the size of a negative surgical margin does not impact prognosis. A close margin achieves the same cure rate as an ample margin; therefore, a close margin should be considered as truly negative.*
   a. Positive surgical margins occur in approximately 3% of patients undergoing PN.
   b. With short term follow up (< 3.5 years), a positive margin does not appear to alter cancer specific or overall survival.
   c. *Patients with a positive margin have a higher risk of local recurrence; however, most patients will remain disease free.* In fact, when ipsilateral radical nephrectomy is performed for a positive margin after partial nephrectomy, residual tumor is found ≤ 16% of the time.
   d. *When a positive margin is found, but there is no gross residual tumor, surveillance is usually appropriate because most of these patients will remain disease free.* However, radical nephrectomy or repeat partial nephrectomy may be considered in patient's with a particularly aggressive tumor (e.g. sarcomatoid, high grade, or collecting duct cancers) because these patients may be at higher risk for a lethal recurrence.
   e. When there is gross residual tumor remaining after PN, consider performing either radical nephrectomy or repeat partial nephrectomy to remove the residual tumor. Ablation may be used in select cases.

6. Renal ischemia time—this is defined as the duration of time that part or all of the kidney is without arterial blood flow because of vascular clamping. Clamping of renal blood flow is done to minimize bleeding while excising the tumor. Ischemia time is designated as either warm (no cooling of the kidney during ischemia) or cold (cooling of the kidney during ischemia). Irreversible renal damage is thought to occur after 20-30 minutes of warm ischemia time and after about 90 minutes of cold ischemia time.

7. Minimizing ischemic renal damage during partial nephrectomy
   a. Avoid hypotension and hypovolemia.
   b. Traditionally, patients received mannitol 12.5 grams IV administered at 5 minutes and 10 minutes prior to clamping the renal artery. *Mannitol reduces ischemic injury by scavenging free radicals and by reducing oxidative cellular damage.* Retrospective data suggests no benefit to using mannitol. In addition, a recent randomized trial by Spaliviero (2018) in patients with preoperative GFR > 45 ml/min showed that using a single 12.5 gram dose of mannitol during PN did not improve postoperative GFR compared to placebo (however, this trial did not examine whether mannitol is beneficial when using the usual regimen of two 12.5 gram doses or when it is used for patients with preoperative GFR < 45 ml/min).
   c. Clamp the renal artery only once (avoid unclamping and re-clamping).
   d. Leaving the renal vein unclamped may permit retrograde renal perfusion; however, it may result in more bleeding.
   e. Rather than clamping the main renal artery, clamp only segmental arteries that feed the region of the tumor.
   f. Minimize renal ischemia time—when the kidney is not cooled, then *warm ischemia time should ideally be less than 20 minutes.* If warm ischemia time is expected to be longer than 20 minutes, then the traditional approach has been to cool the kidney (after clamping the artery, surround the kidney with an ice bath for 15 minutes and cool the kidney to 15° C). Re-cool the kidney at least every 30 minutes). *However, a recent randomized study (Breau et al, 2021) shows that renal hypothermia offers no benefit for the preservation of renal function when clamp time is < 60 minutes.* Although few patients in the study had GFR < 45, the study was able to show that hypothermia did not benefit these patients. *When renal hypothermia is utilized, cold ischemia time should ideally be less than 60 minutes, but the kidney can completely recover after 60-90 minutes of cold ischemia.*
8. Laparoscopic versus open PN
   a. Open and laparoscopic PN achieve equally effective cancer control and survival.
   b. Warm ischemia time is usually longer with laparoscopic PN.
   c. Compared to open PN, laparoscopic PN has a lower intraoperative blood loss, but a higher risk of postoperative hemorrhage. Open and laparoscopic PN have a similar transfusion rate.
   d. Patients undergoing laparoscopic PN have a higher risk of being converted to radical nephrectomy than patients undergoing open PN (2.1% versus 0.05%).
   e. Laparoscopic PN has a higher rate of re-operation for complications than open PN (3.4% versus 1.6%).

Radical Nephrectomy (RN) Versus Partial Nephrectomy (PN)

1. EORTC 30904 was a prospective randomized trial comparing open PN and open RN in patients with a normal contralateral kidney and RCC that was solitary and < 5 cm in diameter. For PN, a macroscopic margin of normal renal tissue was removed (i.e. enucleation was not performed).
2. Complications—EORTC 30904 showed that *partial nephrectomy has a higher rate of complications compared to radical nephrectomy.* The following complications were more likely with PN.
   a. Hemorrhage with > 1 liter of blood loss (3.1% versus 1.2%)
   b. Urine leak/fistula (4.4% versus 0%)
   c. Re-operation for complications (4.4% versus 2.4%)

3. Renal function

    a. *Partial nephrectomy results in a lower risk of chronic renal insufficiency than radical nephrectomy.* Retrospective and randomized (EORTC 30904) data shows that patients undergoing radical nephrectomy have a higher risk of developing a postoperative glomerular filtrate rate (GFR) less than 60 ml/min. However, it appears that the risk of severe renal dysfunction (GFR < 30) is similar after partial and radical nephrectomy.

    b. Retrospective data suggests that partial nephrectomy is less likely to cause proteinuria compared to radical nephrectomy.

4. Oncologic efficacy and survival

    a. *The rate of positive surgical margins is higher with PN than with RN (2-3% versus 1%).*

    b. *Randomized (EORTC 30904) and retrospective studies show that PN and RN achieve equivalent cancer specific survival in patients with stage T1 cancer, but local recurrence is higher with PN (3% versus 1%).*

    c. *Although the data are conflicting, some retrospective studies suggest that patients undergoing PN for clinical stage T1 RCC have a longer overall survival than patients undergoing radical nephrectomy.* Improved overall survival in patients undergoing PN occurs mainly by reducing non-RCC related deaths. Since lower GFR correlates with lower overall survival, partial nephrectomy may achieve its overall survival benefit by preventing a decline in GFR.

    d. EORTC 30904—after a median follow up of 9.3 years, this study was unable to demonstrate equivalent cancer control for RN and PN. It was also unable to confirm the retrospective finding that PN achieves higher overall survival. The inability to show an advantage for PN probably arose because poor accrual forced the study to closed prematurely (< 50% of the required patients were enrolled); therefore, the study was underpowered to adequately assess survival endpoints. The authors state "Oncologic equivalence of NSS [Nephron Sparing Surgery] and RN could not be definitely shown in this randomized study but is nowadays generally accepted" and EORTC 30904 "...supports the recommendation to use NSS in small tumors as a first-line procedure whenever technically feasible..."

5. Erectile dysfunction (ED)—retrospective data suggests that RN leads to a higher rate of postoperative ED than PN. One possible explanation for this is that the renal insufficiency from RN produces endothelial cell dysfunction, which increases the rate of ED.

6. Summary

    a. PN has a higher rate of perioperative complications compared to RN.

    b. PN results in a lower risk of chronic renal insufficiency than RN.

    c. PN achieves equivalent (or possibly better) overall survival compared to RN. The potential overall survival benefit for PN arises from a reduction in non-RCC related deaths (perhaps by preventing renal insufficiency).

    d. The rate of positive surgical margins is higher with PN than with RN (2-3% versus 1%).

    e. PN has a slightly higher local recurrence rate than RN (3% versus 1%).

    f. PN achieves equivalent cancer specific survival compared to RN.

Adrenalectomy During Nephrectomy

1. *Ipsilateral adrenalectomy is recommended when there is suspicion of direct invasion or metastasis to the adrenal gland based on preoperative imaging or based on intraoperative findings.* Adrenalectomy may also be considered when there is a large upper pole tumor. Otherwise, the ipsilateral adrenal gland can be spared. Routine removal the ipsilateral adrenal gland during nephrectomy does not improve survival.

2. Direct invasion or metastasis to the adrenal gland is uncommon.
3. If unilateral adrenalectomy is performed, adrenal insufficiency is rare when the patient has a normal contralateral adrenal gland.
4. For patients undergoing cytoreductive nephrectomy for metastatic RCC, the indications for adrenal sparing are the same as for patients with non-metastatic RCC.

Regional Lymph Node Dissection (LND)

1. Clinical stage N0 patients—*when preoperative imaging and intraoperative findings show no lymphadenopathy, then performing regional LND is optional.*
   a. EORTC 30881 was a prospective randomized trial comparing RN alone to RN with LND in patients with clinical stage T1-T3, N0M0 RCC.
      i. With a median follow up of 12.6 years, there was no difference in overall survival, disease-specific survival, or local progression. Thus, *regional lymph node dissection does not improve survival in patients who undergo RN for clinical stage T1-T3, N0M0 RCC.*
      ii. LND did not increase the risk of surgical complications.
      iii. Regional lymph node metastases were found in 1% of palpably normal nodes and in 17% of palpably enlarged nodes (this is why LND is recommended when palpable nodes are discovered intraoperatively, see below).
   b. Some urologists advocate LND for patients with a high risk of node metastases. The risk of node metastases can be predicted preoperatively using a nomogram (Int J Cancer, 121: 2556, 2007) or intraoperatively using frozen section (high risk has $\geq$ 2 risk factors: stage T3-T4, grade 3-4, tumor size $\geq$ 10 cm, tumor necrosis, or sarcomatoid elements).
2. Clinical stage N1 patients (i.e. preoperative imaging or intraoperative findings show lymphadenopathy)—*LND does not improve survival in patients with clinical stage N1. However, regional LND (including removal of abnormal nodes) is recommended in N1 patients because it helps to accurately stage the tumor.* Some enlarged lymph nodes do not harbor malignancy.
3. The most common location of node metastasis is interaortocaval for right sided tumors, and para-aortic for left sided tumors. Interaortocaval node metastasis can be present in the absence of hilar node metastasis.
4. Crispen et al (2011) recommend the following LND templates.
   a. For left sided tumors, remove the para-aortic and interaortocaval nodes from crus of the diaphragm to the common iliac artery.
   b. For right sided tumors, remove the paracaval and interaortocaval nodes from crus of the diaphragm to the common iliac artery.

Bilateral RCC

1. When possible, renal sparing surgery is preferred for bilateral RCC. In cases where bilateral RN is necessary, the patient is placed on dialysis. Renal transplant may be an option if the patient remains cancer-free.
2. When planning RN on one side and nephron sparing surgery on the other side, consider performing the nephron sparing surgery first and delaying the RN until a later date. This helps avoid dialysis (during recovery from the nephron sparing surgery, the need for dialysis can be avoided if a contralateral kidney is still present to help sustain renal function).

RCC with Tumor Thrombus

1. RCC can grow into the lumen of veins that drain the kidney. Tumor within the venous lumen is called tumor thrombus.
2. Tumor thrombus typically remains attached to and continuous with the primary renal mass.

3. Tumor thrombus growth tends to follow the direction of venous flow; therefore, thrombus that extends into the inferior vena cava (IVC) will usually grow cephalad toward the heart. Once it reaches the heart, it will typically grow into the right atrium rather than into the superior vena cava.

4. Various systems (including TNM stage on page 13) have been proposed to designate the level to which the thrombus extends. Commonly used levels are renal vein only, IVC below the hepatic veins, IVC above the hepatic veins, IVC above the diaphragm, or into the right heart. *A more extensive tumor thrombus is associated with a lower disease specific survival.*

5. The thrombus is usually free-floating in the venous lumen, but it can invade into the vein wall. When the tumor thrombus invades into the vein wall, then the involved vein wall is excised (synthetic graft may be used to reconstruct the vein). *Tumor thrombus invading the caval wall has a worse prognosis than free-floating thrombus.*

6. In surgical candidates, tumor thrombus should be removed during nephrectomy because long term survival has been achieved even when the thrombus extends into the right heart.

7. Cardiopulmonary or veno-venous bypass may be necessary to remove an extensive tumor thrombus, especially if it extends above the diaphragm.

8. Case reports show that systemic therapy can shrink tumor thrombus. When a thoracic incision or cardiopulmonary bypass poses an unacceptable risk, systemic therapy may reduce the thrombus level enough to allow complete resection without a thoracic incision and without cardiopulmonary bypass.

Adjuvant Therapy after Nephrectomy

1. Many randomized studies of adjuvant therapy have been conducted, using agents such as radiation, interferon, interleukin, sunitinib, sorafenib, axitinib, and pazopanib. So far, only one study has shown benefit with adjuvant therapy: the S-TRAC trial.

2. S-TRAC trial—patients with non-metastatic *clear cell RCC* who were at high risk for recurrence after nephrectomy were randomized to either sunitinib or placebo. High risk for recurrence was defined as the presence of any of the following: stage T4, regional lymph node metastasis, or a combination of stage T3N0 + Fuhrman grade ≥ 2 + ECOG performance status ≥ 1. Sunitinib 50 mg po q day was administered on a 4-week-on 2-week-off cycle for 1 year as tolerated, but was stopped sooner if recurrence occurred within 1 year. *Median disease free survival was significantly longer (by 1.2 years) in the sunitinib group.* Data for overall survival were not mature at the time of the report. Grade 3 and 4 adverse events were more common in the sunitinib group. *Based on these results, the FDA approved sunitinib for adjuvant treatment of patients with high risk of recurrence following nephrectomy for RCC.*

3. The randomized ASSURE trial also studied adjuvant sunitinib in patients with a high risk of recurrence after nephrectomy for RCC, *but ASSURE showed no difference in disease free survival between adjuvant sunitinib and placebo.*

4. Given the conflicting data on disease free survival and the lack of proven overall survival benefit, many clinicians are not convinced that sunitinib should be utilized for adjuvant therapy. In fact, the EAU 2021 guideline states "Do not offer adjuvant sunitinib following surgically resected high risk clear renal cell carcinoma." Also, there was major disagreement in the NCCN guideline panel about whether adjuvant sunitinib is appropriate.

5. If adjuvant sunitinib is utilized, it should probably be restricted to patients with clear cell RCC (because S-TRAC only studied clear cell RCC).

Hyperfiltration Renal Injury

1. When functional renal tissue is removed, glomerular hyperfiltration occurs in the remaining tissue to restore filtration capacity.
2. Prolonged glomerular hyperfiltration may cause renal injury. This injury leads to *focal segmental glomerulosclerosis* and progressive renal failure. Hyperfiltration injury may take more than 10 years to develop.
3. *Proteinuria is the harbinger of hyperfiltration renal injury*; therefore, it precedes pathologic and clinical evidence of renal damage.
4. If *more than 75%* of the functional renal tissue is removed, hyperfiltration renal injury is more likely to occur. When ≤ 50% of functional renal tissue is removed, hyperfiltration injury uncommon. For example, after nephrectomy in kidney donors, glomerular filtration rate (GFR) does not decline significantly with 20 years of follow up.
5. Factors that increase the risk of hyperfiltration injury include removal of > 75% of functional renal mass, high protein diet, obesity, steroid use, hypertension, hyperlipidemia, and poorly controlled diabetes mellitus.
6. Ways of reducing the risk of hyperfiltration renal injury
   a. Angiotensin converting enzyme inhibitors (ACEI)—may help prevent hyperfiltration injury by lowering intraglomerular pressure. Some suggest beginning an ACEI if 24 hour urine protein is > 150 mg.
   b. Weight loss in obese patients
   c. Low protein, low sodium diet
   d. Strict control of diabetes, hypertension, and hyperlipidemia.
   e. Avoid steroid use
   f. Avoid nephrotoxins (e.g. NSAIDS)

Follow Up after PN or RN For Localized RCC

1. The majority of recurrences occur within 3 years after nephrectomy.
2. Laboratory tests—BUN, creatinine, estimated glomerular filtration rate, and urinalysis are obtained routinely. Other laboratory tests are obtained at the discretion of the physician, and may include liver function tests, alkaline phosphatase, lactate dehydrogenase, and serum calcium. In patients with less than one whole kidney, perform periodic 24 hour urine for creatinine, protein, and volume to assess for hyperfiltration injury.
3. Bone scan is recommended when alkaline phosphatase is elevated, when the patient has skeletal symptoms such as pain, or when other imaging suggests the presence of bone lesions.
4. Imaging of the central nervous system is recommended when there is an acute onset of neurological signs or symptoms.
5. Follow up during the first 5 years after PN or RN—if a microscopic positive margin is present, increase the risk category at least 1 level higher.
   a. Low risk (pT1 grade 1-2 & N0M0)—history, physical exam, lab tests, abdominal CT or MRI (without and without IV contrast), and chest x-ray at 1, 2, 4, and 5 years after surgery, and when clinically indicated. After 2 years, the clinician may consider alternating between abdominal ultrasound and abdominal cross sectional imaging.
   b. Intermediate risk (pT1 grade 3-4 or pT2 any grade; & N0M0)—history, physical exam, lab tests, abdominal CT or MRI (without and without IV contrast), and chest x-ray at 6 months and at 1, 2, 3, 4, and 5 years after surgery, and when clinically indicated. After 2 years, the clinician may consider alternating between abdominal ultrasound and cross sectional imaging.
   c. High risk (pT3 any grade & N0M0)—history, physical exam, lab tests, abdominal CT or MRI (without and without IV contrast), and chest CT at 6, 12, 18, 24, 30, 36, 48, and 60 months after surgery, and when clinically indicated.

d. Very high risk (pT4, N1M0, sarcomatoid, or macroscopic positive margin)—history, physical exam, lab tests, abdominal CT or MRI (without and with IV contrast), and chest CT at 3, 6, 9, 12, 18, 24, 30, 36, 48, and 60 months after surgery, and when clinically indicated.

6. Follow up beyond 5 years after PN or RN

  a. After 5 years, abdominal and chest imaging are optional, but history, physical exam, and labs should be obtained at 6-7 years and at 8-10 years after surgery. Imaging beyond 5 years may be most appropriate for patients with higher risk cancers.

  b. If chest imaging is continued beyond 5 years in high risk or very high risk patients, then chest x-ray may be considered rather than chest CT.

  c. Additional testing should be obtained when clinically indicated.

7. Patients with a solitary kidney should be advised that participation in contact/collision sports places the kidney at risk for traumatic injury. Need to avoid contact/collision sports is determined on an individual basis.

Treatment of Metastatic RCC

RCC with Oligometastasis

1. Oligometastasis is the presence of a few metastases (e.g ≤ 3).

2. In patients with oligometastases, long term survival has been achieved when the primary and metastatic lesions were treated.

3. When oligometastases present at the same time as the primary RCC, the preferred treatment is excision of the primary tumor and the metastases (for a brain and bone metastasis, radiation therapy is also an option).

4. When oligometastases develop after nephrectomy (local recurrence in renal fossa or other metastasis), the preferred treatment is tumor resection (for a brain and bone metastasis, radiation therapy is also an option).

5. When resection of the metastases is not feasible, then the metastasis may be treated with ablation or radiation (depending on the metastasis location). Another option is systemic therapy.

6. When oligometastases are resected, the prognosis is better when

  a. The metastases occur in the lung rather than in another location.

  b. The metastases arise after nephrectomy (initial stage M0) compared to when the metastases present with the primary tumor (initial stage M1).

RCC with Non-Oligometastases

1. Patients with metastatic renal cell carcinoma can be classified into risk categories using either the Memorial Sloan Kettering Cancer Center Prognostic Model (MSKCC) or the International Metastatic Renal Cell Carcinoma Database Consortium Criteria (IMDC).

2. Cytoreductive nephrectomy—defined as RN in M1 patients before administering systemic therapy (RN is performed to reduce tumor burden). In M1 patients, 2 randomized trials that showed RN followed by interferon (INT) improved time to progression and overall survival compared to INT alone. Currently, INT is rarely used to treat metastatic disease, and there have been no randomized trials specifically addressing cytoreductive nephrectomy with newer agents. However, *data suggests that patients with intermediate risk or high risk metastatic RCC do not benefit from cytoreductive nephrectomy before tyrosine kinase inhibitor therapy compared to tyrosine kinase inhibitor therapy alone.* Cytoreductive nephrectomy is an option for some patients with low risk metastatic RCC. It appears that patients most likely to benefit from cytoreductive nephrectomy have good performance status (e.g. ECOG performance status 0 or 1), no brain metastasis, and metastases only in the lung.

3. Palliative treatment of the primary tumor—when the primary tumor causes significant symptoms (e.g. pain, gross hematuria), nephrectomy or tumor embolization may be performed in order to control cancer related symptoms. Radiation is not effective for primary tumor control.
4. First line systemic treatment for metastatic clear cell RCC
   a. Favorable/low risk
      i. Preferred regimens: pazopanib, sunitinib, cabozantinib + nivolumab, lenvatinib + pembrolizumab, or axitinib + pembrolizumab.
      ii. Other recommended regimens: ipilimumab + nivolumab, or cabozantinib, or axitinib + avelumab.
      iii. Used in select cases: high dose IL-2 or axitinib.
   b. Intermediate or poor risk
      i. Preferred regimens: cabozantinib, cabozantinib + nivolumab, ipilimumab + nivolumab, axitinib + pembrolizumab, or lenvatinib + pembrolizumab.
      ii. Other recommended regimens: pazopanib, sunitinib, or axitinib + avelumab.
      iii. Used in select cases: high dose IL-2, axitinib, or temsirolimus.
5. First line systemic treatment for metastatic non-clear cell RCC
   a. Preferred regimens: clinical trial or sunitinib.
   b. Other recommended regimens: cabozantinib, everolimus, or lenvatinib + everolimus.
   c. Used in select cases: many options are available, including erlotinib, bevacizumab, temsirolimus, etc.
6. For intermediate risk patients who respond well to first line systemic therapy (i.e. a long term sustained response and/or minimal residual metastases), then nephrectomy may be considered. This option is based on data from the SURTIME trial, which randomized patients with metastatic clear cell RCC to immediate cytoreductive nephrectomy followed by sunitinib or to deferred nephrectomy (sunitinib administered first, then nephrectomy if there was no progression on sunitinib). Overall survival was longer for patients in the deferred nephrectomy group.
7. Chemotherapy is ineffective for most types of RCC; however, it has shown modest activity in medullary RCC and collecting duct RCC. Oral targeted therapies (e.g. tyrosine kinase inhibitors) are not effective for renal medullary RCC. Thus, either a clinical trial or systemic chemotherapy is the treatment of choice for metastatic medullary RCC.
8. *Systemic therapies are poorly effective against brain metastases. Brain metastases may be treated with radiation or surgical resection, especially if they are symptomatic or growing.*
9. Radiation may be used for palliation of bone and brain metastasis.

Tyrosine Kinase Inhibitors (TKIs)
1. *Tyrosine kinase inhibitors reduce angiogenesis and cell proliferation.* They inhibit various tyrosine kinases, such as vascular endothelial growth factor receptor (VEGFR), platelet derived growth factor receptor (PDGFR), and stem cell factor receptor (KIT).
2. TKIs are indicated for the treatment of advanced or metastatic RCC.
3. TKIs appear to improve median progression free survival by 2-6 months and improve median overall survival by a few months.
4. Examples of TKIs include sunitinib, sorafenib, pazopanib, axitinib, cabozantinib, lenvatinib, and erlotinib.
5. Compared to sunitinib, pazopanib causes less fatigue, less hand and foot syndrome, less altered taste, less thrombocytopenia, and better quality of life, but a higher risk of elevated LFTs. Both pazopanib and sunitinib are options for first line treatment of low risk metastatic clear cell RCC.

6. Side effects—skin reactions ("hand and foot syndrome"), gastrointestinal (vomiting, diarrhea, elevated amylase, elevated liver function tests, altered taste), hypophosphatemia, hypothyroidism, hypertension, proteinuria, bleeding, hematologic (thrombocytopenia, neutropenia), alopecia, headache, fatigue, and embolic events (e.g. stroke and myocardial infarction). Low ejection fraction, cardiac ischemia, and prolonged QT have been reported.

7. During therapy, check blood pressure, complete blood count, urinalysis for protein, thyroid function tests, and serum chemistries (sodium, potassium, phosphate, creatinine, liver function tests, amylase, lipase). Monitoring of ejection fraction can be considered.

8. Since these medications impair angiogenesis, they can interfere with wound healing. To avoid poor wound healing, stop the TKI before elective surgery. Do not resume the TKI until wound healing is adequate. The time frame in which the TKI is stopped before and after surgery depends on the TKI being used.

Immune Check Point Inhibitors

1. Immune check point inhibitors are medications that block an important regulatory step of the immune system. These medications typically reduce the tumor's ability to evade the immune system, which allows the immune system to more effectively attack the cancer.

2. PD-1/PD-L1 pathway inhibitors—examples include pembrolizumab, nivolumab, and avelumab. For details on these medicines, see page 82 (pembrolizumab), page 83 (nivolumab), and page 83 (avelumab).

   a. The programmed death receptor-1 (PD-1) is located on lymphocytes. When certain proteins bind to PD-1, the immune system has a reduced capacity to attack normal tissues (decreasing auto-immune reactions) and a reduced capacity to attack malignant tissues (hindering the body's ability to kill cancer). PD-L1 (programmed death ligand 1) is a protein that binds to the PD-1 receptor. Many cancers evade the body's defenses by expressing a high level of PD-L1, which binds to PD-1 and inhibits the immune system's ability to kill cancer.

   b. Medicines can block the binding of PD-L1 to PD-1 by attaching to PD-L1 (PD-L1 inhibitors) or by attaching to the PD-1 receptor (PD-1 inhibitors). However, both PD-1 inhibitors and PD-L1 inhibitors achieve their anticancer effects by inhibiting the PD-1/PD-L1 pathway.

   c. The increased immune activity from blocking the PD-1/PD-L1 pathway can also result in an attack on normal tissue (which leads to some of the side effects). Since all PD-1 inhibitors and PD-L1 inhibitors block the same pathway, they all tend to have similar side effects.

3. CTLA-4 pathway inhibitor—examples include ipilimumab.

   a. CTLA-4 (cytotoxic T lymphocyte antigen 4) is a protein receptor on activated T cells. Under normal circumstances, a ligand binds to the CTLA-4 receptor and down-regulates the cytotoxic activity of T-cells.

   b. Ipilimumab is a monoclonal antibody that binds to the CTLA-4 receptor and blocks the down-regulation of cytotoxic activity, which increases the immune system's ability to kill the cancer.

Mammalian Target of Rapamycin (mTOR) Inhibitor

1. mTOR is a protein that regulates hypoxia inducible factor (HIF) and vascular endothelial growth factor (VEGF). When mTOR is inhibited, VEGF decreases (which reduces angiogenesis) and HIF decreases (which reduces cell proliferation). *Thus, mTOR inhibitors reduce angiogenesis and cell proliferation.*

2. Temsirolimus and everolimus inhibit mTOR.
3. Temsirolimus is FDA approved for the treatment of advanced RCC in patients with predictors of short survival.
4. Everolimus is FDA approved for the treatment of advanced RCC after failure of sorafenib or sunitinib. Everolimus is also FDA approved to shrink angiomyolipoma (AML) in patients with tuberous sclerosis whose AML does not require surgery.
5. Side effects—include rash, stomatitis (e.g. mouth ulcers), infections, asthenia (weakness), peripheral edema, gastrointestinal (nausea, vomiting, diarrhea, anorexia), hematologic (thrombocytopenia, neutropenia, anemia), hyperglycemia, hyperlipidemia, elevated creatinine, elevated liver function tests, and hypophosphatemia. Rare side effects include bowel perforation and interstitial pneumonitis (cough, dyspnea, hypoxia).

Interleukin

1. Interleukin-2 (IL-2)—a cytokine that stimulates cell mediated immunity. It was one of the first FDA approved treatments for advanced RCC, but it is rarely used now because of its toxicity and its limited effectiveness in most patients.
   a. IL-2 is used to treat clear cell RCC (other types of RCC usually do not respond to IL-2).
   b. To be a candidate for IL-2, the patient must have no brain metastasis and have adequate cardiac, renal, and pulmonary function. Good performance status (ECOG PS < 2), predominantly clear cell carcinoma, and absence of sarcomatoid features are preferred.
   c. The most effective regimen is "high dose bolus IL-2". Each cycle consists of intravenous IL-2 (600,000 or 720,000 IU/kg) q 8 hours x 14 doses. 2 cycles are given with 5-9 days of rest in between cycles. In responding patients, this 2 cycle course is repeated every 6-12 weeks.
   d. Side effects—include fever, chills, weight gain, fluid retention, reversible renal and hepatic insufficiency, and hypotension.
   e. Response rate = 16% (5% complete response; 11% partial response).
   f. Criteria that predict a better response to IL-2: ECOG PS of 0, absence of metastases in multiple organs, no bone metastasis, lung only metastasis, prior nephrectomy, and no sarcomatoid features in the primary tumor.
2. Interferon—interferon is less effective than IL-2.

Bevacizumab with Interferon Alfa-2a

1. Bevacizumab, a recombinant monoclonal antibody, inhibits angiogenesis and tumor growth by binding to and neutralizing vascular endothelial growth factor A (VEGF-A).
2. Bevacizumab with interferon alfa-2a is FDA approved for treatment of metastatic RCC.
3. In patients with clear cell RCC, bevacizumab with interferon alfa-2a improves progression free survival by 3-5 months compared to interferon alone, but it did not improve overall survival. *Thus, bevacizumab with interferon is more effective than interferon alone.* Most patients that were studied had a previous nephrectomy.
4. Side effects—include dry mouth, headache, hypertension, stomatitis (e.g. mouth ulcers), gastrointestinal (dyspepsia, anorexia, constipation), dyspnea, voice changes, minor bleeding, and poor wound healing. Rare side effects include bowel perforation and hemorrhage.
5. To avoid poor wound healing, stop bevacizumab at least 28 days before elective surgery. It may be resumed at least 28 days after surgery.

Treatment for RCC (Adapted from the NCCN, AUA, & EAU Guidelines)

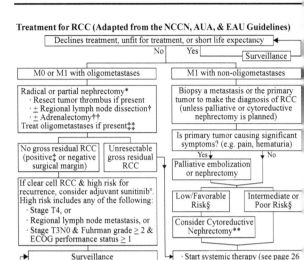

CNS = central nervous system; RCC = renal cell carcinoma;
ECOG = Eastern Cooperative Oncology Group

* Partial nephrectomy is the preferred treatment for most clinical stage T1 tumors. Ablation may be utilized for select T1 tumors (mainly tumors < 3 cm).

** Patients that are most likely to benefit from cytoreductive nephrectomy have good performance status (e.g. ECOG performance status 0 or 1), no brain metastasis, and metastases only in the lung.

† Regional lymph node dissection (LND) does not improve survival. LND is unnecessary in patients with clinical N0 disease, but should be considered in patients at high risk for regional node metastases. LND is recommended in patients with clinical N1 disease (enlarged lymph nodes found on imaging or intraoperatively) because it helps to accurately stage the tumor (some enlarged lymph nodes do not harbor malignancy).

†† Perform adrenalectomy when there is an abnormal ipsilateral adrenal gland on preoperative imaging or when there is an intraoperative suspicion of adrenal involvement.

‡ When a positive margin is present, repeat resection may be considered in patient's with an aggressive tumor.

‡‡ Excision of the metastasis is usually preferred (for a brain and bone metastasis, radiation therapy is also an option).

° Adjuvant sunitinib is continued for 1 year as tolerated.

°° Local recurrence includes tumor in the renal fossa after radical nephrectomy and tumor in the ipsilateral kidney after renal sparing therapy.

§ Risk is assigned based on the Memorial Sloan Kettering Cancer Center Prognostic Model (MSKCC) or the International Metastatic Renal Cell Carcinoma Database Consortium Criteria (IMDC).

Recurrence and Survival

Recurrence After Curative Treatment for Primary RCC

1. After partial or radical nephrectomy, local recurrence in the renal fossa is rare (< 2%). Resection of a local recurrence (in the absence of metastatic disease) can achieve long term survival.
2. In the absence of genetic and familial RCC syndromes, recurrence in the contralateral kidney is rare (2-4%).
3. *Lung is the most common site of distant recurrence.*
4. Most recurrences occur within 3 years of treatment.

Poor Prognostic Factors of RCC

1. Higher ECOG performance status
2. Symptomatic tumor
3. High stage tumor
4. Large tumor size
5. Collecting system invasion
6. High grade tumor
7. Sarcomatoid features
8. Tumor necrosis
9. Microvascular invasion
10. Histology—the prognosis is worse for collecting duct, medullary, type II papillary, and unclassified RCC.
11. Higher level of tumor thrombus
12. Tumor thrombus invading the vena cava wall
13. Residual tumor—incomplete resection or positive margin.
14. Presence of metastases

ECOG PS	Activity
0	Normal Activity
1	Symptomatic but ambulatory
2	Bedridden < 50% of the time
3	Bedridden > 50% of the time
4	Completely bedridden

ECOG PS = Eastern Cooperative Oncology Group performance status

Survival Based on Nomograms

Nomograms can predict metastasis free survival and cancer specific survival for patients who undergo partial or radical nephrectomy for RCC.
   a. Preoperative—J Urol, 179(6): 2146, 2008; Eur Urol, 55(2): 287, 2009.
   b. Postoperative—J Clin Oncol, 25: 1316, 2007.

Survival Based on the UCLA Integrated Staging System (UISS)

2017 TNM Stage	ECOG PS	Fuhrman Grade	5-Year Disease Specific Survival	When Treated With
T1 N0M0	0	1-2	91%	Radical Nephrectomy*
	0	3-4		
	≥1	Any		
T2 N0M0	Any	Any	80%	
T3 N0M0	0	Any		
	≥1	1		
	≥1	≥2	55%	
T4 N0M0	Any	Any		
N1M0 (only one node metastasis)	Any	Any	32%	Radical Nephrectomy* ± Immunotherapy
N1M0 (> 1 node metastasis) or M1	0	1-2		
	0	3-4	20%	
	≥1	1-3		
	≥1	4	0%	

* Tumor thrombectomy was performed when tumor thrombus was present.
ECOG PS = ECOG performance status (see page 31)

Survival Based on TNM Stage

Pathologic Stage (AJCC 2017)	Treatment	5-Year *Disease Specific* Survival
T1aN0M0	RN or PN	95-100%
T1bN0M0	RN or PN	88-92%
T2N0M0	RN	88%

Pathologic Stage (AJCC 2017)	Treatment	5-Year *Overall* Survival
T3aN0M0 in perirenal or sinus fat, but no venous tumor thrombus	RN	47-68%
T3N0M0 with tumor thrombus in the renal vein or vena cava°	RN & thrombectomy	43-72%
T4 not into contiguous organs	RN	28%
T4 into contiguous organs	RN	< 5%
N1M0	RN	0-33%
Solitary recurrence develops after nephrectomy for M0 tumor	Treatment of recurrence†	13-54*
Solitary metastasis present at initial diagnosis	RN & treatment of metastasis†	0-20%**
Multiple unresectable metastases	Any therapy	0%‡

RN = radical nephrectomy, PN= partial nephrectomy
° A more extensive tumor thrombus is associated with a lower disease specific survival. Tumor thrombus invading the caval wall has a worse prognosis than free floating thrombus.
* Survival is from time of metastasis resection. Pulmonary metastasis probably have better prognosis than other metastatic locations. A longer interval between RN and the development of a metastasis (especially > 2 years) is associated with a longer survival from the time of metastasis resection.
** Most die within 2 years of diagnosis. These patients have a worse survival than patients that develop a solitary metastasis after RN.
† Options include resection, cryotherapy, or radiation. Resection is often preferred.
‡ Most die within one year of diagnosis.

REFERENCES

Renal Tumors - General
Modlin CS, Novick AC: Hyperfiltration renal injury: urologic implications. AUA Update Series, Vol. 20, Lesson 6, 2001.

Renal Biopsy
Alle N, et al: Percutaneous image guided core biopsy of solid renal masses: analysis of safety, efficacy, pathologic interpretation, and clinical significance. Abdom Radiol (NY), 43(7): 1813, 2018.
Dechet CB, et al: Prospective analysis of computerized tomography and needle biopsy with permanent sectioning to determine the nature of solid renal masses in adults. J Urol, 169: 71, 2003.
Marconi L, et al: Systematic review and meta-analysis of diagnostic accuracy of percutaneous renal tumor biopsy. Eur Urol, 69(4): 660, 2016.
Neuzillet Y, et al: Accuracy and clinical role of fine needle percutaneous biopsy with computerized tomography guidance of small (less than 4.0 cm) renal masses. J Urol, 171:1802, 2004.
Patel HD, et al: Diagnostic accuracy and risks of biopsy in the diagnosis of a renal mass suspicious for localized renal cell carcinoma: systematic review of the literature. J Urol, 195(5): 1340, 2016.
Posielski NM, et al: Risk factors for complications and non-diagnostic results following 1155 consecutive percutaneous core renal mass biopsies. J Urol, 201(6): 1080, 2019.

Renal Biopsy - Tumor Seeding Along the Biopsy Tract

Busset C, et al: A case report of papillary renal cell carcinoma seeding along a percutaneous biopsy tract. Open Journal of Pathology, 8: 139, 2018.

Chang DTS, et al: Needle tract seeding following percutaneous biopsy of renal cell carcinoma. Korean J Urol, 56(9): 666, 2015.

Herts BR, et al: The current role of percutaneous biopsy in the evaluation of renal masses. Semin Urol Oncol, 13(4): 254, 1995.

Macklin PS, et al: Tumor seeding in the tract of percutaneous renal tumor biopsy: a report on seven cases from a UK tertiary referral center. Urology, 75(5): 861, 2019.

Mullins JK, et al: Renal cell carcinoma seeding of a percutaneous biopsy tract. Can J Assoc J, 7: e176, 2013.

Renshaw AA, et al: Needle tract seeding in renal mass biopsies. Cancer Cytopathol, 127(6): 358, 2019.

Singer E, et al: Tumor seeding from a percutaneous renal mass biopsy. Urol Case Rep, 23: 32, 2018.

Soares D, et al: Papillary renal cell carcinoma seeding along a percutaneous biopsy tract. Case Rep Urol, 2015: 925254, 2015.

Hereditary Disorders Associated with Renal Tumors

Cybulski C, et al: CHEK2 is a multi-organ cancer susceptibility gene. Am J Hum Genet, 75: 1131, 2004.

Haas NB, et al: Hereditary renal cancer syndromes. Adv Chronic Kidney Dis, 21(1): 81, 2014.

Klein EA, Novick AC: Urologic manifestations of von Hippel Lindau disease. AUA Update Series, Vol. 19, Lesson 33, 1990.

Lendvay TS, Marshall FF: The tuberous sclerosis complex and its highly variable manifestations. J Urol, 169: 1635, 2003.

Maher ER: Hereditary renal cell carcinoma syndromes: diagnosis, surveillance and management. World J Urol, 36: 1891, 2018.

Pavlovich CP, et al: Evaluation and management of renal tumors in the Birt-Hogg-Dubé syndrome. J Urol, 173: 1482, 2005.

Benign Tumors

Bissler JJ, et al: Everolimus for angiomyolipoma associated with tuberous sclerosis complex or sporadic lymphangioleiomyomatosis (EXIST-2): a multicenter, randomized, double blind, placebo controlled trial. Lancet, 381: 817, 2013.

Dechet CB, et al: Renal oncocytoma: multifocality, bilateralism, metachronous tumor development and coexistent renal cell carcinoma. J Urol, 162: 40, 1999.

Feldman AE, Pollack HM, Perri Jr AJ, et al: Renal pseudotumors: an anatomic-radiographic classification. J Urol, 120: 133, 1978.

Nelson CP, Sanda M: Contemporary diagnosis and management of renal angiomyolipoma. J Urol, 168: 1315, 2002.

Steiner MS, Goldman SM, Fishman EK, et al: The natural history of renal angiomyolipoma. J Urol, 150: 1782, 1993.

Surveillance & Relation of Tumor Size to Aggressiveness

Alam R, et al: Comparative effectiveness of management options for patients with small renal masses: a prospective cohort study. BJU Int, 123: 42, 2019.

Chawla SN, et al: The natural history of observed enhancing renal masses: a meta-analysis and review of the world literature. J Urol, 175(2): 425, 2006.

Corcoran AT, et al: A review of contemporary data on surgically resected small renal masses - benign or malignant. Urology, 81(4): 707, 2013.

Crispen PL, et al: Natural history, growth kinetics, and outcomes of untreated clinically localized renal tumors under active surveillance. Cancer, 115: 2844, 2009.

Crispen PL, et al: Delayed intervention of sporadic renal masses undergoing active surveillance. Cancer, 112: 1051, 2008.

Frank I, et al: Solid renal tumors: an analysis of pathological features related to tumor size. J Urol, 170: 2217, 2003.

Guo RQ, et al: Comparison of survival benefits of nephron sparing intervention or active surveillance for patients with localized renal masses: a systematic review and meta-analysis. BMC Urology, 19: 74, 2019.

Jewett MAS, et al: Active surveillance of small renal masses: progression patterns of early stage kidney cancer. Eur Urol, 60: 39, 2011.

Kates M, et al: Predictors of locally advanced and metastatic disease in patients with small renal masses. BJU Int, 109(10): 1463, 2012.

Klatte T, et al: Tumor size does not predict risk of metastatic disease or prognosis of small renal cell carcinomas. J Urol, 179(5): 1719, 2008.

Ku JH, et al: Metachronous metastatic potential of small renal cell carcinoma: dependence on tumor size. Urology, 74(6): 1271, 2009.

McIntosh AG, et al: Active surveillance for localized renal masses: tumor growth, delayed intervention rates, and >5 years clinical outcomes. Eur Urol, 74(2): 157, 2018.

Nguyen MM, Gill IS: Effect of renal cancer size on the prevalence of metastasis at diagnosis and mortality. J Urol, 181(3): 1020, 2009.

Pahernik S, et al: Small renal tumors: correlation of clinical and pathological features with tumor size. J Urol, 178: 414, 2007.

Remzi M, et al: Are small renal tumors harmless? Analysis of histopathological features according to tumors 4 cm or less in diameter. J Urol, 176: 896, 2006.

Rosales JC, et al: Active surveillance for renal cortical neoplasms. J Urol, 183(5): 1698, 2010.

Rothman J, et al: Histopathological characteristics of localized renal call carcinoma correlate with tumor size: a SEER analysis. J Urol, 181(1): 29, 2009.

Smaldone M, et al: Small renal masses progressing to metastasis under active surveillance. Cancer, 118: 997, 2012.

Thompson RH, et al: Tumor size is associated with malignancy potential in renal cell carcinoma cases. J Urol, 181: 2033, 2009.

Thompson RH, et al: Metastatic renal cell carcinoma risk according to tumor size. J Urol, 182(1): 41, 2009.

Zini L, at al: A population based comparison of survival after nephrectomy vs. nonsurgical management for small renal masses. BJU Int, 103: 899, 2009.

Renal Cell Carcinoma - Types of RCC

Cindolo L, et al: Chromophobe renal cell carcinoma: comprehensive analysis of 104 cases from multicenter European database. Urology, 65: 681, 2005.

Crispen PL, et al: Unclassified renal cell carcinoma: impact on survival following nephrectomy. J Urol, 76(3): 580, 2010.

Crotty TB, Farrow GM, Lieber MM: Chromophobe cell renal carcinoma: clinicopathological features of 50 cases. J Urol, 154: 964, 1995.

Davis CJ Jr., Mostofi FK, Sesterhen IA: Renal medullary carcinoma. The seventh sickle cell nephropathy. Am J of Surg Pathol, 19: 1, 1995.

Leibovich BC, et al: Histologic subtype is an independent predictor of outcome for patients with renal cell carcinoma. J Urol, 183(4): 1309, 2010.

Patard JJ, et al: Prognostic value of histologic subtypes in renal cell carcinoma: a multicenter experience. J Clin Oncol, 23(12): 2763, 2005.

Pignot G, et al: Survival analysis of 130 patients with papillary renal cell carcinoma: prognostic utility of type 1 and type 2 subclassification. Urology, 69(2): 230, 2007.

Pirich LM, et al: Prolonged survival of a patient with sickle cell trait and metastatic renal medullary carcinoma. J Pediatr Hematol Oncol, 21: 67, 1999.

Zambrano NR, et al: Histopathology and molecular genetics of renal tumors: toward unification of a classification system. J Urol, 162: 1246, 1999.

Zisman A, et al: Unclassified renal cell carcinoma: clinical features and prognostic impact of a new histological subtype. J Urol, 168: 950, 2002.

Renal Cell Carcinoma - General

AUA—Campbell S, et al: Renal mass and localized renal cancer: evaluation, management, and follow up: AUA guideline. AUA Education and Research, Inc., 2021. (www.auanet.org).

EAU—Ljundberg B, et al: Guidelines on renal cell carcinoma. European Association of Urology, 2021. (www.uroweb.org).

Fuhrman SA, Lasky LC, Limas C: Prognostic significance of morphologic parameters in renal cell carcinoma. Am J Surg Pathol, 6: 655, 1982.

Gelfond J, et al: Modifiable risk factors to reduce renal carcinoma incidence: insight from the PLCO trial. Urol Oncol, 36(7): 340.e1, 2018.

MacLennan S, et al: Systematic review of oncological outcomes following surgical management of localized renal cancer. Eur Urol, 61(5): 972, 2012.

NCCN—National Comprehensive Cancer Network clinical practice guidelines in oncology: kidney cancer. V.4.2021, 2021. (www.nccn.org).

Zisman A, Pantuck AJ, Wieder J, et al: Risk group assessment and clinical outcome algorithm to predict the natural history of patients with surgically resected renal cell carcinoma. J Clin Oncol, 20: 4559, 2002.

Partial Nephrectomy Versus Ablation

Alam R, et al: Comparative effectiveness of management options for patients with small renal masses: a prospective cohort study. BJU Int, 123: 42, 2019.

Go AS, et al: Chronic kidney disease and the risks of death, cardiovascular events, and hospitalization. New Engl J Med, 351: 1296, 2004.

Huang WC, et al: Chronic kidney disease after nephrectomy in patients with renal cortical tumors: a retrospective study. Lancet Oncol, 7(9): 735, 2006.

Klatte T, et al: Perioperative, oncologic, and functional outcomes of laparoscopic cryoablation and open partial nephrectomy. J Endourol, 25(6): 991, 2011.

Klatte T, et al: Systematic review and meta-analysis of perioperative and oncologic outcomes of laparoscopic cryoablation versus laparoscopic partial nephrectomy for the treatment of small renal tumors. J Urol, 191(5, part 1): 1209, 2014.

Kunkle DA, et al: Excise, ablate, or observe: the small renal mass dilemma - a meta-analysis and review. J Urol, 179: 1227, 2008.

Pan XW, et al: Radiofrequency ablation versus partial nephrectomy for treatment of renal masses: a systematic review and meta-analysis. Kaohsiung J Med Sci, 31: 649, 2015.

Pierorazio PM, et al: Management of renal masses and localized renal cancer: systematic review and meta-analysis. J Urol, 196(4): 989, 2016.

Rivero JR, et al: Partial nephrectomy versus thermal ablation for clinical stage T1 renal masses: systematic review and meta-analysis of more than 3900 patients. J Vasc Interv Radiol, 29(1): 18, 2018.

Weight CJ, et al: Nephrectomy induced chronic renal insufficiency is associated with increased risk of cardiac death and death from any cause in patients with localized cT1b renal masses. J Urol, 183(4): 1317, 2010.

Whitson JM, et al: Population based comparative effectiveness of nephron sparing surgery vs ablation for small renal masses. BJU Int, 110: 1438, 2012.

Partial Nephrectomy - General

Minervini A, et al: Simple enucleation is equivalent to traditional partial nephrectomy for renal cell carcinoma: results of a non-randomized, retrospective, comparative study. J Urol, 185(5): 1604, 2011.

Minervini A, et al: Endoscopic robot assisted simple enucleation (ERASE) for clinical T1 renal masses: description of the technique and early postoperative results. Surg Endosc, 29(5): 1241, 2015.Pahernik, S, et al: Elective nephron sparing surgery for renal cell carcinoma larger than 4 cm. J Urol, 179(1): 71, 2008.

Mir MC, et al: Partial nephrectomy versus radical nephrectomy for clinical T1b and T2 renal tumors: a systematic review and meta-analysis of comparative studies. Eur Urol, 71(4): 606, 2017.

Pahernik, S, et al: Nephron sparing surgery for renal cell carcinoma with normal contralateral kidney: 25 years of experience. J Urol, 175: 2027, 2006.

Uzzo RG, Novick AC: Nephron sparing surgery for renal tumors: indications, techniques, and outcomes. J Urol, 166: 6, 2001.

Partial Nephrectomy - Renal Ischemia Time & Preservation of Renal Function

Becker F, et al: Assessing the impact of ischemia time during partial nephrectomy. Eur Urol, 56(4): 625, 2009.

Breau RH, et al: Hypothermia during partial nephrectomy for patients with renal tumors: a randomized controlled trial. J Urol, 205(5): 1303, 2021.

Cooper CA, et al: Intraoperative mannitol not essential during partial nephrectomy.J Endourol, 32(4): 354, 2018.

Funahashi Y, et al: Comparison of warm and cold ischemia on renal function after partial nephrectomy. Urology, 84(6): 1408, 2014.

Spaliviero M, et al: Intravenous mannitol versus placebo during partial nephrectomy in patients with normal kidney function: a double blind clinically integrated randomized trial. Eur Urol, 73(1): 53, 2018.

Partial Nephrectomy - Surgical Margins

Bensalah K, et al: Positive surgical margin appears to have negligible impact on survival of renal cell carcinomas treated by nephron sparing surgery. Eur Urol, 57(3): 466, 2010.

Castilla EA, et al: Prognostic importance of resection margin width after nephron sparing surgery for renal cell carcinoma. Urology, 60(6): 993, 2002.

Kwon EO, et al: Impact of positive surgical margins in patients undergoing partial nephrectomy for renal cortical tumors. BJU Int, 99(2): 286, 2007.

Marszalek M, et al: Positive surgical margins after nephron sparing surgery. Eur Urol, 61(4): 757, 2012.

Sutherland SE, et al: Does the size of the surgical margin in partial nephrectomy for renal cell cancer really matter? J Urol, 167: 61, 2002.

Timsit MO, et al: Prospective study of safety margins in partial nephrectomy. Urology, 67(5): 923, 2006.

Yossepowitch O, et al: Positive surgical margins at partial nephrectomy: predictors and oncological outcomes. J Urol, 179(6): 2158, 2008.

Nephron Sparing Therapy Versus Radical Nephrectomy

Alam R, et al: Comparative effectiveness of management options for patients with small renal masses: a prospective cohort study. BJU Int, 123: 42, 2019.

Badalato GM, et al: Survival after partial and radical nephrectomy for the treatment of stage T1bN0M0 renal cell carcinoma in the USA. BJU Int, 109(10): 1457, 2012.

Crepel M, et al: Nephron sparing surgery is equally effective to radical nephrectomy for T1bN0M0 renal cell carcinoma. Urology, 75(2): 271, 2010

Crepel M, et al: A population based comparison of cancer control rates between radical and partial nephrectomy for T1a renal cell carcinoma. Urology, 76(4): 883, 2010.

EORTC 30904—Scosyrev E, et al: Renal function after nephron sparing surgery versus radical nephrectomy: results from the EORTC randomized trial 30904. Eur Urol, 65: 372, 2014.

EORTC 30904—Van Poppel H, et al: A prospective randomized EORTC Intergroup phase 3 study comparing the complications of elective nephron sparing surgery and radical nephrectomy for low stage renal cell carcinoma. Eur Urol, 51: 1606, 2007.

EORTC 30904—Van Poppel H, et al: A prospective randomized EORTC Intergroup phase 3 study comparing the oncologic outcome of elective nephron sparing surgery and radical nephrectomy for low stage renal cell carcinoma. Eur Urol, 59: 543, 2011.

Huang WC, et al: Partial nephrectomy versus radical nephrectomy in patients with small renal tumors: is there a difference in mortality and cardiovascular disease? J Urol, 181(1): 55, 2009.

Hung-jui T, et al: Long term survival following partial versus radical nephrectomy among older patients with early stage kidney cancer. JAMA, 307(15): 1629, 2012.

Weldres C, et al: Partial versus radical nephrectomy in patients with adverse clinical or pathologic characteristics. Urology, 73(6): 1300, 2009.

Kopp RP, et al: Does radical nephrectomy increase the risk of erectile dysfunction compared with partial nephrectomy. BJU Int, 111: E98, 2013.

Lau WK, et al: Matched comparison of radical nephrectomy vs. nephron sparing surgery in patients with unilateral renal cell carcinoma and a normal contralateral kidney. Mayo Clin Proc, 75(12): 1236, 2000.

Lee H, et al: Outcomes of pathologic stage T3a renal cell carcinoma up staged from small renal tumor: emphasis on partial nephrectomy. BMC Cancer, 18: 427, 2018.

MacLennan S, et al: Systematic review of oncological outcomes following surgical management of localized renal cancer. Eur Urol, 61(5): 972, 2012.

McKiernan J, et al: Natural history of chronic renal insufficiency after partial and radical nephrectomy. Urology, 59(6): 816, 2002.

Mir MC, et al: Partial nephrectomy versus radical nephrectomy for clinical T1b and T2 renal tumors: a systematic review and meta-analysis of comparative studies. Eur Urol, 71(4): 606, 2017.

Patard JJ, et al: The use of nephron sparing surgery may favorably impact the risk of non-cancer related death in renal cell carcinoma. J Urol, 181(4, suppl): 322 (abstract 901), 2009.

Pierorazio PM, et al: Management of renal masses and localized renal cancer: systematic review and meta-analysis. J Urol, 196(4): 989, 2016.

Scosyrev E, et al: Overall survival after partial versus radical nephrectomy for a small renal mass: systematic review of observational studies. Urology Practice, 1(1): 27, 2014.

Sun M, et al: A non-cancer related survival benefit is associated with partial nephrectomy. Eur Urol, 61(4): 725, 2012.

Tan HJ, et al: Long term survival following partial vs radical nephrectomy among older patients with early stage kidney cancer. JAMA, 307(15): 1629, 2012.

Thompson RH, et al: Radical nephrectomy for pT1a renal masses may be associated with decreased overall survival compared to partial nephrectomy. J Urol, 179(2): 468, 2008.

Weight CJ, et al: Elective partial nephrectomy in patients with clinical T1b renal tumors is associated with improved overall survival. Urology, 76: 631, 2010.

Zini L, et al: Radical versus partial nephrectomy: effect on overall survival and non-cancer mortality. Cancer, 115(7): 1465, 2009.

Lymph Node Dissection

Bhindi B, et al: The role of lymph node dissection in the management of renal cell carcinoma: a systematic review and meta-analysis. BJU Int, 121(5): 684, 2018.

Blute ML, et al: A protocol for performing extended lymph node dissection using primary tumor pathological features for patients treated with radical nephrectomy for clear cell renal carcinoma. J Urol, 172(2): 465, 2004.

Canfield SE, et al: Renal cell carcinoma with nodal metastases in the absence of distant metastatic disease (clinical stage TxN1-2M0): the impact of aggressive surgical resection on patient outcome. J Urol, 175: 864, 2006.

Crispen PL, et al: Lymph node dissection at the time of radical nephrectomy for high risk clear cell renal cell carcinoma: indications and recommendations for surgical templates. Eur Urol: 59: 18, 2011.

EORTC 30881—Blom JH, et al: Radical nephrectomy with and without lymph node dissection: final results of the European Organization for Research and Treatment of Cancer (EORTC) randomized phase 3 trial 30881. Eur Urol, 55(1): 28, 2009. [Update of Eur Urol 36: 570, 1999].

Hutterer GC, et al: Patients with renal cell carcinoma nodal metastases can be accurately identified: external validation of a new nomogram. Int J Cancer, 121: 2556, 2007.

Karakiewicz PI, et al: Renal cell carcinoma with nodal metastases in the absence of distant metastatic disease. Eur Urol, 51: 1616, 2007.

Leibovich BC, Blute ML: Lymph node dissection in the management of renal cell carcinoma. Urol Clin North Am, 35: 673, 2008.

Minervini A, et al: Regional lymph node dissection in the treatment of renal cell carcinoma: is it useful in patients with no suspected adenopathy before or during surgery? BJU Int 88: 16, 2001.

Pantuck AJ, et al: Renal cell carcinoma with retroperitoneal lymph nodes: role of lymph node dissection. J Urol, 169(6): 2076, 2003.

Vasselli JR, et al: Lack of retroperitoneal lymphadenopathy predicts survival of patients with metastatic renal cell carcinoma. J Urol 166: 68, 2001.

Whitsin JM, et al: Lymphadenectomy improves survival of patients with renal cell carcinoma and nodal metastases. J Urol, 185(5): 1615, 2011.

Adrenal Sparing

Lane BR, et al: Management of the adrenal gland during partial nephrectomy. J Urol, 181(6), 2430, 2009.

O'Malley RL, et al: The necessity of adrenalectomy at the time of radical nephrectomy: a systematic review. J Urol, 181: 2009, 2009.

Tumor Thrombus and Caval Wall Invasion

Ciancio G, et al: Liver transplantation techniques for the surgical management of renal cell carcinoma with tumor thrombus in the inferior vena cava: step by step description. Eur Urol, 59(3): 401, 2011.

Ciancio G, et al: Management of renal cell carcinoma with level III thrombus in the inferior vena cava. J Urol, 168(4, part 1): 1374, 2002.

Dominik J, et al: Long term survival after radical surgery for renal cell carcinoma with tumor thrombus extension into the right atrium. BJU Int, 111: E59 2013.

Glazer AA, Novick AC: Long-term follow up after surgical treatment for renal cell carcinoma extending into the right atrium. J Urol, 155: 448, 1996.

Hatcher PA, Anderson EE, et al: Surgical management and prognosis of renal cell carcinoma invading the vena cava. J Urol, 145: 20, 1991.

Horn T, et al: Presurgical treatment with sunitinib for renal cell carcinoma with a level III/IV vena cava tumor thrombus. Anticancer Res, 32(5): 1729, 2012.

Libertino JA, Zinman L, Watkins, E: Long-term results of resection of renal cell carcinoma with extension into inferior vena cava. J Urol, 137: 21, 1987.

Martinez-Salamanca JI, et al: Prognostic impact of the 2009 UICC/AJCC TNM staging system for renal cell carcinoma with venous extension. Eur Urol, 59(1): 120, 2011.

Nesbitt JC, Soltero ER, et al: Surgical management of renal cell carcinoma with inferior vena cava tumor thrombus. Ann Thorac Surg, 63: 1592, 1997.

Polascik TJ, et al: Frequent occurrence of metastatic disease in patients with renal cell carcinoma and intrahepatic or supradiaphragmatic intracaval extension treated with surgery: an outcome analysis. Urology, 52: 995, 1998.

Sano F, et al: Presurgical downstaging of vena caval tumor thrombus in advanced clear cell renal cell carcinoma using temsirolimus. Int J Urol, 20: 637, 2013.

Skinner DG, Pritchett TR, Lieskovsky G, et al: Vena caval involvement by renal cell carcinoma. Ann Surg, 210: 387, 1989.

Suggs WD, Smith RB III, Dodson TF, et al: Renal cell carcinoma with inferior vena cava involvement. J Vasc Surg, 14: 413, 1991.

Swierzewski DJ, et al: Radical nephrectomy in patients with renal cell carcinoma with venous, vena caval and atrial extension. Am J Surg, 168: 205, 1994.

Takeda H, et al: Downsizing a thrombus of advanced renal cell carcinoma in a presurgical setting with sorafenib. Urol Int, 88(2): 235, 2012.

Tongaonkar HB, Dandekar NP, Dalal AV, et al: Renal cell carcinoma extending to the renal vein and inferior vena cava: results of surgical treatment and prognostic factors. J Surg Oncol, 59: 94, 1995.

Vaidya A, Ciancio G, Soloway M: Surgical techniques for treating a renal neoplasm invading the inferior vena cava. J Urol, 169(2): 435, 2003.

Wieder JA, et al: Renal cell carcinoma with tumor thrombus extension into the pulmonary artery. J Urol, 169: 2296, 2003.

Zisman A, Wieder JA, et al: Renal cell carcinoma with tumor thrombus extension: biology, role of nephrectomy and response to immunotherapy. J Urol, 169: 909, 2003.

Adjuvant Therapy After Nephrectomy

ASSURE—Haas NB, et al: Adjuvant sunitinib or sorafenib for high risk non-metastatic renal cell carcinoma (ECOG-ACRIN E2805): a double blind placebo controlled randomized phase III trial. Lancet, 387(10032): 2008, 2016.

Gross-Goupil M, et al: Axitinib versus placebo as an adjuvant treatment of renal cell carcinoma: results from the phase II randomized ATLAS trial. Ann Oncol, 29(12): 2371, 2018.

Harshman LC, et al: Evaluation of disease free survival as an intermediate metric of overall survival in patients with localized renal cell carcinoma: a trial level meta-analysis. Cancer, 124: 925, 2018.

Motzer RJ, et al: Randomized phase III trial of adjuvant pazopanib versus placebo after nephrectomy in patients with localized or locally advanced renal cell carcinoma. J Clin Oncol, 35(35): 3916, 2017.

S-TRAC—Ravaud A, et al: Adjuvant Sunitinib in high risk renal cell carcinoma after nephrectomy. N Engl J Med, 375: 2246, 2016.

Survival

Karakiewicz PI, et al: A preoperative prognostic model for patients treated with nephrectomy for renal cell carcinoma. Eur Urol, 55(2): 287, 2009.

Karakiewicz PI, et al: Multi-institutional validation of a new cancer specific survival nomogram. J Clin Oncol, 25(11): 1316, 2007.

Raj GV, et al: Preoperative nomogram predicting 12 year probability of metastatic renal cancer. J Urol, 179(6): 2146, 2008.

Zisman A, Pantuck AJ, et al: Improved prognostication using of RCC using an integrated staging system (UISS). J Clin Oncol, 19: 1649, 2001.

Metastatic and Recurrent Renal Cell Carcinoma - Metastasis Resection

Dineen MK, Patore RD, Emrich LJ, et al: Results of surgical treatment of renal cell carcinoma with solitary metastasis. J Urol, 140: 277, 1988.

Durr HR, Maier M, Pfahler M, et al: Surgical treatment of osseous metastasis in patients with renal cell carcinoma. Clin Orthop, 367: 283, 1999.

Friedel G, Hurtgen M, Penzenstadler M, et al: Resection of pulmonary metastasis from renal cell carcinoma. Anticancer Res, 19: 1593, 1999.

Giehl JP, Kluba T: Metastatic spine disease in renal cell carcinoma - indication and results of surgery. Anticancer Res, 19: 1619, 1999.

Margulis V, et al: Predictors of oncological outcome after resection of locally recurrent renal cell carcinoma. J Urol, 181: 2044, 2009.

Middleton R: Surgery for metastatic renal cell carcinoma. J Urol, 97: 973, 1967.

O'Dea MJ, Zincke H, Utz DC, et al: The treatment of renal cell carcinoma with solitary metastasis. J Urol, 120: 540, 1978.

Tolia BM and Whitmore Jr. WF: Solitary metastasis from renal cell carcinoma. J Urol, 114: 836, 1975.

Metastatic Renal Cell Carcinoma - Cytoreductive Nephrectomy

Flanigan RC, Salmon SE, Blumenstein BA, et al: Nephrectomy followed by interferon alfa-2b compared with interferon alfa-2b alone for metastatic renal-cell carcinoma. N Engl J Med, 345: 1655, 2001.

Mejean A, et al: Sunitinib alone or after nephrectomy in metastatic renal cell carcinoma. N Engl J Med, 379(5): 417, 2018.

Mickisch GH, Garin A, van Poppel H, et al: Radical nephrectomy plus interferon-alfa-based immunotherapy compared with interferon alfa alone in metastatic renal-cell carcinoma: a randomized trial. Lancet 358: 966, 2001.

Pantuck AJ, Zisman A, Belldegrun AS: The changing history of renal cell carcinoma. J Urol, 166: 1611, 2001.

SURTIME—Bex A, et al: Comparison of immediate vs delayed cytoreductive nephrectomy in patients with synchronous metastatic renal cell carcinoma receiving sunitinib. JAMA Oncol, 5(2): 164, 2019.

Metastatic Renal Cell Carcinoma - Systemic Therapy

Escudier B, et al: Bevacizumab plus interferon alfa-2a for treatment of metastatic renal cell carcinoma: a randomized phase III trial. Lancet, 370: 2103, 2007.

Escudier B, et al: Randomized phase II trial of first line treatment with sorafenib versus interferon alfa-2a in patients with metastatic renal cell carcinoma. J Clin Oncol, 27(8): 1280, 2009 [Update of N Engl J Med, 356: 125, 2007].

Escudier B, et al: Sorafenib for treatment of renal cell carcinoma: final efficacy and safety results of the phase III treatment approaches in renal cancer global evaluation trial. J Clin Oncol, 27(20): 3312, 2009.

Motzer RJ, et al: Axitinib versus sorafenib as second line treatment for advanced renal call carcinoma: overall survival analysis and updated results from a randomised phase 3 trial. Lancet Oncol, 14(6): 552, 2013.

Motzer RJ, et al: Overall survival and updated results for sunitinib compared with interferon-alfa in patients with metastatic renal cell carcinoma. J Clin Oncol, 27(22): 3584, 2009.

Motzer RJ, et al: Pazopanib versus sunitinib in metastatic renal cell carcinoma. N Engl J Med, 369(8): 722, 2013.

Hudes G, et al: Temsirolimus, interferon alfa, or both for advanced renal cell carcinoma. N Engl J Med, 356(22): 2271, 2007.

Motzer RJ, et al: Sunitinib in patients with metastatic renal cell carcinoma. JAMA, 295(21): 2516, 2006.

Motzer RJ, et al: Phase 3 trial of everolimus for metastatic renal cell carcinoma: final results and analysis of prognostic factors. Cancer, 116: 4256, 2010. [update of Lancet, 372: 449, 2008].

Rini BI, et al: Phase III trial of bevacizumab plus interferon alfa versus interferon alfa monotherapy in patients with metastatic renal cell carcinoma: CALGB 90206. J Clin Oncol, 28(13): 2137, 2010 [update of J Clin Oncol, 26(33): 5422, 2008].

WILMS' TUMOR & OTHER PEDIATRIC RENAL TUMORS

Wilms' Tumor

Presentation

1. *Wilms' tumor is the most common primary malignant renal tumor in children.*
2. Mean age of presentation is 3.5-4.0 years old. Bilateral cases usually present earlier at a mean age of 2.5 years old. *Wilms' tumor is rare in the newborn (a solid renal tumor in the newborn is more likely to be congenital mesoblastic nephroma or neuroblastoma).*
3. The most common presenting symptom is an *abdominal mass.* Hypertension occurs in up to 65%. Microscopic hematuria may be seen, but gross hematuria is rare.
4. Physical examination often reveals a large, smooth, firm flank mass that *rarely crosses the midline.*
5. Congenital anomalies occur with 15% of Wilms' tumors.
   a. Genitourinary anomalies (5% of cases)—including renal anomalies (ectopia, fusion, hypoplasia), ureteral duplications, hypospadias, cryptorchidism, and ambiguous genitalia.
   b. Hemihypertrophy (3% of cases)—may be ipsilateral or contralateral to the tumor. Isolated hemihypertrophy (i.e. not accompanied by other congenital abnormalities) is associated with chromosome 11p disorders.
   c. Aniridia (1% of cases)—abnormal development of the iris of the eye. Isolated aniridia is associated with chromosome 11p disorders. Up to 33% of patients with aniridia develop Wilms' tumor.
6. Gross renal vein invasion occurs in up to 20% of cases.
7. Acquired von Willebrand disease occurs in 5-10% of cases (a bleeding disorder characterized by the deficiency of a platelet adhesion factor).

Etiology

1. Wilms' tumor is thought to arise from abnormal persistence of the metanephric blastema (the metanephric blastema is the embryologic structure that contains the nephrogenic cells).
2. Premalignant lesions
   a. Nephrogenic rest—a focus of abnormally persistent nephrogenic cells. Wilms' tumor and nephrogenic rests are indistinguishable histologically. The only way to differentiate them is by following their clinical course. Most nephrogenic rests do *not* develop into Wilms' tumor. Nevertheless, patients with nephrogenic rests must be followed closely.
   b. Nephroblastomatosis—diffuse or multi-focal nephrogenic rests.
3. Wilms' tumor genes (WT)
   a. WT1—tumor suppressor gene on chromosome 11p13. Inactivation of WT1 results in Wilms' tumor.
   b. WT2—on chromosome 11p15. Inactivation of WT2 causes Wilms' tumor.
   c. 16q—Loss of heterozygosity at this site results in Wilms' tumor.

Metastasis

Location of metastasis (from most to least common):
   Pulmonary, hepatic, other sites (including bone and rarely brain)

Disease Associations

1. WAGR syndrome (*W*ilms' tumor, *A*niridia, *G*enitourinary abnormalities, mental *R*etardation)—associated with WT1. Up to 30% develop Wilms' tumor.
2. Denys-Drash syndrome (Wilms' tumor, intersex disorder, glomerulopathy with proteinuria)—associated with WT1.
3. Beckwith-Wiedemann syndrome (multiple growth abnormalities which may include visceromegaly, gigantism, hemihypertrophy, omphalocele, and macroglossia)—associated with WT2. Up to 5% with this syndrome develop Wilms' tumor.
4. Mixed gonadal dysgenesis
5. Trisomy 18
6. Perlman syndrome
7. Congenital syndromes such as aniridia (see Presentation, page 41)

Bilateral Wilms' Tumor

1. Approximately 5% of patients present with bilateral tumors.
2. Bilateral cases usually present earlier (at a mean age of 2.5 years) than unilateral Wilms' tumor.
3. *Nephrogenic rests are always present in bilateral Wilms' tumor.* Thus, the presence of nephrogenic rests should raise the suspicion of bilateral Wilms' tumor.
4. Bilateral tumors are generally treated with preoperative chemotherapy followed by renal sparing surgery.
5. When nephrectomy is performed for a unilateral Wilms' tumor, the presence of an ipsilateral nephrogenic rest or nephroblastomatosis increases the patient's risk of developing a metachronous Wilms' tumor in the contralateral kidney. Therefore, these patients are followed more frequently regardless of histology and stage.

Work Up

1. History and physical (including search for aniridia, hemihypertrophy, hypospadias, cryptorchidism, ambiguous genitalia, etc.)
2. Blood pressure measurement
3. CBC with platelets, PT/PTT, bleeding time, BUN, serum creatinine, liver function tests, serum calcium, and urinalysis. Obtain urinary catecholamines if neuroblastoma is suspected. Platelets, bleeding time, PT, and PTT are obtained because 5-10% of patients with Wilms' tumor develop acquired von Willebrand disease (a bleeding disorder).
4. Abdominal ultrasound is often the initial imaging study. It can visualize the liver as well as tumor thrombus in the vena cava. Wilms' tumor usually has a heterogeneous echo texture. CT scan may be obtained if a solid renal mass is suspected based on ultrasound.
5. Chest x-ray to assess for pulmonary metastasis.
6. Bone scan if the patient has bone pain, elevated alkaline phosphatase, or elevated serum calcium.

Initial Exploratory Surgery

1. After a complete work up, the initial therapy for a suspected Wilms' tumor is usually surgical exploration. However, preoperative chemotherapy is indicated in certain circumstances (see #8 below).
2. In general, a transverse supra-umbilical abdominal incision is made.
3. Peritoneal exploration is performed to rule out metastasis. Biopsies should be taken of suspicious lesions and resectability is determined. If the tumor is unresectable, close and administer chemotherapy.
4. Palpate the renal vein for tumor thrombus.

5. *When the preoperative CT or MRI shows a normal contralateral kidney, exploration of the contralateral kidney is unnecessary.* When preoperative imaging shows an abnormal contralateral kidney, the *entire* contralateral kidney is exposed and inspected. Biopsy any suspicious lesions (a cleft or discoloration suggests a nephrogenic rest). If the contralateral kidney was abnormal on preoperative imaging but appears grossly normal during surgery, intraoperative ultrasound may localize lesions for biopsy. After inspection of the contralateral kidney, close Gerota's fascia. If bilateral Wilms' tumor is present, close the patient and treat accordingly.
6. Inspect the retroperitoneal lymph nodes. Biopsy abnormal nodes and obtain random node biopsies. Regional lymph node dissection does not improve survival but may provide prognostic information.
7. If the tumor is unilateral, perform a nephrectomy (and tumor thrombectomy if indicated). Resect the adrenal gland if it is grossly involved, the tumor is in the upper pole of the kidney, or the adrenal is adherent to the kidney.
8. Preoperative chemotherapy has not improved survival, but may reduce the morbidity of surgery by shrinking the tumor. It is administered when the mass has any of the following characteristics:
   a. Unresectable at initial presentation
   b. Bilateral renal involvement
   c. Extensive intracaval involvement

Stage

I   Tumor confined to kidney and completely excised (margins negative, no capsular penetration, no tumor spillage). No nodal or hematogenous metastases.

II   Local extension of tumor outside the kidney and completely excised (invasion into perinephric tissue or presence of tumor thrombus in the renal vein or vena cava; margins negative, tumor thrombus completely removed). No nodal or hematogenous metastases.

III   Incompletely resected intra-abdominal tumor (tumor spillage, positive margins), non-hematogenous intra-abdominal spread (positive regional lymph nodes, peritoneal invasion, peritoneal implants), or tumor was biopsied before excision. No non-regional nodal or hematogenous metastases.

IV   Hematogenous metastasis or non-regional nodal metastases

V   Bilateral tumor at diagnosis (an attempt should be made to stage each side by the above criteria before biopsy)

Pathology and Histology

1. Gross features—tan tumor with a pseudocapsule. Cysts may be present.
2. Microscopic features—three tissue elements must be present: *stroma*, *epithelial cells*, and *blastema*.
3. Histology—favorable histology is most common.
   a. Unfavorable (anaplastic) histology (5% of cases)—nuclear enlargement ($\geq$ 3 fold larger than adjacent cells), nuclear hyperchromasia, and abnormal mitoses. This histology is rare when Wilms' is diagnosed at < 2 years of age. *Unfavorable histology has a worse prognosis.* Clear cell sarcoma and rhabdoid tumor are no longer classified as unfavorable histology Wilms' tumor. They are classified as non-Wilms' tumors.
   b. Favorable histology (95% of cases)—no characteristics of unfavorable histology.

Treatment

Treatment After Removal of Wilms' Tumor (based on NWTS V)

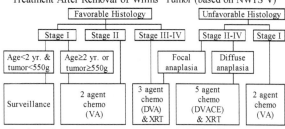

D = doxorubicin   C = cyclophosphamide
V= vincristine   E = etoposide
A = actinomycin D (dactinomycin)   XRT= external beam radiation therapy
NTWS V = National Wilms' Tumor Study 5

Survival

Tumor	Histology	Stage	4-Year Relapse-Free Survival*	4-Year Overall Survival*
Wilms' Tumor	FH	I	92%	98%
		II	85%	96%
		III	90%	95%
		IV	80%	90%
		V	65%	56-87%†
	UH	Any	60%	66%
Clear cell sarcoma	Any	Any	65%	75%
Rhabdoid sarcoma	Any	Any	25%	26%

FH = favorable histology; UH = unfavorable histology
* Data is from National Wilms' Tumor Studies 3-5.
† Survival is better in those with negative lymph nodes, favorable histology,
  younger age, and lower tumor stage of each kidney.

Follow Up
1. Initially, obtain follow up tests at least every 3 months.
   a. History and physical (especially abdominal exam).
   b. Serum BUN, creatinine, liver function tests, and urinalysis.
   c. Abdominal ultrasound—every 3 months for any stage with unfavorable
      histology, stage III-IV with favorable histology, and any stage with
      nephrogenic rests. Favorable histology stage I-II without nephrogenic
      rests may be imaged less often.
   d. Chest x-ray—every 3 months.
2. When nephrectomy is performed for a unilateral Wilms' tumor, the
   presence of an ipsilateral nephrogenic rest or nephroblastomatosis
   increases the patient's risk of developing a metachronous Wilms' tumor in
   the contralateral kidney. Therefore, these patients are followed more
   frequently regardless of histology and stage.
3. If metastases were present, the metastatic locations should be monitored
   with routine imaging.
4. In patients receiving radiation to bones, imaging studies of these areas
   should be conducted at least each year until bone growth is complete, and
   then at least every 5 years thereafter. Secondary malignancies (such as
   osteosarcomas) have been reported after radiation for Wilms' tumor.

5. Side effects of doxorubicin include a 4-17% long-term risk of congestive heart failure. Consider monitoring the patient for heart disease.
6. Most recurrences occur within 2 years of diagnosis. Therefore, follow up should be intensive during this interval and may be less frequent thereafter.
7. Patients with a solitary kidney should be advised that participation in contact/collision sports places the kidney at risk for traumatic injury. Need to avoid contact/collision sports is determined on an individual basis.

Relapse

1. *The lung is the most common site of relapse.*
2. Relapses usually occur within 2 years of diagnosis.
3. Treatment of relapse often consists of a combination of surgery, radiation, and chemotherapy. Patients that have not had doxorubicin (i.e. patients who have not had chemotherapy or who have had chemotherapy without doxorubicin) are given doxorubicin based chemotherapy. There is no consensus regarding a chemotherapy regimen for patients that relapse after receiving doxorubicin.
4. Factors that increase the risk of relapse
   a. Age > 2 years
   b. Higher stage
   c. Unfavorable histology—*histology is the most important prognostic factor.*
   d. Lymph node metastasis
   e. Hematogenous metastasis
5. No apparent influence on survival
   a. Level of caval involvement
   b. Lymph node dissection
6. Factors that increase local recurrence
   a. Unfavorable histology
   b. Tumor spillage
   c. Positive surgical margins
   d. Incomplete tumor resection
   e. Lymph node metastasis

Other Malignant Pediatric Renal Tumors

Relative Frequency of Malignant Pediatric Renal Tumors

Wilms' Favorable Histology	89%
Wilms' Unfavorable Histology	5%
Rhabdoid Tumor	4%
Clear Cell Sarcoma	2%

Clear Cell Sarcoma of the Kidney

1. This tumor is *not* classified as a Wilms' tumor. It is a sarcoma.
2. Mean age of diagnosis = 3-4 years of age.
3. This tumor been called the "bone-metastasizing renal tumor of childhood" because *bone is the most common site of metastases.* 50% of patients present with bone metastases. If this tumor is discovered, a bone scan must be performed.
4. This tumor has a worse prognosis than Wilms' tumor.
5. Treatment—nephrectomy followed by chemotherapy and external beam radiation. In NWTS 5, the chemotherapy regimen consisted of doxorubicin, vincristine, actinomycin, cyclophosphamide, and etoposide.
6. The 4-year relapse-free and overall survival with treatment is 65% and 75%, respectively (see Survival table, page 44).

Rhabdoid Tumor of the Kidney
1. This tumor is *not* classified as a Wilms' tumor. It is a sarcoma.
2. Mean age of diagnosis is 13 months.
3. *The most common metastatic site is the brain.* All patients that have this tumor should undergo a brain CT or MRI.
4. *Rhabdoid tumor has the worst prognosis of all childhood renal masses.*
5. Treatment is nephrectomy followed by chemotherapy and external beam radiation. In NWTS 5, the chemotherapy regimen consists of carboplatin, etoposide, and cyclophosphamide.
6. The 4-year relapse-free and overall survival with treatment is 25% and 26%, respectively (see Survival table, page 44).

Benign Pediatric Renal Tumors

Multilocular Cystic Nephroma
1. Multilocular cystic nephroma is a benign cystic renal mass.
2. Presentation
   a. It is virtually always *unilateral*.
   b. Incidence is highest in two populations
      i. Male child (usually age <2)—presents with painless abdominal mass
      ii. Female adult (usually age >40)—presents with pain or hematuria.
3. Pathology
   a. Gross—well-circumscribed non-calcified mass with fibrous capsule surrounding non-communicating cysts.
   b. Microscopic—cysts separated by fibrous septa.
4. Imaging—imaging cannot differentiate between multilocular cystic nephroma and malignant cystic masses (e.g. cystic Wilms'). *Renal scan usually shows that the affected kidney does function.*
5. Treatment—nephrectomy is curative. If nephron sparing surgery is performed, consider intraoperative frozen sections to rule out malignancy.

Mesoblastic Nephroma
1. *Mesoblastic nephroma is the most common solid renal tumor in the newborn.* It is considered benign, but may be locally invasive. Metastases are rare and are usually associated with the cellular variant.
2. Presentation
   a. Mean age of presentation = 3.5 months. It is uncommon after the age of 6 months. It is more common in males.
   b. Usually discovered as a unilateral abdominal mass.
   c. It is associated with *polyhydramnios* in utero.
   d. 14% of patients have associated congenital anomalies.
3. Pathology
   a. Gross—*resembles a leiomyoma* (firm, rubbery, light colored).
      i.   It interdigitates with the surrounding kidney.
      ii. There is no capsule and calcifications are absent.
      iii. These tumors may be friable and *prone to rupture.*
   b. Microscopic—*spindle cells that infiltrate the renal parenchyma.*
      i. Classic variant—rare mitotic figures.
      ii. Cellular variant—densely cellular mass with many mitotic figures.
4. Imaging—imaging studies cannot reliably differentiate this mass from other solid renal masses.
5. Treatment—nephrectomy with wide local excision is usually curative. Complete resection and avoiding tumor spillage are imperative to prevent local recurrence. Patients diagnosed at < 3 months of age may have a lower recurrence rate. Although local recurrence is uncommon, it does occur; therefore, surveillance after nephrectomy is recommended.

Multicystic Dysplastic Kidney (MCDK)

1. MCDK is a congenital benign cystic dysplasia of the kidney.
2. Presentation
   a. Usually presents as a childhood abdominal mass or is found incidentally on prenatal ultrasound.
   b. MCDK is associated with contralateral vesicoureteral reflux (VUR) in 20-40% of cases and contralateral ureteropelvic junction (UPJ) obstruction in 3-12% of cases. *VUR is the most common defect associated with MCDK; therefore, patients with MCDK should undergo voiding cystourethrogram.*
3. Gross appearance—cysts with minimal renal parenchyma ("bunch of grapes" appearance). *The ureter is usually atretic.*
4. Histologic appearance—primitive tubules that are not organized into nephrons (disorganized architecture). *Ectopic cartilage is often present.*
5. Imaging
   a. Ultrasound shows non-communicating cysts and minimal parenchyma (small communications may exist, but they are not visible on ultrasound), whereas hydronephrosis usually shows fluid filled areas that have visible communications.
   b. *Renal scan usually shows that the affected kidney does not function.*
6. Sometimes MCDK may involute into a "nubbin" or disappear completely.
7. Hypertension can develop in up to 8% of patients with MCDK.
8. Treatment
   a. Patients with UPJ obstruction and VUR should be treated accordingly.
   b. Patients with MCDK should be observed with a yearly blood pressure measurement. A repeat renal ultrasound can be performed at age 1 year (and perhaps another ultrasound around age 6).
   c. If the kidney enlarges or becomes symptomatic (e.g. the patient develops hypertension), nephrectomy should be performed.

Differentiating Cystic Renal Masses

Cystic Mass	Ultrasound Shows Grossly Visible Communication Between Fluid Spaces	Functioning Kidney on Renal Scan
MCDK	No	No
MLCN	No	Yes
Cystic Wilms'	No	Yes
Hydronephrosis	Yes	Sometimes

MCDK = multicystic dysplastic kidney
MLCN = multilocular cystic nephroma

Survival For Pediatric Renal Tumors

Tumor	2-Year Relapse-Free Survival (all stages combined)
Multilocular cystic nephroma	100%
Mesoblastic nephroma	98%
Wilms' tumor FH	84%
Clear cell sarcoma	75%
Wilms' tumor UH	63%
Rhabdoid sarcoma	25%

FH = favorable histology; UH = unfavorable histology

REFERENCES

Argani P, Perlman EJ, Breslow NE, et al: Clear cell sarcoma of the kidney. Am J Surg Pathol, 24: 4, 2000.

Clericuzio CL, Johnson C: Screening for Wilms' tumor in high-risk individuals. Hematol Oncol Clin North Am, 9: 1253, 1995.

D'Angio GJ, Breslow N, Beckwith JB, et al: Treatment of Wilms' tumor - results of the Third National Wilms' Tumor Society. Cancer, 64: 349, 1989.

Dome JS, et al: Treatment of anaplastic histology Wilms' tumor: results from the fifth National Wilms' Tumor Study. J Clin Oncol, 24(6): 2352, 2006.

Green DM, et al: Comparison between single dose and divided dose administration of dactinomycin and doxorubicin for patients with Wilms' tumor: a report from the National Wilms' Tumor Study group. J Clin Oncol, 16(1): 237, 1998.

Green DM, et al: Treatment of children with stage II to IV anaplastic Wilms' tumor: a report from the National Wilms' Tumor Study group. J Clin Oncol, 12(10): 2126, 1994.

Green DM, et al: Effect of duration of treatment on treatment outcome and cost of treatment for Wilms' tumor: a report from the National Wilms' Tumor Study group. J Clin Oncol, 16(12): 3744, 1998.

Green DM, D'Angio GJ, et al: Wilms' tumor. CA Cancer J Clin, 46: 46, 1996.

Howell CG, Othersen HB, Kiviat NE, et al: Therapy and outcome in 51 children with mesoblastic nephroma: a report of the National Wilms' Tumor Study. J Pediatr Surg, 17: 826, 1982.

Kirsch AJ, Snyder III HM: What's new and important in pediatric urologic oncology. AUA Update Series, Vol. 17, Lesson 11, 1998.

Metzger ML, Dome JS: Current therapy for Wilms' tumor. The Oncologist, 10: 815, 2005.

Montgomery BT, et al: Extended follow up of bilateral Wilms' tumor: results of the National Wilms' Tumor Study. J Urol, 146 (2, part 2): 514, 1991.

National Cancer Institute: Wilms' tumor and other childhood kidney tumors treatment (PDQ) - health professional version. Accessed 4/20/2021. (https://www.cancer.gov/types/kidney/hp/wilms-treatment-pdq).

Peters CA, Badwan K: The multicystic dysplastic kidney. AUA Update Series, Vol. 24, Lesson 37, 2005.

Ross JH: Wilms' tumor: updated strategies for evaluation and management. Contemp Urol, 18(11): 18, 2006.

Shamberger RC, et al: Surgery-related factors and local recurrence of Wilms' tumor in National Wilms' Tumor Study 4. Ann Surg, 229: 292, 1999.

BLADDER TUMORS

Types of Bladder Cancer
1. Primary tumors
   a. Urothelial carcinoma (UC)—more than 90% of cases in the U.S.
   b. Non-urothelial cancers
      i. Squamous cell carcinoma (SCC)—5% of cases in the U.S.
      ii. Adenocarcinoma—1% of cases in the U.S.
      iii. Other—small cell carcinoma, rhabdomyosarcoma (most commonly seen in children), bladder lymphoma.
2. Secondary tumors (metastatic to bladder)—from most to least common: melanoma, colon, prostate, lung, breast.

Risk Factors for Bladder Cancer
1. Smoking—*smoking is the most common cause of bladder cancer.* The carcinogen in tobacco smoke is thought to be an *aromatic amine.* Smoking increases the risk of bladder cancer 2 to 4 fold. A higher risk of cancer is associated with more frequent smoking and a longer duration of smoking. The risk of bladder cancer declines within 1 year of smoking cessation, and continues to decline thereafter.
2. Chronic cystitis—associated with an increased risk of squamous cell carcinoma (SCC). Causes of chronic cystitis that have been associated with SCC include
   a. Chronic urinary tract infection.
   b. Indwelling bladder catheter—SCC is the most common type of bladder cancer in patients with long-term indwelling catheters.
   c. Schistosoma haematobium (bilharzial) infection.
   d. Chronic bladder stones.
3. Chemical exposure—*aromatic amines, aniline dye, benzene, and toluene* are among the carcinogens that increase the risk of bladder cancer. Certain occupations are more likely to be exposed to these carcinogens; thus, they have an increased risk for bladder cancer. These occupations include

Textile workers	Dye workers	Drill press operators
Tire/rubber workers	Leather workers	Petroleum workers
Bootblacks	Painters	Dry cleaners
Truck drivers	Hairdressers (hair dye)	Chemical workers

4. Phenacetin—an analgesic with a chemical structure similar to aniline dyes. Phenacetin has been removed from the market.
5. Radiation exposure of the bladder
6. Pioglitazone (Actos)—taking this diabetes drug for more than 1 year may increase the absolute risk of bladder cancer by 0.03% (the risk increases from 7 in 10,000 among non-users to 10 in 10,000 among users).
7. Cyclophosphamide and ifosfamide—acrolein, a urinary metabolite of these chemotherapy agents, causes hemorrhagic cystitis and an increased risk of bladder cancer. The latency period for acrolein induced bladder cancer is 6-13 years. *Mesna, which binds to acrolein in the urine, is often administered with cyclophosphamide or ifosfamide to reduce the risk of hemorrhagic cystitis. Mesna may also reduce the risk of bladder cancer.*
8. Prior history of bladder cancer

Presentation

1. *Painless hematuria (microscopic or gross) is the most common symptom of bladder cancer.* Urinary frequency, urgency, and dysuria are more common with invasive or high grade tumors (especially carcinoma in situ)
2. Patients with advanced cancer may have bone pain (from bone metastases) or flank pain (from ureteral obstruction or retroperitoneal metastases).
3. 75% of bladder cancers are non-muscle invasive at initial diagnosis.
4. The average age of diagnosis is 65.

Diagnosis

General Information

1. Most cases of bladder cancer are discovered during office based cystoscopy when evaluating the patient for hematuria, unexplained voiding symptoms, or incidental bladder mass on imaging.
2. If a bladder tumor is discovered on cystoscopy, upper tract imaging using CT urogram (if not done already) is recommended before proceeding to transurethral resection of the bladder tumor (TURBT). See Upper Urinary Tract Imaging, page 51.
3. Urine cytology or other urine tumor markers may be helpful for diagnosis; however, they cannot replace cystoscopy or upper tract imaging.
4. If a urine tumor marker suggests malignancy, but upper tract imaging and cystoscopy are normal, then conduct the evaluation described on page 117

Cystoscopy

1. White light cystoscopy—this is the standard method for examining the urethra and the bladder.
2. Enhanced visualization cystoscopy (also called "enhanced cystoscopy")— Examples include blue light cystoscopy and narrow band imaging.
   a. Compared to cystoscopy using white light alone, *cystoscopy using both white light and enhanced visualization has the following advantages:*
      i. *Improves detection of non-muscle invasive urothelial cancer (especially CIS).*
      ii. *Allows for a more complete resection of tumor during TURBT, which decreases the recurrence rate* (but it does not reduce progression to muscle invasive disease).
   b. During enhanced cystoscopy, *urothelial inflammation generates a significant number of false positive detections.*
   c. Enhanced cystoscopy techniques are used with white light cystoscopy, and may be most useful in any of the following scenarios.
      i. Patients suspected of having a non-muscle invasive bladder cancer (at either initial or repeat transurethral resection).
      ii. Patients undergoing a repeat transurethral resection (to help achieve complete tumor resection and to minimize the risk of residual tumor)
      iii. To assess for complete response after intravesical therapy.
      iv. To assess patients who have a positive urinary tumor marker and whose white light cystoscopy shows no visible tumor.
3. Blue light cystoscopy (fluorescence cystoscopy)—after instilling a photoactive agent into the bladder, visualization is performed using a blue light (wavelength 360-450 nm).
   a. Photoactive agent—hexaminolevulinate (HAL) is the only FDA approved intravesical agent for detection of bladder cancer during blue light cystoscopy. 5-aminolevulinic acid has also been studied.
   b. Mechanism of action—after intravesical instillation of HAL (a heme precursor), it is absorbed into the urothelial cells, where it enters the heme metabolism pathway and is converted to photoactive porphyrins

(including protoporphyrin IX). These photoactive porphyrins tend to accumulate in rapidly proliferating cells (such as cancer cells), which causes the abnormal cells to fluoresce a red color when exposed to blue light (normal cells appear blue). Other rapidly proliferating cells (e.g. inflammatory cells) may also fluoresce, leading to false positive results.

c. False positive results may occur from benign conditions such as inflammation, cystoscopic trauma, scar tissue, previous bladder biopsy, or recent intravesical treatment with BCG or chemotherapy.

d. False negative results also occur. For example, many muscle invasive cancers do not fluoresce because cells on their surface are necrotic.

e. Before transurethral resection, HAL is instilled into the bladder, where it remains for 1 to 3 hours. Then, it is emptied out by catheterization or by voiding. Within 30 minutes of emptying HAL from the bladder, perform a white light cystoscopy, followed by a blue light cystoscopy. Perform transurethral biopsy/resection of abnormal areas that are seen under blue light, white light, or both (do not use only blue light to direct biopsies). Then, repeat the white light and blue light cystoscopy to ensure that suspicious areas have been completely resected and/or fulgurated.

f. Do not use HAL in patients with gross hematuria or porphyria.

g. Side effects of HAL include bladder spasm/pain, dysuria, and hematuria.

4. Narrow band imaging (NBI)—NBI helps differentiate areas of increased vascularity. It does not require an intravesical instillation.

a Mechanism of action—NBI filters white light into two narrow bands of light: blue (wavelength 451 nm) and green (wavelength 540 nm). These bands are absorbed by hemoglobin, which enhances the visibility of blood vessels. The blue band (shorter wavelength) can assess mucosa vascularity, whereas the green band (longer wavelength) penetrates deeper to assess submucosal vascularity. NBI detects bladder cancers because they tend to be more vascular than normal tissue. However, benign processes (such as inflammation) can also be more vascular than normal tissue, leading to false positive results.

b. False positive results may occur from benign conditions such as inflammation or recent intravesical therapy.

c. False negative results also occur.

d. NBI can also be used with ureteroscopy.

Upper Urinary Tract Imaging

1. Less than 2.5% of patients with bladder cancer have a synchronous upper tract urothelial cancer.

2. *The preferred test for upper urinary tract imaging is CT urogram (CTU).* CTU is more accurate than other imaging modalities for diagnosing upper urinary tract abnormalities. If CTU is contraindicated, inconclusive, or not available, then the following options may also be used.

a. Magnetic resonance urogram (MRU)—uses intravenous Gadolinium. MRU may be most appropriate in patients with a glomerular filtration rate (GFR) > 30 cc/min who have an allergy to iodinated contrast or who have mild to moderate renal insufficiency. For details, see page 459.

b. Intravenous urogram (IVU) with either renal ultrasound or non-contrast cross sectional imaging of the abdomen and pelvis (CT or MRI).

c. Pyelogram (retrograde or antegrade) with either renal ultrasound or non-contrast cross sectional imaging of the abdomen & pelvis (CT or MRI).

d. Ureteroscopy with either renal ultrasound or non-contrast cross sectional imaging of the abdomen and pelvis (CT or MRI).

e. Non-contrast cross sectional imaging of the abdomen and pelvis (CT or MRI)—this option is only used if intravenous contrast, retrograde pyelogram, and ureteroscopy cannot be utilized.

Transurethral Resection of Bladder Tumors (TURBT)

1. Perform a bimanual exam before *and* after TURBT when invasive tumor is suspected. *Clinical stage is based on the bimanual exam after TURBT.* Include a prostate exam in males if it was not done recently.

2. *During TURBT for non-invasive bladder cancer, using enhanced visualization techniques (blue light or NBI) with white light cystoscopy improves tumor detection, allows for a more complete resection, and reduces recurrence compared to using white light alone.*

3. If the patient's medical condition permits, all grossly visible tumor should be completely removed, except when
   a. Extensive CIS is present—extensive resection or fulguration may cause a contracted bladder. CIS may be treated with intravesical therapy.
   b. The tumor appears to be unresectable by the transurethral approach.

4. *When carcinoma in situ (CIS) is known or suspected, biopsy the area adjacent to papillary tumors and biopsy the prostatic urethra.* Prostatic urethra biopsies are also prudent when there are tumors at the bladder neck or multiple bladder tumors (especially if they are high grade).

5. In most cases, TURBT should remove enough tissue to determine depth of invasion. For high grade or stage T1 tumors, understaging is nearly 4 times more likely when muscularis propria is absent from the pathology specimen compared to when it is present (49% versus 14%).

6. TURBT completely excises muscle invasive cancer in 10% of cases (when cystectomy is performed for muscle invasive cancer, 10% are pT0).

7. Restaging TURBT for non-muscle invasive cancer ("repeat TURBT")–this is a second TURBT (performed within 6 weeks after the previous TURBT) that helps to ensure accurate staging and complete tumor resection. *Restaging TURBT should include re-resection of the previous tumor sites and resection of new tumor sites. For tumors that are stage T1, high grade, or variant histology, restaging TURBT should include muscular propria in the resected specimen (except when the cancer is in a diverticulum).*
   a. For tumors not in a diverticulum, perform restaging TURBT in the following scenarios (for tumors in a diverticulum, see page 65).
      i. There was incomplete eradication of all grossly visible tumor during the prior TURBT (except when diffuse CIS was present or when the tumor was unresectable by the transurethral approach).
      ii. Presence of variant histology—these tumors usually turn out to be high grade and muscle invasive.
      iii. Stage T1 cancers—*restaging TURBT should be performed for all stage T1 cancers (regardless of whether muscularis propria was present in the initial pathology) and the restaging TURBT should sample the muscular propria.* A randomized trial in stage T1 urothelial cancer showed that restaging TURBT improved 3-year recurrence free survival by over 30% compared to no restaging TURBT (68.7% versus 37.0%) even though muscularis propria was present in the initial specimen. Retrospective data on stage T1 cancer shows that restaging TURBT reduces recurrence and progression. After initial TURBT for T1 cancers, the risk of residual cancer is greater for high grade tumors (63% for high grade versus 6% for low grade) and the risk of upstaging is greater when muscular propria was not sampled (45% when absent versus 15% when present).
      iv. High grade stage Ta tumor—*restaging TURBT for high grade Ta cancer should be performed when the previous TURBT did not contain muscularis propria or did not resect all grossly visible tumor. However, restaging TURBT should be considered for any high grade Ta tumor, especially when the tumor is large (e.g. ⏵ 3 cm in size) or*

multifocal. *Restaging TURBT should include muscular propria in the sample.* For high grade Ta tumor, restaging TURBT finds residual cancer in 50% of cases and upstages 15% of cases.

8. Obturator reflex—when electrical current from the resectoscope stimulates the obturator nerve, the obturator reflex (sudden adduction of the patient's ipsilateral leg) can push the bladder onto the resectoscope, causing bladder perforation. *The obturator reflex is most likely to occur when resecting tumors on the lateral bladder because this part of the bladder is closest to the nerve.* Methods to minimize the risk of obturator reflex include

a. Avoid bladder over-distention—bladder over-distension can move the bladder wall closer to the obturator nerve.

b. Consider using bipolar instead of monopolar resection—although most data shows no difference in the risk of obturator reflux between monopolar and bipolar resection, a few studies that show that bipolar resection significantly reduces the risk of the obturator reflex.

c. Lower the resection current.

d. Obturator nerve block using local anesthesia.

e. General anesthesia with neuromuscular blockade—the obturator nerve can still be stimulated, but the impulse is not transmitted to the muscles.

9. *Bladder perforation should be avoided because it increases the risk of bleeding, urinary tract infection, sepsis, and death from bladder cancer.* Methods to decrease the risk of bladder perforation include

a. Use caution when resecting tumors in a diverticulum—the diverticulum wall lacks muscularis propria & is thinner than the normal bladder wall.

b. Avoid the obturator reflex.

c. Avoid bladder over-distention.

d. Avoid deep resection of tumors that appear low grade and non-invasive.

10. Tumors at the ureteral orifice

a. *Extensive cauterization of the ureteral orifice should be avoided because it causes distal ureteral stricture.* If cautery near the orifice is required, use minimal low current, focal "pin-point" cautery.

b. *When cutting current is used to resect the ureteral orifice, postoperative ureter obstruction (from edema or stricture) is unlikely. In most cases, placing a ureteral stent should be avoided after resection of the ureteral orifice because it does not appear to reduce the risk of stricture and it increases the risk of upper urinary tract cancer by 3 fold.*

c. Perform a urogram, renal scan, or renal ultrasound 3-6 weeks after resection of the ureteral orifice to check for ureteral obstruction (consider obtaining one of these tests sooner in patients with a solitary kidney or poor overall renal function).

d. Resection of the ureteral orifice can cause vesicoureteral reflux (VUR). When urothelial carcinoma (UC) of the bladder occurs in the presence of VUR, the risk of subsequent upper tract UC increases by 15 to 22 fold. Thus, surveillance of the upper tracts is performed more frequently in patients with VUR and a history of bladder cancer.

11. *Simultaneous TURP for BPH and TURBT for stage Ta or T1 UC does not appear to increase the risk subsequently developing UC in the prostatic urethra compared to TURBT alone.*

Random Bladder Biopsies

1. Routine random bladder biopsies are not recommended.

2. Random bladder biopsies are indicated in any of these circumstances.

a. Partial cystectomy is planned.

b. Abnormal urine tumor marker with no visible tumor in the bladder. See page 117.

c. Urine cytology shows high grade cells, but biopsy shows low grade UC.

d. After intravesical therapy for CIS to evaluate for complete response.

Prostatic Urethra Biopsies
1. Prostatic urethra biopsies are indicated in any of these circumstances:
   a. Multifocal UC of the bladder (especially high grade tumors).
   b. Tumor at the bladder neck.
   c. CIS of the bladder (known or suspected).
   d. An abnormality in the prostatic urethra that is suspicious for tumor.
   e. Unexplained abnormal urine tumor marker. See page 117.
2. When prostate invasion is suspected, obtain prostatic urethra biopsies using loop resection at 5 and 7 o'clock just cephalad to the verumontanum (the diagnostic yield is lower for cold cup biopsies and for biopsies taken from other areas of the prostatic urethra). When prostate invasion is not suspected, cold cup biopsies may be used.
3. Resect visible tumors in the prostatic urethra.

Benign Bladder Tumors

Nephrogenic Adenoma
1. Nephrogenic adenoma is a rare benign lesion. It is a metaplastic response to trauma or inflammation. Histologically, it has a *single layer of cuboidal epithelium* (which resembles renal collecting tubules) with few mitosis and minimal atypia. The classic microscopic finding is *hobnail* epithelial cells.
2. Presentation—patients often have dysuria, frequency, and a history of UTI.
3. Nephrogenic adenoma has a high recurrence rate.
4. Treatment—transurethral resection, followed by an optional long term course of antibiotics.

Other Benign Bladder Tumors
1. Malacoplakia—see page 717.
2. Pheochromocytoma—approximately 90% of bladder pheochromocytomas are benign and 10% are malignant. Most patients present with hematuria and hypertension. *Some symptoms are triggered during or immediately following urination (e.g. micturition syncope, headache, palpitations, flushing, dizziness, sweating)*. The usual treatment is partial cystectomy.
3. Other benign tumors include inverted papilloma and hemangioma.

Non-Urothelial Cancer of the Bladder

Squamous Cell Carcinoma (SCC) of the Bladder
1. SCC of the bladder is associated with chronic inflammation and cigarette smoking.
2. SCC often presents at a higher stage than UC.
3. SCC is more common in Egypt than in the U.S. because Egypt has a higher incidence of Bilharzial (Schistosoma haematobium) infections.
4. SCC has a worse prognosis than UC, except SCC arising from Bilharzial infections. Bilharzial bladder SCC is usually well differentiated and has a low incidence of metastasis. The average age of diagnosis is 45-55 for Bilharzial bladder SCC and 60-70 for non-Bilharzial SCC.
5. SCC is less responsive to chemotherapy and radiation than UC. Intravesical therapy is not effective.
6. Treatment of localized bladder SCC is usually radical cystectomy and pelvic lymphadenectomy (with urethrectomy if indicated). Pelvic radiation is also an option.

Adenocarcinoma of the Bladder

1. Classification of bladder adenocarcinoma
   a. Primary—arises from the bladder.
   b. Urachal—arises from the urachus (see Urachal Tumors, below).
   c. Metastatic—adenocarcinoma that has metastasized to bladder.
2. Evaluate for an adenocarcinoma that may have metastasized to the bladder
   (e.g. colon, stomach, lung, prostate, breast, endometrium, ovary). Testing
   generally includes
   a. CT or MRI of the abdomen and pelvis with contrast
   b. Chest imaging
   c. Upper and lower gastrointestinal endoscopy
   d. In males: PSA and prostate examination.
   e. In females: pelvic examination, CA-125, and mammogram.
3. Primary adenocarcinoma of the bladder
   a. Adenocarcinoma is the most common tumor in exstrophic bladders.
   b. Serum carcinoembryonic antigen (CEA) may be elevated.
   c. Bladder adenocarcinoma has a worse prognosis than UC and responds
      poorly to chemotherapy and radiation. Intravesical therapy is not
      effective.
   d. Treatment of localized bladder adenocarcinoma—radical cystectomy
      (with en block removal of the urachus) and pelvic lymphadenectomy.
4. Adenocarcinoma metastatic to bladder—treat the primary cancer.

Urachal Adenocarcinoma

1. Gross hematuria is the most common presenting symptom. In 15-33% of
   cases, mucin is identified in the urine.
2. Pathology—adenocarcinoma is the most common type of urachal tumor.
   These tumors are usually high grade and cystic.
3. Patients with urachal adenocarcinoma may have an elevated serum CEA.
4. Most cases involve the lower third of the urachus and extend through the
   bladder wall. *Tumors usually occur at the bladder dome*, but may also
   occur on the anterior bladder wall.
5. Urachal adenocarcinoma is poorly responsive to chemotherapy and
   radiation. Intravesical therapy is not effective.
6. Treatment of localized disease—partial or radical cystectomy with en
   block removal of the urachus and umbilicus, and pelvic lymphadenectomy.
7. Mean 5-year cancer free survival is 55% (range 33-88%).
8. After excision, local recurrence occurs in 20-50% of patients.

Small Cell Carcinoma of the Bladder

1. Small cell carcinoma is an aggressive neuroendocrine tumor.
2. Presentation—the mean age of diagnosis is 66. The most common
   presenting symptom is hematuria. Small cell carcinoma usually presents
   with a locally advanced stage (stage T2-T4) and/or metastases.
3. Diagnosis
   a. Small cell carcinoma stains positive for chromogranin A and
      synaptophysin (whereas negative staining is seen with urothelial
      carcinoma, adenocarcinoma, and squamous cell carcinoma).
   b. *All patients whose bladder tumor contains small cell carcinoma should
      undergo metastatic evaluation because of the high risk of metastasis.*
4. *The initial treatment for small cell carcinoma is systemic chemotherapy.*
   a. Non-metastatic (M0)—usually treated with systemic etoposide and
      cisplatin. In patients who respond to chemotherapy, administer
      consolidation therapy with radical cystectomy and/or pelvic radiation.
   b. Metastatic (M1)—usually treated with systemic chemotherapy alone.
5. Prognosis—overall survival is usually < 50% at 5 years follow up.

Urothelial Carcinoma (UC) of Bladder

General Information
1. UC was previously called transitional cell carcinoma.
2. At presentation, 75% of bladder UC are low grade and stage Ta or T1.
3. Among patients with muscle invasive bladder UC, 60% have muscle invasion at initial presentation, while 40% progress from non-muscle invasive tumors.
4. *The presence of tumor on cystoscopy at 3 months after TURBT is a strong prognostic predictor of future recurrence and progression.* Therefore, surveillance cystoscopy is recommended at 3 months after TURBT.
5. Sites of bladder cancer metastasis (from most to least common): pelvic lymph nodes, liver, lung, bone.

Stage, Grade, and Risk Category of Urothelial Cancer

Imaging for Staging of Bladder Cancer
1. Upper tract and abdominal pelvic cross sectional imaging—if not done recently, upper urinary tract imaging and abdominal pelvic cross sectional imaging (CT or MRI) should be done for all patients with bladder cancer. See Upper Urinary Tract Imaging, page 51.
2. Local and regional staging—clinical T stage is determined using bimanual examination and TURBT pathology. Clinical N stage is determined by imaging. Although neither CT nor MRI are highly accurate for local and regional staging, MRI with and without gadolinium is better than CT for detecting depth of muscle invasion and metastasis into the regional lymph nodes. MRI of the pelvis can be performed in addition to CTU in patients with muscle invasive disease to help better define the local and regional extent of the cancer.
3. Evaluate for metastases when symptoms or laboratory tests suggest the presence of metastases or when there is a significant risk for metastasis based on tumor characteristics (e.g. muscularis propria invasion, prostate stroma invasion, variant histology, non-urothelial cancer).
4. Evaluation used in all patients at risk for metastasis
   a. Chest imaging—chest CT (with or without IV contrast) is preferred over chest x-ray because is has a higher sensitivity for detecting metastasis.
   b. Abdominal pelvic imaging with and without contrast (CT or MRI)—this imaging is usually obtained when the upper urinary tracts are assessed.
   c. Blood tests—should include creatinine, alkaline phosphatase, liver function tests, and complete blood count.
5. Evaluation used in select patients at higher risk for metastasis
   a. Bone imaging—bone imaging is recommended for patients with bone pain, elevated alkaline phosphatase, or at high risk for bone metastasis (e.g. patients with multiple soft tissue metastasis). Bone scan is usually the initial test; however, MRI or FDG-PET/CT may also be used.
   b. Brain imaging—brain MRI (with and without gadolinium) is recommended for patients with symptoms suggestive of a central nervous system metastasis or in patients at higher risk of brain metastasis (e.g. small cell carcinoma or multiple metastasis outside the central nervous system). CT scan with intravenous contrast may be used if MRI with gadolinium is contraindicated.
6. FDG-PET/CT may be useful to assess for metastasis in the bones, nodes, chest, abdomen, and pelvis; however, its use is often restricted to when initial imaging is inconclusive. FDG-PET/CT does not provide enough detail to determine local T stage or to assess the upper urinary tracts.

Stage (AJCC 2017)

This TNM classification refers to both clinical and pathological staging.
Bimanual exam under anesthesia should be performed before and after
transurethral resection. Clinical stage is determined by using a combination
of bimanual exam *after* transurethral resection and the pathologic assessment
of the transurethral resection. Pathologic staging requires partial or radical
cystectomy. Higher stage lesions progress more often, recur more often, and
have a worse prognosis.

Primary Tumor (T)

Tx	Primary tumor cannot be assessed
T0	No evidence of primary tumor
Ta	Non-invasive papillary carcinoma
Tis	Urothelial carcinoma in situ: "flat tumor"
T1	Tumor invades lamina propria (subepithelial connective tissue)
T2	Tumor invades muscularis propria
T2a	Tumor invades superficial muscularis propria (inner half)
T2b	Tumor invades deep muscularis propria (outer half)
T3	Tumor invades perivesical soft tissue
T3a	Microscopically
T3b	Macroscopically (extravesical mass)
T4	Extravesical tumor directly invades any of the following: prostatic stroma, seminal vesicles, uterus, vagina, pelvic wall, abdominal wall
T4a	Extravesical tumor invades directly into prostatic stroma, seminal vesicles, uterus, vagina
T4b	Extravesical tumor invades pelvic wall, abdominal wall

Regional Lymph Nodes (N)

Laterality does not affect the N classification. Regional lymph nodes are
common iliac nodes and nodes in the true pelvis. Nodes above the aortic
bifurcation are considered distant lymph nodes.

Nx	Lymph nodes cannot be assessed
N0	No lymph node metastasis
N1	Single regional lymph node metastasis in the true pelvis (perivesical, obturator, internal and external iliac, or sacral lymph node)
N2	Multiple regional lymph node metastasis in the true pelvis (perivesical, obturator, internal and external iliac, or sacral lymph node metastasis)
N3	Lymph node metastasis to the common iliac lymph nodes

Distant Metastasis (M)

M0	No distant metastasis
M1	Distant metastasis
M1a	Distant metastasis limited to lymph nodes beyond the common iliacs
M1b	Non-lymph-node distant metastases

Grade

High grade tumor is more likely to progress and recur.

Grade	Histologic Description
PUNLUMP†	Well differentiated, negligible risk of progression
Low Grade	Well differentiated
High Grade	Poorly differentiated or undifferentiated

PUNLUMP = papillary urothelial neoplasm of low malignant potential
† PUNLUMP can be assigned only to stage Ta tumors.

Terminology for Urothelial Cancer

1. "Muscle invasive" means that cancer has invaded into the muscularis propria of the bladder.
2. Stage Tis, Ta, or T1—referred to as "non-muscle invasive tumors." The previously used term ("superficial tumor") should not be used anymore.
3. Stage T2, T3, or T4—referred to as "muscle invasive tumors."

Risk Categories for Non-Muscle Invasive Urothelial Cancer

These risk categories correlate with the risk of recurrence and the risk of progression to a higher stage.

Adapted from the AUA/SUO 2016 and the EAU 2021 guidelines		Risk Category† for Non-muscle Invasive Urothelial Bladder Cancer		
		Low Risk	Intermediate Risk	High Risk
Urothelial carcinoma with no variant histology, no lymphovascular invasion, & no prostatic urethra involvement	PUNLMP	All cases		
	Stage Ta Low grade	Solitary & ≤ 3 cm & not recurrent within 1 year	Multifocal or > 3 cm or recurrent within 1 year	Multifocal & > 3 cm & recurrent within 1 year
	Stage Ta High grade	—	Solitary & ≤ 3 cm & not recurrent & did not fail BCG	Multifocal or > 3 cm or recurrent or failed BCG
	Stage T1 Low Grade‡	—	0 or 1 of the factors below: Prognostic factors: multifocal, tumor > 3 cm, or age > 70 years	2 or 3 of the factors below§:
	Stage T1 High Grade	—	—	All cases
CIS		—	—	All cases
Variant histology present		—	—	All cases
Lymphovascular invasion present		—	—	All cases
Non-invasive (mucosal &/or ductal) prostatic urethra involvement*		—	—	High grade

PUNLMP = papillary urothelial neoplasm of low malignant potential;
cm = centimeter; CIS = carcinoma in situ; BCG = Bacillus Calmette-Guerin
† If multiple risk levels are present, then assign the category of greatest risk.
* Non-invasive means no invasion of the prostate stroma (i.e. cancer is confined to the prostatic urethra mucosa and/or within the prostatic ducts). The AUA and EAU did not specify a risk category for low grade prostatic urethra involvement. Prostate stroma invasion is treated similar to muscle invasive bladder cancer.
‡ The AUA categorized all T1 low grade tumors as intermediate risk, whereas the EAU categorized the risk of T1 low grade tumors based on the presence of additional prognostic factors (multifocal tumor, tumor > 3 cm, age > 70 years): low risk = 0 factors, intermediate risk = 1 factor, and high risk = 2 or 3 factors. To account for the different methods of assigning risk, the T1 low grade category in the table above utilizes an amalgamation of EAU and AUA risk criteria.
§ Although not specified by either the AUA or EAU guideline, recurrent T1 low grade tumors could be considered high risk.

Carcinoma In Situ (CIS)

1. *CIS is a urothelial cancer that is flat, high grade, and non-invasive.*
2. CIS often appears as a velvety patch of erythematous urothelium, but it may look like normal urothelium.
3. CIS is more common in patients with multiple or high grade tumors.
4. *CIS often produces irritative voiding symptoms.*
5. *Urine cytology is positive in approximately 95% of patients with CIS* because of the poor cohesiveness of the cells.
6. CIS has a propensity for recurrence and progression.
   a. Progression occurs in 20% after a complete response to BCG.
   b. Recurrence occurs in 30% after treatment with BCG.
7. The first line of treatment for CIS is BCG (see Intravesical Therapy, page 65 and Intravesical Immunotherapy with BCG, page 69). External beam radiation and systemic chemotherapy for CIS are not effective.

Treatment of Urothelial Carcinoma

General Information

1. *All smokers should be advised to stop smoking.*
2. After TURBT for non-muscle invasive UC, *the initial surveillance cystoscopy is always done at 3 months after the TURBT. The result of this 3 month cystoscopy is an important prognostic indictor: patients with tumor at 3 months are more likely to have subsequent recurrences and to progress to a higher stage compared to patients without tumor.*
3. Tumor characteristics that increase the risk of recurrence and progression include high grade, higher stage, greater number of concurrent tumors (multifocal tumors), size ≥ 3 cm, and recurrence with 1 year. *The EORTC calculator can predict recurrence and progression for non-muscle invasive bladder cancer (www.eortc.be/tools/bladdercalculator/default.htm)*

Stage Tis—Carcinoma in Situ (CIS)

1. Recurrence—30% after a complete response to BCG.
2. Progression—20% after a complete response to BCG.
3. TURBT, bladder biopsy, and/or tumor fulguration for CIS
   a. Biopsy the prostatic urethra (see page 54).
   b. Non-diffuse CIS—for focal bladder lesions that are suspicious for CIS, biopsy the lesions and then completely eradicate the lesions (by either resection or fulguration).
   c. Diffuse CIS—when CIS is diffuse, avoid extensive fulguration or resection because it can cause bladder contracture. Diffuse CIS can be treated with intravesical BCG.
4. For treatment of CIS in the prostatic urethra, see page 65.
5. Treatment of CIS in the bladder
   a. Induction intravesical therapy—*a 6-week course of intravesical induction BCG is recommended* starting 3-4 weeks after TURBT. Intravesical chemotherapy is less effective for CIS (see Intravesical Therapy, page 65). Six weeks after finishing the course of BCG, perform bladder biopsy and bladder wash cytology to check for persistent tumor.
      i. If CIS is eradicated after a 6-week course of BCG, then a second 6-week course of BCG is optional. If CIS is not eradicated after a 6-week course of BCG, then administer a second 6-week course of BCG.
      ii. If a second 6-week course of BCG is given, perform bladder biopsy and bladder wash cytology six weeks after finishing the second course.

       iii. If two 6-week courses of BCG fail to eradicate CIS, cystectomy is the preferred treatment. If the patient is not eligible for cystectomy or elects not to undergo cystectomy, there are two FDA approved alternatives to treat CIS that is refractory to BCG: intravesical valrubicin or intravenous pembrolizumab. See page 72.

    b. Maintenance BCG—if CIS is eradicated after one or two 6-week courses of induction BCG, then maintenance BCG is recommended.

6. Example follow up regimen after CIS is eradicated

    a. Cystoscopy and urine cytology at 3 months post-TURBT, then every 3 months for 2 years, then every 6 months for 3 years, then annually. Using other urinary tumor markers is optional.

    b. CT urogram every 1-2 years. CT urogram should also be performed when there are frequent recurrences or when symptoms develop that may be cancer related (e.g. gross hematuria, flank pain, etc.). CT urogram is preferred in most cases, but other imaging alternatives are available (see page 51).

Stage Ta, Low Grade

1. TURBT—try to eliminate all grossly visible tumor.

2. Immediate postoperative intravesical chemotherapy—*a single dose of intravesical chemotherapy within 24 hours of TURBT (ideally within 6 hours) is recommended because it reduces the risk of recurrence (absolute reduction of 14% in 5-year recurrence).*

3. Induction intravesical therapy

    a. When risk factors for recurrence are absent—avoiding induction therapy is reasonable when the risk of recurrence is low. Options include surveillance versus intravesical induction chemotherapy.

    b. When risk factors for recurrence are present—consider administering a 6 week induction course of intravesical chemotherapy (starting 3-4 weeks after TURBT) when any of the following risk factors are present
      i. Multiple tumors
      ii. Recurrence of tumor within 1 year
      iii. Large bladder tumor (e.g. > 3 cm)

    c. *For low grade Ta tumors, chemotherapy is preferred over BCG because toxicity is less and the risk of tumor progression is low.*

    d. BCG may be considered for higher risk cancers, such as diffuse tumor, tumor with multiple risks for recurrence (e.g. several tumors > 3 cm), or rapid recurrence after previous intravesical induction chemotherapy.

4. Surveillance or office fulguration of recurrent tumor—this is only an option when all of the following criteria are met.

    a. The patient has a history of only low grade Ta tumors that have been confirmed pathologically (i.e. no history high grade or stage $\geq$ T1 tumors.)

    b. Urine cytology shows no high grade cells.

    c. The current tumors appear to be few in number, < 1 cm in size, low grade, and stage Ta.

5. Example follow up regimen

    a. Cystoscopy at 3 months post-TURBT, then at 12 months post-TURBT, then every 12 months. Urine tumor markers are not recommended for follow up of treated stage Ta low grade tumors, but cytology should be performed for surveillance of an untreated tumor.

    b. CT urogram when there are frequent recurrences or when symptoms develop that may be cancer related (e.g. gross hematuria, flank pain, etc.). CT urogram is preferred in most cases, but other imaging alternatives are available (see page 51).

Stage Ta, High Grade

1. TURBT—if high grade or invasive bladder cancer is suspected, resection should be deep enough to remove muscularis propria (except when the cancer is in a diverticulum. For tumors in a diverticulum, see page 65).

2. Restaging TURBT—restaging TURBT (within 6 weeks after the previous TURBT) is an option for all patients with Ta high grade cancer, but it is strongly recommended for any of the following situations.
   a. The prior resection did not remove all grossly visible tumor.
   b. The prior resection did not contain muscularis propria (except when the cancer is in a diverticulum.)
   c. The tumor was large or multifocal.

3. Immediate postoperative intravesical chemotherapy—*a single dose of intravesical chemotherapy within 24 hours of TURBT (ideally within 6 hours) is recommended because it reduces the risk of recurrence (absolute reduction of 14% in 5-year recurrence).*

4. Induction therapy—administer a 6-week induction course of intravesical therapy (preferably BCG) starting 3-4 weeks after TURBT. *BCG is preferred for high grade Ta tumors because it is more effective at preventing recurrence and progression than chemotherapy.* Intravesical chemotherapy may be used for induction when BCG is not feasible. Six weeks after finishing a 6-week induction course, perform cystoscopy (with or without biopsy) and bladder wash cytology to check for persistent tumor.
   a. If TURBT after the first 6-week induction course shows high grade T1 cancer, then radical cystectomy is the preferred management.
   b. If TURBT after the first 6-week induction course shows persistent Ta tumor (low or high grade) or no tumor, treatment typically consists of a second 6-week induction course of intravesical BCG. Six weeks after finishing the second course of BCG, perform cystoscopy (with or without biopsy) and bladder wash cytology.
   c. If two 6-week courses of intravesical therapy fail to eradicate the tumor, options include cystectomy or change to a different intravesical agent.

5. Maintenance BCG—if the tumor is eradicated after one or two 6-week courses of induction therapy, then maintenance BCG is recommended.

6. Example follow up regimen after induction BCG
   a. Cystoscopy and urine cytology
      i. For intermediate risk cancer—cystoscopy and urine cytology at 3 months post-TURBT, then every 3-6 months for 2 years, then every 6-12 months for 2 years, then annually.
      ii. For high risk cancer—cystoscopy and urine cytology at 3 months post-TURBT, then every 3 months for 2 years, then every 6 months for 2 years, then annually.
      iii. Using other urinary tumor markers is optional.
   b. CT urogram every 1-2 years (every two years may be more appropriate for intermediate risk cancers, whereas every year more be more appropriate for high risk cancers). CT urogram should also be performed when there are frequent recurrences or when symptoms develop that may be cancer related (e.g. gross hematuria, flank pain, etc.). CT urogram is preferred in most cases, but other imaging alternatives are available (see page 51).

Stage T1

1. TURBT—resection should be deep enough to sample muscularis propria (except when the cancer is in a diverticulum. For tumors in a diverticulum, see page 65).

2. Restaging TURBT—a second TURBT within 6 weeks after the previous TURBT should be performed in all patients with stage T1 cancer (even when muscularis propria was present in the prior TURBT specimen).

3. Immediate postoperative intravesical chemotherapy—*a single dose of intravesical chemotherapy within 24 hours of TURBT (ideally within 6 hours) is recommended because it reduces the risk of recurrence (absolute reduction of 14% in 5-year recurrence).*

4. Stage T1 can only be assigned when the pathology specimen contains muscularis propria that is free of cancer. In other words, stage T1 should not be assigned when muscularis propria is absent from the specimen.

5. Very high risk T1 cancers—the following cancers have a higher risk of progressing to a more advanced stage; therefore, the preferred treatment for these higher risk cancers is early cystectomy.
   a. Low grade T1 cancer with *all* of the following characteristics: size > 3 cm, multifocal, and recurrent.
   b. High grade T1 cancers with *any* of the following characteristics: size > 3 cm, multifocal, recurrent, associated with CIS in the bladder, or associated with CIS in the prostatic urethra.
   c. Any T1 cancer exhibiting lymphovascular invasion or variant histology.
   d. Any T1 cancer that cannot be completely resected by the transurethral approach.

6. T1 cancers not at very high risk—for these cancers, intravesical BCG is generally the preferred treatment.
   a. Induction intravesical therapy—administer a 6-week induction course of intravesical therapy (preferably BCG) starting 3-4 weeks after TURBT. *BCG is preferred in stage T1 tumors because it is more effective at preventing recurrence and progression than chemotherapy.* Intravesical chemotherapy may be used for induction when BCG is not feasible. Six weeks after finishing a 6-week induction course, perform cystoscopy (with or without biopsy) and bladder wash cytology to check for persistent tumor.
      i. If TURBT after the first 6-week induction course shows high grade T1 cancer, then radical cystectomy is the preferred management.
      ii. If TURBT after the first 6-week induction course shows low grade papillary tumor or no tumor, treatment typically consists of a second 6-week induction course of intravesical therapy. Six weeks after finishing the second course, perform cystoscopy (with or without biopsy) and bladder wash cytology.
      iii. If two 6-week courses of intravesical therapy fail to eradicate the tumor, then cystectomy is recommended.
   b. Maintenance BCG—if the tumor is eradicated after one or two 6-week courses of induction therapy, then maintenance BCG is recommended.

7. Example follow up regimen after induction BCG
   a. Cystoscopy and urine cytology at 3 months post-TURBT, then every 3 months for 2 years, then every 6 months for 2 years, then annually. Using other urinary tumor markers is optional.
   b. CT urogram every 1-2 years. CT urogram should also be performed when there are frequent recurrences or when symptoms develop that may be cancer related (e.g. gross hematuria, flank pain, etc.). CT urogram is preferred in most cases, but other imaging alternatives are available (see page 51).

Stage T2-T4a, N0-N1, M0

1. *Intravesical therapy is not effective for stages T2-T4.*
2. Radical cystectomy—radical cystectomy is the preferred treatment for most patients with M0 muscle invasive bladder cancer (it is the "gold standard"). Radical cystectomy is performed with a urinary diversion and with a bilateral pelvic lymphadenectomy. Neoadjuvant systemic chemotherapy before radical cystectomy is recommended. In select cases, postoperative pelvic radiation may be utilized.

   a. *Neoadjuvant systemic chemotherapy with a cisplatin based regimen is recommended before cystectomy* because randomized trials have shown that it achieves a 5% absolute improvement in 5-year overall survival and a 9% absolute improvement in 5-year disease free survival. *Initiate neoadjuvant chemotherapy within 8 weeks of the cancer diagnosis. After neoadjuvant chemotherapy, perform radical cystectomy as soon as possible (ideally within 8-12 weeks after finishing chemotherapy).* If the patient is not eligible for cisplatin based chemotherapy, proceed directly to radical cystectomy (do not administer a carboplatin based regimen instead). Neoadjuvant radiation is not recommended.

   b. If neoadjuvant systemic chemotherapy is not given
      i. *Radical cystectomy should be performed within 3 months of the cancer diagnosis* because operating beyond 3 months increases the risk of progression and the risk of death from bladder cancer.
      ii. Consider adjuvant chemotherapy when surgical pathology shows extravesical extension (stage $\geq$ pT3), lymphovascular invasion, or lymph node metastasis. For adjuvant systemic chemotherapy, there are no randomized trials of adequate size to prove a benefit, but non-randomized studies show that it lowers recurrence rate and improves overall survival. *Neoadjuvant chemotherapy is preferred over adjuvant chemotherapy based on a higher quality of evidence.* Radical cystectomy without chemotherapy can be utilized for patients not eligible for cisplatin based chemotherapy.

   c. The preferred chemotherapy regimen (for either neoadjuvant or adjuvant therapy) is either ddMVAC (dose dense methotrexate, vinblastine, adriamycin, cisplatin) or GC (gemcitabine and cisplatin). Substituting carboplatin for cisplatin in this setting is not recommended because it reduces response rate and survival (i.e. only cisplatin containing regimens should be utilized).

   d. Postoperative pelvic radiation—patients with extravesical extension (stage $\geq$ pT3) have a high risk of pelvic recurrence and a lower overall survival, even when perioperative chemotherapy is added to radical cystectomy. There is minimal data on the use of post-operative radiation, but some data suggests that it may decrease local recurrence and improve disease free survival. *The NCCN 2021 guideline states "While there are no conclusive data demonstrating improvement in overall survival, it is reasonable to consider adjuvant radiation in patients with pT3/pT4 pN0-2 urothelial bladder cancer following radical cystectomy..."* Pelvic radiation may also be considered in patients with positive surgical margins. Post-cystectomy pelvic radiation is typically restricted to patients with a conduit urinary diversion. A neobladder or catheterizable continent diversion would likely suffer too much radiation damage to make radiation a feasible option.

3. Bladder sparing treatments—these treatments preserve most or all of the bladder; thus, urinary diversion is unnecessary. Bladder sparing treatments are typically used for patients who elect not to undergo radical cystectomy or patients who are unfit for either radical cystectomy or urinary diversion.

a. Bladder sparing therapy is less effective in patients with any of the following criteria: large tumors in which TURBT cannot resect all grossly visible tumor, stage T3-T4 cancers, multifocal CIS, extensive CIS, or hydronephrosis caused by bladder cancer. For these patients, bladder sparing therapy results in a relatively low cure rate and a substantial risk of needing salvage cystectomy.

b. Maximal TURBT with chemoradiation (trimodality therapy)—*trimodality therapy is more effective than other forms of bladder sparing therapy. Therefore, if a patient wants to retain their bladder and is eligible for chemoradiation, then trimodality therapy is the preferred form of bladder sparing treatment.* See page 79 for details.

c. Partial cystectomy—only an option in select patients (see page 78). Based on studies of patients undergoing radical cystectomy, neoadjuvant chemotherapy is recommended for patients undergoing partial cystectomy. Partial cystectomy alone may be used in patients who are not eligible for systemic cisplatin based chemotherapy. Also, postoperative pelvic radiation may be considered in situations that are similar to when its used for radical cystectomy.

d. Maximal TURBT with pelvic radiation—used when patients are not eligible for systemic chemotherapy.

e. Maximal TURBT with systemic chemotherapy—used when patients are not eligible for pelvic radiation.

f. TURBT alone—less effective than trimodality therapy; however, TURBT alone can help control local symptoms in patients who do not want or cannot tolerate systemic chemotherapy and pelvic radiation.

4. Example follow up regimen

a. Chest imaging (CT or x-ray), CT urogram, and urine cytology every 3-6 months for 2 years, then annually. CT urogram is preferred in most cases, but other imaging alternatives are available (see page 51).

b. Serum LFTs, electrolytes, BUN, and creatinine (and CBC if the patient had systemic chemotherapy) every 3-6 months for 1 year, then annually

c. After radical cystectomy

i. If the urinary diversion contains a significant length of ileum, obtain a vitamin B12 level each year.

ii. For patients with a retained urethra, perform a urethral wash cytology (with or without urethroscopy) every 6-12 months.

iii. Consider visualization of the urinary diversion (e.g. endoscopy or pouchogram) when urine cytology or imaging suggests recurrence within the urinary system.

d. After bladder sparing–cystoscopy and urine cytology every 3 months for 2 years, then every 6 months for 2 years, then annually.

Stage T4b, N2-N3, M0

1. Initial treatment typically consists of systemic chemotherapy.

2. When systemic chemotherapy sufficiently downstages the disease, then radical cystectomy or trimodality therapy may be offered.

3. When the local tumor is causing problematic symptoms (such as significant gross hematuria), then external beam radiation may be utilized for local tumor control.

Stage M1

1. Initial treatment typically consists of systemic chemotherapy.

2. External beam pelvic radiation may be used to control cancer related symptoms (such as significant gross hematuria).

3. For patients who are without rapid cancer progression and who have few residual metastatic lesions following systemic chemotherapy, limited data suggest that excision of the metastases can achieve long term survival.

Urothelial Cancer with Mixed or Variant Histology
1. Mixed histology UC—UC can mutate into a different histology (e.g. squamous differentiation, glandular differentiation, etc.), yielding a mixture of urothelial cancer and other histologic types of cancer.
   a. Mixed histology UC must be distinguished from pure non-urothelial cancers because pure non-urothelial cancers are often treated differently.
   b. *In most cases mixed histology UC it is treated the same way as a pure urothelial carcinoma of similar stage, grade, and risk;* however, it has a worse prognosis than pure urothelial carcinoma and the clinician should have a lower threshold for proceeding to cystectomy.
2. *The micropapillary, plasmacytoid, and sarcomatoid variants of UC are very aggressive.* Intravesical therapy is typically ineffective. Resectable disease may be best treated with immediate radical cystectomy.

Urothelial Cancer Arising in a Bladder Diverticulum
1. Aggressive transurethral resection of these tumors has a higher risk of bladder perforation because diverticula typically have a thin wall and no muscularis propria. Restaging TURBT is avoided if the patient will be undergoing partial or radical cystectomy. Otherwise, a restaging TURBT is done for the same indications as a tumor not in bladder diverticulum (see page 52). However, restaging TURBT for tumors in a diverticulum should not attempt to sample muscularis propria (since muscularis propria is usually not present in the wall of the diverticulum) and resection depth should be limited to reduce the risk of perforation.
2. CIS in a diverticulum may be treated with transurethral fulguration followed by intravesical BCG.
3. Low grade Ta UC may be treated with TURBT with or without subsequent intravesical therapy.
4. Recurrent, high grade, or stage T1 to T4 tumors are probably best treated with partial cystectomy (i.e diverticulectomy) or radical cystectomy.

Urothelial Cancer of the Prostatic Urethra
1. Mucosal UC in the prostatic urethra—initially treated by transurethral resection of the tumor. If the tumor is high grade, large, or recurrent, then perform a transurethral resection of the prostate (TURP) and start intravesical BCG (TURP improves penetration of BCG into the prostate). Recurrence is generally treated with radical cystectomy and urethrectomy (especially if the recurrence is high grade or invasion).
2. UC inside the prostatic ducts (no stroma invasion)—treatment options include TURP followed by intravesical BCG or radical cystectomy with urethrectomy. TURBT with intravesical BCG is often preferred initial treatment.
3. UC invading the prostatic stroma—for M0 disease, treatment is neoadjuvant chemotherapy, then radical cystectomy and urethrectomy.

Intravesical Therapy for Urothelial Carcinoma
General Information
1. *Intravesical therapy is indicated for stage Ta, T1, or CIS urothelial carcinoma of the bladder.* Intravesical therapy is not effective for muscle invasive UC (stage T2-T4) or for non-urothelial tumors.
2. There are two types of intravesical therapy: chemotherapy (mitomycin, thiotepa, gemcitabine, etc.) and immunotherapy (BCG, interferon, etc.).
3. The three main indications for intravesical therapy are
   a. Eradication of CIS with or without associated papillary tumor.
   b. Eradication of residual papillary tumor after incomplete resection.
   c. To reduce the recurrence and progression of completely resected tumors.

4. Terms used to describe the timing of administration.
   a. Immediate postoperative dose—one dose of intravesical *chemotherapy* administered within 24 hours (ideally within 6 hours) after TURBT. *BCG should never be given intravesically within 2 weeks of TURBT.*
   b. Induction course—induction intravesical therapy is administered starting 3-4 weeks after TURBT. The first cycle typically consists of an intravesical dose once per week for 6 weeks. The induction course should not exceed two 6-week cycles (total of 12 doses).
   c. Maintenance therapy—intravesical therapy administered every several months after induction therapy.

Comparison of Intravesical Chemotherapy and BCG

1. BCG reduces tumor recurrence and progression. Intravesical chemotherapy reduces recurrence, but does *not* alter progression.
2. An induction course of intravesical therapy achieves a similar decrease in recurrence whether BCG or chemotherapy is used. Adding maintenance therapy with BCG reduces recurrence further. Maintenance therapy with chemotherapy does not appear to reduce recurrence when including all chemotherapy agents in the analysis; however, when analyzing each chemotherapy agent separately, maintenance therapy with mitomycin C may reduce recurrence.
3. *BCG is superior to intravesical chemotherapy for treating CIS, high grade tumors, and stage T1 tumors.*
4. One dose of intravesical chemotherapy may be used within 24 hours (ideally within 6 hours) of TURBT in the absence of bladder perforation. *BCG should never be given intravesically within 2 weeks of TURBT.*
5. Side effects are greater with BCG than with intravesical chemotherapy.

	Intravesical BCG	Intravesical Chemotherapy
Used for single dose after TURBT	No	Yes
Absolute reduction in recurrence rate	–	14%
6-12 week induction course reduces recurrence	Yes	Yes
Maintenance therapy reduces recurrence	Yes	No†
Maintenance therapy reduces progression	Yes	No
Mean absolute reduction in progression	5%	–
Side effects/toxicity	Moderate-High	Low-Moderate

TURBT = transurethral resection of bladder tumor; BCG = Bacillus Calmette Guerin
† When analyzing all chemotherapy agents together, chemotherapy did not reduce recurrence (Eur Urol Focus 4: 512, 2018). When analyzing the chemotherapy agents separately, only mitomycin C reduced recurrence (J Urol 197: 1189, 2017).

Intravesical Chemotherapy

1. Intravesical chemotherapy agents are *DNA synthesis inhibitors* that have a direct cytotoxic effect. Inhibition of DNA synthesis results in cell death, particularly in cells with a higher growth rate (such as cancer cells). Intercalating agents insert into DNA (after DNA is cut) and prevent topoisomerase II from resealing the cut.
2. *Intravesical chemotherapy does not change progression, time to metastasis, or overall survival; however it does reduce recurrence rate.*
3. Intravesical chemotherapy is usually utilized for low grade stage Ta urothelial carcinoma (UC) of the bladder when risk factors for recurrence are present (multiple tumors, tumor > 3 cm, or recurrence within 1 year). For high grade tumors and stage T1 tumors, BCG is more effective.

4. *In the United States, mitomycin and gemcitabine are the most frequently used agents for intravesical chemotherapy. The NCCN prefers gemcitabine because it causes less side effects and is less expensive.*

5. Treatment regimens
   a. Postoperative dose—a single dose is administered intravesically within 24 hours (ideally within 6 hours) after TURBT. *For stage Ta and T1 tumors, one postoperative dose of mitomycin C, gemcitabine, or epirubicin is recommended (when not contraindicated) because it reduces the risk of recurrence (absolute reduction of 14% in 5-year recurrence).*
      i. A single postoperative intravesical dose of chemotherapy is most effective in low volume, low grade, stage Ta cancer.
      ii. There is no benefit for patients with ≥ 2 recurrences per year, ≥ 8 tumors in the bladder simultaneously, large volume high grade T1 cancer (≥ 3 cm or multifocal), or an EORTC recurrence risk score ≥ 5. Also, there is no proven benefit in patients with only CIS.
      iii. Valrubicin and thiotepa are not used in this setting.
   b. Induction course—a cycle of intravesical chemotherapy starting 3-4 weeks after TURBT. The initial induction course typically consists of one intravesical instillation every week for 6 weeks.
   c. Maintenance therapy—may be used after induction. The regimen is usually one instillation every 1-3 months for up to one year.

6. Contraindications to intravesical chemotherapy—when urothelial integrity is disrupted, local and systemic toxicity are more likely. Therefore, these agents should not be administered when any of the following are present:
   a. Known or suspected bladder perforation—*intravesical chemotherapy should not be administered when bladder perforation or extravasation from the bladder is present or suspected.*
   b. Recent extensive transurethral resection (within the past 1 week).
   c. Current urinary tract infection
   d. Gross hematuria
   e. Clots that may hinder drainage of the bladder
   f. Traumatic catheterization.

7. Before starting a course of therapy
   a. Ensure that the patient does not have a urinary infection.
   b. Advise the patient to limit fluid intake for 8 hours before each instillation to avoid rapid dilution of the chemotherapy agent.
   c. When using mitomycin, consider oral methods to alkalinize the urine before each instillation (mitomycin is more effective at pH > 6). For example, administer 1.3 grams of oral sodium bicarbonate the night before, the morning of, and 30 minutes before each instillation.

8. Instillation technique immediately after TURBT
   a. Do not instill chemotherapy if it is contraindicated (see above).
   b. Empty the bladder. Place a catheter and instill the chemotherapy agent into the bladder. The agent is held in the bladder (ideally by raising the catheter drainage bag above the patient) for 2 hours or until the patient becomes uncomfortable. After draining the bladder, the catheter may be removed.

9. Instillation technique for subsequent therapeutic and maintenance cycles
   a. Before each instillation
      i. The patient voids before each instillation. Perform a urinalysis to check for gross hematuria and urinary infection.
      ii. When the catheter is placed, a post void residual is measured.
      iii. The bladder should be emptied completely before each instillation.
   b. Instillation—infused through a catheter and into the bladder.

    c. After each instillation
        i. Attempt to hold the agent in the bladder for at least 2 hours. The body position may be varied to ensure thorough distribution in the bladder.
        ii. If the patient has a high post void residual, consider catheterizing the patient 2 hours after instillation to prevent prolonged exposure.
        iii. Patients should wash their hands and genitals after voiding.
        iv. Refraining from sex for 48 hours.

10. Mitomycin C—not FDA approved for intravesical use.
    a. Mechanism of action—alkylating agent.
    b. *Systemic absorption is rare because mitomycin C has a high molecular weight.* Systemic absorption can cause myelosuppression.
    c. Mitomycin C is more effective at urine pH > 6 (consider alkalinization of the urine during therapy) and when its concentration is high (mix mitomycin C in 20 ml of water rather than 40 ml).
    d. Usual dose—40 mg in 20 ml sterile water intravesically [Vials: 40 mg].
    e. Side effects—*contact dermatitis* (minimized by washing the hands and genitals after instillation and after voiding), irritative voiding symptoms.

11. Gemcitabine—not FDA approved for intravesical use.
    a. Mechanism of action—a cytosine analogue and anti-metabolite that gets incorporated into DNA, where it inhibits further DNA synthesis and causes death of the cell.
    b. *Systemic absorption is rare because gemcitabine has a high molecular weight.* Systemic absorption can cause myelosuppression.
    c. Usual dose—for postoperative instillation: 2000 mg in 100 ml normal saline intravesically. For induction or maintenance: 2000 mg in 50 to 100 ml of normal saline intravesically [Vials: 1000 mg].
    d. Side effects—dysuria, urgency, frequency, hematuria.

12. Thiotepa—FDA approved for Ta, T1, and CIS bladder cancer.
    a. Mechanism of action—alkylating agent.
    b. Therapeutic course—60 mg in 30-60 ml of sodium chloride instilled intravesically each week for 6 weeks. Therapy is often continued with a single instillation each month for one year. [Vials: 15 mg].
    c. *Systemic absorption may occur when thiotepa is given intravesically because of its lower molecular weight.* Systemic absorption can cause myelosuppression. Check complete blood count before each instillation.
    d. Side effects—myelosuppression (10%) and irritative voiding symptoms.

13. Epirubicin—not FDA approved for intravesical use.
    a. Epirubicin is an anthracycline.
    b. Mechanism of action—intercalating agent.
    c. *Systemic absorption is rare because epirubicin has a high molecular weight.* Systemic absorption can cause myelosuppression.
    d. Usual dose—40-100 mg in 40-100 ml of sterile normal saline instilled intravesically [Vials: 50 mg].
    e. Side effects include—irritative voiding symptoms.

14. Valrubicin (Valstar™)—FDA approved for the treatment of patients with CIS (with or without papillary tumors) that is refractory to BCG and who are not candidates for radical cystectomy. All visible stage Ta and T1 papillary tumors should be resected before treatment.
    a. Valrubicin is an anthracycline.
    b. Mechanism of action—intercalating agent.
    c. *Systemic absorption is rare because valrubicin has a high molecular weight.* Systemic absorption can cause myelosuppression.
    d. Therapeutic course—800 mg (20 ml) in 55 ml of sterile normal saline instilled intravesically each week for 6 weeks. [Vials: 200 mg/5 ml].
    e. Complete response rate is 18% at 6 months follow up.
    f. Side effects include—irritative voiding symptoms.

Intravesical Immunotherapy with Bacillus Calmette-Guerin (BCG)
1. BCG is an attenuated live bacillus vaccine (Mycobacterium bovis).
2. The three main indications for intravesical BCG are
   a. Eradication of bladder CIS with or without associated papillary tumor.
   b. Eradication of residual bladder UC because of incomplete resection.
   c. Reduce recurrence in completely resected Ta, T1, or CIS bladder UC.
3. Intravesical induction BCG decreases tumor recurrence. Maintenance BCG reduces tumor recurrence and progression, and it may also reduce cystectomy rate and death from bladder cancer.
4. *BCG is superior to intravesical chemotherapy for treatment of carcinoma is situ (CIS) and high grade urothelial cancer (UC)*.
5. Mechanism of action—BCG activates the immune system, which causes T-cells to attack abnormal urothelium. BCG may inhibit tumor invasion.
6. Minor side effects—cystitis, dysuria, frequency, urgency, hematuria, malaise, fatigue, and low grade fever (usually resolve in 24-48 hours). Options for managing these side effects include:
   a. Oral quinolone antibiotic—randomized trials showed that administering a quinolone with each dose of BCG reduces side effects, increases the chance of completing the entire course of BCG, and reduces need for anti-tuberculosis treatment. The oral quinolone is started 6 hours after the first post-BCG urination, followed by 1 or 2 more doses at the appropriate interval for the chosen quinolone. Administration of the quinolone in this fashion did not hinder the anti-cancer effects of BCG.
   b. NSAIDS, medications for overactive bladder, and urinary analgesics (e.g. phenazopyridine) may help reduce BCG related symptoms.
   c. Isoniazid does not reduce the side effects of BCG.
   d. If symptoms are intense or last > 24 hours, consider the following:
      i. Delay additional instillations until symptoms improve or abate.
      ii. Lower the BCG dose—using one-third of the usual dose may reduce local side effects (data are conflicting), but it does not reduce the risk of severe systemic toxicity. Reducing the dose may decrease efficacy, especially if less than one-third of the full dose is used.
7. Major side effects
   a. Fever—if a patient has moderate fever (e.g. 101-102°F) for > 12-24 hours without signs of sepsis, stop the BCG instillations, obtain a urine culture for bacteria and acid fast bacilli, start broad spectrum antibiotics and isoniazid 300 mg po q day. Continue isoniazid for 3 months if BCG infection is suspected. Resume BCG when the patient is asymptomatic.
   b. BCG sepsis (0.4%)—admit patients with very high fever (e.g. $\geq$ 102°F) or signs of sepsis. Obtain urine and blood cultures for bacteria and acid fast bacilli. Administer prednisolone 40 mg IV q day, broad spectrum antibiotics, and anti-tuberculosis drugs (isoniazid 300 mg po q day, rifampin 600 mg po q day, ethambutol 1200 mg po q day, adjust medications based on sensitivity from cultures). Cycloserine may be added for very ill patients because it works faster than other anti-tuberculosis drugs (24 hours versus one week). The adult dose is cycloserine 250 mg or 500 mg po BID (adjust the dose for renal insufficiency). Cycloserine's major toxicity is neurologic (seizures, psychosis, confusion, etc.). A lower dose decreases the risk of side effects. Monitor blood cycloserine levels (at least weekly) and adjust the dose to keep peak blood levels at 20-35 ug/ml. Taper the prednisolone when sepsis has resolved. Continue antituberculosis drugs for 6 months. After BCG sepsis, the patient should not receive BCG again. For patients taking isoniazid or cycloserine, administer pyridoxine (vitamin B6) 50 mg po q day to prevent neurotoxicity.

    c. Other rare side effects—granulomatous prostatitis, contracted bladder, hepatitis, arthritis, pneumonia, myelosuppression, skin rash, ureteral obstruction, and epididymitis/orchitis. Symptomatic BCG epididymitis, orchitis, or granulomatous prostatitis may be treated with isoniazid 300 mg po q day and rifampin 600 mg po q day for 3-6 months. Asymptomatic BCG granulomatous prostatitis requires no therapy.

    d. Most patients convert to a positive protein purified derivation (PPD). This does not require treatment. Patients that convert to positive PPD have a higher chance of complete response to BCG.

    e. There are no known reports of mycobacterial infection caused by close contact with patients receiving BCG.

8. Contraindications to BCG therapy
    a. Gross hematuria (BCG may be given during microscopic hematuria)
    b. Within 2 weeks after TURBT
    c. Recent traumatic catheterization
    d. Urinary tract infection, sepsis, or high fever
    e. Severely immunosuppressed (lymphoma, leukemia, steroids, HIV, etc.)
    f. Previous severe BCG reaction (such as BCG sepsis)

9. Before starting a course of therapy
    a. Ensure that the patient does not have a urinary infection.
    b. Advise the patient to limit fluid intake before each instillation to avoid rapid dilution of BCG and the need to void too soon after instillation.

10. Instillation technique
    a. Dose—the recommended dose is 1 vial of BCG (50 mg Tice or 81 mg Theracys) in 50 ml normal saline instilled intravesically.
    b. Before each instillation
       i. Check the patient's temperature (BCG is contraindicated with fever).
      ii. The patient voids before each instillation. Perform a urinalysis to check for gross hematuria and urinary infection.
     iii. When the catheter is placed, a post void residual is measured.
     iv. If traumatic catheterization is suspected, do not give BCG. Consider waiting at least 1 week before attempting the next instillation.
      v. The bladder should be emptied completely before each instillation.
    c. Instillation—infused through a catheter and into the bladder.
    d. After instillation
       i. Attempt to hold the BCG in the bladder for at least 2 hours. The body position may be varied to thoroughly distribute BCG in the bladder.
      ii. Patients with a high post void residual may be catheterized 2 hours after instillation to prevent excessive exposure to BCG.
     iii. For 24 hours after the BCG instillation, the patient may consider voiding into dilute bleach, voiding into a single toilet and then cleaning it with bleach, hand and genital washing after voiding, and refraining from sex for 48 hours. It is unknown if these actions prevent BCG from affecting people in contact with the patient.

11. Induction therapy—no more than 12 doses are administered.
    a. Administer BCG intravesically once a week for 6 weeks. Six weeks after the last treatment, re-evaluate the bladder with urine tumor marker and cystoscopy (with TURBT if tumor is suspected).
    b. If there is a recurrence after the initial 6-week course of BCG:
       i. If recurrence is stage Ta or CIS—administer another 6-week course of BCG (one dose per week for 6 weeks). *Approximately 50% of these patients will respond to the second course of BCG.*
      ii. If recurrence is stage $\geq$ T2 or high grade stage T1—the preferred treatment is radical cystectomy.
     iii. If recurrence is low grade stage T1—options include radical cystectomy or another course of induction BCG.

c. If there is no recurrence after the initial 6-week course of BCG, then options include no further induction therapy versus another 6-week course of BCG induction.

d. If 12 doses of BCG have been administered, six weeks after the last treatment, re-evaluate the bladder with urine tumor marker and cystoscopy (with TURBT if tumor is suspected). If tumor has recurred at this point, radical cystectomy is usually the preferred option.

12. Two 6 week courses of BCG has a higher response rate than one course.

Reason for Intravesical BCG	CR at 1 Year		CR at 4-5 Years	
	Mean	Range	Mean	Range
Eradication of residual papillary tumor	60%	35-73%	-	-
Eradication of CIS (bladder only)	70%	46-100%	64%	52-71%
Eradication of CIS (prostatic urethra)*				
Response in prostate only	83%	70-100%	-	-
Response in bladder & prostate	68%	47-80%	-	-
Prophylaxis for tumor recurrence	80%	35-91%	58%	28-86%

CR = complete response to 1 or 2 six-week courses of BCG.
* Before starting BCG, TURP is usually performed to remove tumor and to facilitate contact between BCG and the prostatic ducts.

13. Cytology may be positive for up to 3 months after induction BCG. *Inflammation caused by recent intravesical therapy can impair the accuracy of cytology, but it does not impair the accuracy of FISH. The presence of an abnormal FISH shortly after induction BCG is associated with a higher risk of recurrence and progression. Therefore, FISH can be used to identify patients at risk for early failure after BCG.*

14. Maintenance therapy

a. In patients with CIS and/or completely resected recurrent Ta or T1 bladder UC who are disease free at 3 months after a 6-12 week induction course of BCG, *maintenance BCG improves complete response rate, improves disease-free survival, and decreases recurrence rate compared to the 6-12 week induction course of BCG alone.* Maintenance BCG does not improve overall survival.

Patients with CIS and/or Completely Resected Ta or T1 Bladder UC	6 Week Induction Course of BCG	6 Week Induction Course of BCG + Maintenance BCG
Complete response rate (CIS only)†	57%	84%
5-year recurrence-free survival†	41%	60%
5-year overall survival	78%	83%

† Statistically significant difference.

b. Maintenance regimen—one intravesical BCG instillation each week for 3 weeks is administered at 3 and 6 months after the BCG induction course, and then every 6 months thereafter for a total duration of 1-3 years. *Maintenance BCG should be administered for at least 1 year if tolerated.*

   i. *For high risk tumors, 3 years of full dose maintenance BCG is recommended* because it reduces recurrence more than 1 year of maintenance BCG. However, a 3-year course increases side effects. The benefit of continuing BCG for 3 years must be weighed against the increased side effects.

   ii. *For intermediate risk tumors, 1 year of maintenance BCG is recommended* (longer regimens do not improve outcome).

   iii. Reducing the BCG dose (from full dose to a fraction of the full dose) may decrease the efficacy of maintenance therapy, but it can be considered if the patient has substantial BCG related symptoms.

Intravesical Immunotherapy with Interferon
1. Interferon is not FDA approved for intravesical use.
2. Mechanism of action—stimulates the immune system to destroy tumor.
3. Response appears to be better when at least 50 million units of interferon are used and when interferon is combined with BCG.
4. Interferon alone to treat residual tumor
   a. For stage Ta, T1, and Tis, complete response rate is 20-40% at 1-2 years.
   b. For BCG-refractory CIS, complete response rate is 10-20% at 1-2 years.
5. After a combination of intravesical interferon and BCG (6 week induction followed by maintenance) for stage Ta, T1, and Tis, cancer free rate at 24 months is 57% in BCG naive patients and 42% in patients who failed BCG.
6. Dose: 50-100 million units interferon α-2b in 50 ml normal saline. For combination therapy, mix BCG directly into the interferon. Instillation schedule is similar to BCG alone.
7. Side effects include flu like symptoms.
8. The AUA/SUO 2016 guideline states "There is insufficient evidence to recommend using BCG in combination with other intravesical agents"; thus, interferon is typically used in select situations.

Treatment of Non-muscle Invasive UC That Failed BCG

1. *If a patient has persistent urothelial cancer after 12 doses of induction BCG, then radical cystectomy is the preferred management.*
2. If the patient is unfit or unwilling to undergo radical cystectomy, then the following treatment options are available.
   a. When CIS is not present—consider using an intravesical agent that the patient has not yet received (e.g. gemcitabine, docetaxel, nanoparticle albumin bound paclitaxel), a combination of agents, or a clinical trial.
   b. For treatment of CIS (when any associated papillary tumors have been completely resected)
      i. Intravesical valrubicin—this is FDA approved for the treatment patients with CIS (with or without papillary tumors) that is refractory to BCG and who are not candidates for radical cystectomy. All visible stage Ta and T1 papillary tumors should be resected before treatment. Complete response rate is 10% at 12 months follow up. For more details on valrubicin, see page 68.
      ii. Intravenous pembrolizumab—this is FDA approved for the treatment of patients with BCG unresponsive carcinoma in situ (with or without papillary tumors) who are not eligible for or have elected not to undergo cystectomy. All visible stage Ta and T1 papillary tumors should be resected before treatment. Complete response rate at 1 year is 20%. For more details on pembrolizumab, see page 82.
      iii. If the above options are not feasible, then consider administering an intravesical agent that the patient has not yet received (e.g. gemcitabine, docetaxel, nanoparticle albumin bound paclitaxel), a combination of agents, or a clinical trial.

Radical Cystectomy
General Information
1. Radical cystectomy is the gold standard for treating for non-metastatic, muscle invasive primary bladder UC. Radical cystectomy removes the bladder and pelvic lymph nodes. In men, the prostate and seminal vesicles are typically removed. In women, the anterior vagina, uterus, fallopian tubes, and ovaries are typically removed. The reproductive organs can be spared in patients who wish to preserve sexual or reproductive function.

2. *If no neoadjuvant systemic chemotherapy is given, radical cystectomy should be performed within 3 months of cancer diagnosis* because it reduces the risk of progression and the risk of death from bladder cancer.
3. Radical cystectomy reveals incidental prostate cancer in 28-61% of men.
4. Without neoadjuvant chemotherapy, 10% of cystectomy specimens are pT0. Thus, TURBT completely excises 10% of muscle invasive tumors.
5. The worst prognostic finding in a primary bladder tumor is prostatic stromal invasion. The 5-year survival is 22-36%.
6. Unless contraindicated, a peripherally acting mu-opioid (μ-opioid) receptor antagonist (such as alvimopan) should be used to accelerate recovery of postoperative gastrointestinal function.
7. Side effects and complications
   a. Perioperative complications occur in 50-60% of patients and include infection, bleeding requiring transfusion, ileus, deep venous thrombosis, intra-abdominal urine leakage, and leak from the bowel anastomosis. Perioperative mortality is approximately 4%.
   b. Other side effects include sexual dysfunction, infertility, urinary infection, and renal dysfunction.
   c. Long term complications of urinary diversion—see page 77.
8. Recurrence after cystectomy
   a. Local (pelvic) recurrence occurs in ≤ 12% of cases.
   b. Upper tract UC develops in 2-4% of cases when there was no CIS in the bladder and up to 20% of cases when CIS was present in the bladder.
   c. A positive ureteral margin increases the risk of upper tract recurrence.
   d. Recurrence usually occurs within 2 years after cystectomy.

Preserving Sexual Function

1. Attempts at preserving sexual function should only be conducted when it does not compromise cancer control.
2. Nerve sparing—nerve sparing reduces the risk of sexual dysfunction.
   a. Parasympathetic nerves in the neurovascular bundles (NVBs) are important for sexual function. In men, these nerves are involved in generating an erection. In women, these nerves are involved in vaginal lubrication, clitoral engorgement, and labial engorgement.
   b. In males, urethrectomy decreases the potency rate after nerve sparing.
   c. Nerve sparing techniques avoid removal of the NVBs and minimize injury to the NVBs. Nerve sparing techniques can be combined with preservation of the reproductive organs.
3. Preservation of reproductive organs in females—during standard radical cystectomy, the anterior vagina, uterus, fallopian tubes, and ovaries are typically removed. These reproductive organs can be spared to preserve sexual or reproductive function if it does not compromise cancer control. *To be a candidate for reproductive organ sparing, the patient must have negative screening for cancer of the reproductive organs.*
   a. Anterior vaginal wall—the anterior vaginal wall is in direct contact with the posterior bladder; thus, tumors in the posterior bladder (including the trigone) can more easily invade the vaginal wall. Also, the lymphatic vessels that drain the bladder neck traverse along the lateral vaginal wall before they enter the pelvic lymph nodes, therefore, cancer can spread through these lymphatics to the vagina. If the anterior vagina is resected, then vaginal reconstruction may be performed. *Vaginal sparing is typically avoided when any of the following criteria are present.*
      i. *Non-organ confined cancer (stage ≥ T3)*
      ii. *Tumor in the bladder neck, trigone, or urethra.*
      iii. *Suspicion of direct invasion of the vaginal wall.*

b. Uterus, fallopian tubes, and ovaries—when there is no suspicion for spread of cancer to these organs, then they may be spared. The ovaries may be spared to preserve hormone balance, even if preservation of sexual and reproductive function are not important.

4. Preservation of reproductive organs in males—during standard radical cystectomy, the prostate and seminal vesicles are typically removed. These reproductive organs can be spared to preserve sexual or reproductive function if it does not compromise cancer control.

 a. Reproductive organ preservation—this includes "prostate capsule sparing" and "prostate sparing" procedures. Reproductive organ preservation in men removes a variable portion of the prostate and the prostate capsule, but it preserves the NVBs, seminal vesicles, ejaculatory ducts, and the vas deferens. Preserving these organs reduces the risk of postoperative erectile and ejaculatory dysfunction. *To be a candidate for reproductive organ sparing, the patient must have benign prostate biopsies and benign prostatic urethra biopsies. Reproductive organ sparing in men is typically avoided when any of the following criteria are present*
   i. *Non-organ confined bladder cancer (stage ≥ T3)*
   ii. *Tumor in the bladder neck, prostatic urethra, or anterior urethra.*
   iii. *Prostate cancer is present.*

 b. Nerve sparing (without reproductive organ preservation) and prostate sparing are equally effective for achieving postoperative erectile function. However, prostate sparing can also preserve fertility and ejaculatory function. Even with nerve or prostate sparing, erectile dysfunction occurs in more than 40% of cases.

Pelvic Lymph Node Dissection (PLND)

1. *Perform bilateral PLND with radical cystectomy.* Cancer can spread to nodes that are contralateral to the tumor; thus, PLND is always bilateral.

2. Standard PLND—the limits of dissection are the bifurcation of the common iliac artery superiorly, the inguinal ligament inferiorly, the bladder medially, and the genitofemoral nerve and pelvic side wall laterally. Standard PLND removes the obturator, internal iliac, and external iliac nodes.

3. Extended PLND—extending the superior dissection to the aortic bifurcation (to remove the common iliac nodes) may reduce pelvic recurrence and may improve cancer specific and overall survival (although data are conflicting). Therefore, *most guidelines state that either a standard PLND or an extended PLND may be performed.*

4. Lymphocele is rare after radical cystectomy because the intraperitoneal approach allows lymph fluid to be absorbed by the peritoneum.

Urethrectomy

1. An orthotopic neobladder cannot be performed after urethrectomy.

2. After cystectomy without urethrectomy, urethral tumor recurrence occurs in up to 10% of patients, usually within 2 years postoperatively.

 a. In females, the risk of urethral recurrence is highest in patients with tumor at the bladder neck.

 b. In males, the risk of urethral recurrence is highest in patients with prostatic stroma invasion (approximately 23%) and prostatic ductal invasion (approximately 15%).

Prostate Involvement in Men Undergoing Radical Cystectomy for UC	Anterior Urethral Recurrence	
	Mean	Range
Prostatic Urethral Mucosa	5%	0-8%
Prostatic Ducts	15%	0-25%
Prostatic Stroma	23%	0-64%

3. Perform urethrectomy if any of the following criteria exist:
   a. In a female, UC in any part of the urethra.
   b. In a male, UC in the anterior urethra.
   c. UC at the urethral margin during cystectomy (based on frozen section).
4. Consider performing urethrectomy in patients at higher risk for urethral recurrence (especially patients not receiving an orthotopic neobladder).
   a. Males with ductal or stromal invasion of the prostate.
   b. Females with tumors involving the bladder neck.
5. In females who are not receiving a neobladder, urethrectomy should be performed because it adds minimal morbidity to cystectomy.
6. Urethrectomy decreases the potency rate of nerve sparing cystectomy.
7. If the urethra is retained, perform urethral wash cytology every 6-12 months. Place a catheter or cystoscope to the proximal most extent of the urethra. Flush ≥ 20 ml of normal saline through the catheter/scope. Collect the saline as it drains from the meatus. Wash cytology is the preferred method of evaluating the urethra for recurrence because it is more sensitive than urethroscopy. Urethroscopy may be used as an adjunct to wash cytology. Patients with urethral symptoms (pain, bleeding) tend to have higher stage of recurrence than asymptomatic patients.
   a. For a resectable urethral recurrence, perform a total urethrectomy.
   b. For CIS recurring in the urethra, intra-urethral BCG may be utilized.

Survival After Radical Cystectomy for UC

Pathologic Stage (AJCC 2017)	Mean Disease-Free Survival* (Range)			
	5-Year		10-Year	
pT0N0	92%	—	86%	—
pTaN0	79%	(79-100%)	74%	(74-80%)
pTisN0	91%	(85-92%)	89%	—
pT1N0	83%	(80-93%)	78%	(72-78%)
pT2N0	83%	(62-89%)	81%	(76-87%)
pT3N0	62%	(57-62%)	61%	—
pT4N0	50%	(50-62%)	45%	(41-45%)
N1-N3	35%	(28-48%)	34%	(21-34%)
All stages	68%	(55-79%)	66%	(65-69%)

* Without adjuvant or neoadjuvant therapy.

Urinary Diversion (also see page 742)

1. Diversion options
   a. Non-continent cutaneous diversion—urine drains continuously from an ostomy and into a collection bag. Examples include ileal conduit, colon conduit, and cutaneous ureterostomy.
   b. Continent cutaneous diversion—a *continent* reservoir that is emptied by catheterizing through a stoma on the skin. A segment of bowel is detubularized, reconfigured into a pouch, and then connected to the ureters. A catheterizable limb (constructed from bowel) extends from the pouch to the skin. Continence mechanisms include pressure equilibration (intussuscepted bowel) and flap valve (tunnelled implant).
   c. Orthotopic bladder replacement (neobladder)—a *continent* reservoir that allows voiding per urethra. A segment of bowel is detubularized and reconfigured into a pouch, which is then connected to the ureters and to the urethra. The *urethral sphincter* is the continence mechanism. [by strict definition, neobladder is not a diversion (see page 742), but it is included in this section for the sake of simplicity].
   d. Ureterosigmoidostomy and variations—*continent* diversions that divert the urine into the gastrointestinal tract. The *anal sphincter* is the continence mechanism.

2. For continent diversions, a spherical pouch of detubularized bowel minimizes the internal pressure (based on Laplace's law) and minimizes the surface area. Low pressure reduces the risk of incontinence, reflux, and diversion rupture. Low surface area reduces the length of bowel required to make the diversion and the risk of metabolic complications.
3. Ureteral anastomosis to the diversion
   a. For conduits and neobladders, a refluxing anastomosis has a lower stricture rate than an anti-refluxing anastomosis. Thus, a refluxing anastomosis is often recommended. For a conduit, the Bricker and Wallace techniques have a similar stricture rate.
   b. For catheterizable continent diversions and for ureterosigmoidostomy variations, an anti-refluxing ureteral anastomosis is recommended.
4. The most commonly performed diversions are ileal conduit, orthotopic neobladder, and continent cutaneous diversion.
5. *The type of urinary diversion does not affect the cure rate of cystectomy.*
6. *All urinary diversions have a similar patient reported quality of life.*
7. Absolute contraindications for a continent diversion
   a. Limited life expectancy
   b. Stage N2-N3 or positive surgical margin (including a positive urethral margin)—these patients have a high risk of pelvic recurrence and may require postoperative radiation.
   c. The patient is unlikely to be compliant with care for their diversion and with follow up appointments—patients must be motivated to comply with the postoperative management.
   d. The patient is unwilling or unable to catheterize—patients must have sufficient manual dexterity to catheterize.
   e. The patient lacks sufficient cognitive function to care for their diversion—patients should have sufficient psychiatric and mental function to comply with postoperative management.
   f. The presence of a progressive condition that would, in the near future, impair the patient's ability to catheterize or care for their diversion (e.g. progressive neurologic disease, early stage dementia).
   g. Impaired liver or renal function that is severe enough to pose significant risk for a postoperative metabolic abnormality—these patients have an increased risk of developing a metabolic complication caused by the reabsorption of urine from the diversion (see page 742). Continent urinary diversions are best avoided when creatinine clearance is less than 45-60 ml/min or when there is severe liver dysfunction.
   h. Gastrointestinal conditions that may be exacerbated when bowel is used to create the urinary diversion (e.g. Crohn's disease, severe irritable bowel syndrome, fat malabsorption, short bowel syndrome, etc.).
   i. High-dose radiotherapy to the abdomen and/or pelvis—some surgeons consider this to be a relative contraindication. Regardless, performing a continent diversion after abdominal or pelvic radiation has a significantly higher complication rate.
8. Absolute contraindications specific to neobladder
   a. Presence of cancer in the anterior urethra (this requires urethrectomy).
   b. Uncorrectable or unmanageable urethral stricture.
9. Relative contraindications specific to neobladder
   a. Cured or well managed urethral stricture disease
   b. Incompetent urethral sphincter causing stress incontinence.
   c. High risk for urethral recurrence (females with tumor at the bladder neck; males with prostatic ductal or stroma invasion)—if the urethral margin is free of tumor, these patients can undergo continent diversion; however, their risk of subsequent urethral recurrence is higher.

10. Long term complications of urinary diversion include:
   a. All diversions—urine tract infection, metabolic abnormalities, stenosis at the ureteral anastomosis, declining renal function, etc. For a more complete list of complications, see page 742. Also see Stricture at the Ureterointestinal Anastomosis, page 446. *After urinary diversion, life long surveillance of the upper tracts (with imaging and creatinine) is mandatory because the risk of renal dysfunction increases over time.*
   b. Conduits—stoma stenosis, stoma prolapse, peristomal hernia, dermatitis of peristomal skin.
   c. Continent cutaneous diversions—difficulty catheterizing, stoma stenosis, urine leak from stoma, stones in the diversion, pouchitis.
   d. Orthotopic neobladders—urine incontinence, urine retention (10% of men and 40% of women require catheterization for retention).

Neoadjuvant and Adjuvant Therapies with Cystectomy

1. *Neoadjuvant systemic chemotherapy with a cisplatin based regimen is recommended before cystectomy* because randomized trials have shown that it achieves a 5% absolute improvement in 5-year overall survival and a 9% absolute improvement in 5-year disease free survival.
   a. *Initiate neoadjuvant chemotherapy within 8 weeks of the cancer diagnosis. After neoadjuvant chemotherapy, perform radical cystectomy as soon as possible (ideally within 8-12 weeks after finishing chemotherapy).*
   b. If the patient is not eligible for cisplatin based chemotherapy, proceed directly to radical cystectomy (do not administer a carboplatin based regimen instead). Neoadjuvant radiation is not recommended.
2. If neoadjuvant systemic chemotherapy is not given, consider administering adjuvant chemotherapy when surgical pathology shows extravesical extension (stage $\geq$ pT3), lymphovascular invasion, or lymph node metastasis. Although non-randomized studies show that adjuvant chemotherapy lowers recurrence rate and improves overall survival, *neoadjuvant chemotherapy is preferred based on a higher quality of evidence.* Radical cystectomy without chemotherapy can be utilized for patients not eligible for cisplatin based chemotherapy.
3. The preferred chemotherapy regimen (for either neoadjuvant or adjuvant therapy) is either ddMVAC (dose dense methotrexate, vinblastine, adriamycin, cisplatin) or GC (gemcitabine and cisplatin). Substituting carboplatin for cisplatin in this setting is not recommended because it reduces response rate and survival.
4. Postoperative pelvic radiation—patients with extravesical extension (stage > pT3) have a high risk of pelvic recurrence and a lower overall survival, even when perioperative chemotherapy is added to radical cystectomy. There is a paucity of data regarding the use of post-operative radiation in these patients, but some data suggests that it may decrease local recurrence and improve disease free survival. *The NCCN 2021 guideline states "While there are no conclusive data demonstrating improvement in overall survival, it is reasonable to consider adjuvant radiation in patients with pT3/pT4 pN0-2 urothelial bladder cancer following radical cystectomy..." Pelvic radiation may also be considered in patients with positive surgical margins.* Post-cystectomy pelvic radiation is typically restricted to patients with a conduit urinary diversion. A neobladder or catheterizable continent diversion would likely suffer too much radiation damage to make radiation a feasible option.

Partial Cystectomy

Partial Cystectomy for Urothelial Bladder Cancer

1. Partial cystectomy is an attractive option because it preserves the bladder and maintains potency. However, it may be associated with a higher risk of all-cause mortality than radical cystectomy or trimodality therapy. *Therefore, partial cystectomy is usually restricted to patients who are unable or unwilling to undergo radical cystectomy or trimodality therapy.*

2. Partial cystectomy and pelvic lymphadenectomy may be performed for primary bladder cancer if all of the following criteria are met.
   • Solitary cancer that is stage T1 or higher—for stage T1, partial cystectomy is often reserved for high grade tumors. Low grade tumors are usually treated with TURBT and intravesical therapy.
   • No CIS
   • Negative random bladder biopsies
   • No prior history of bladder tumors
   • No prostate invasion
   • Ability to maintain adequate bladder capacity after resection.
   • Ability to achieve negative margins—tumors at the bladder dome or in a diverticulum are good candidates. Resection of the ureteral orifice with ureteral reimplant may be performed when necessary.

3. *During partial cystectomy, bilateral pelvic lymph node dissection should always be performed* (use the same PLND template that is used during radical cystectomy; see page 74).

4. Retrospective data shows that cancer specific survival is similar for partial and radical cystectomy; however, partial cystectomy has a higher all-cause mortality than radical cystectomy. A randomized prospective study comparing radical and partial cystectomy has not been performed.

5. Older studies report rates of up to 18% for tumor implantation along the incision or suprapubic tube tract. With current surgical techniques, tumor recurrence in the incision or suprapubic tract is rare. Some surgeons recommend leaving only a urethral catheter postoperatively to avoid tumor implantation along a suprapubic tube tract.

6. Recurrence in the bladder occurs in approximately 32% of patients; nearly two-thirds of these recurrences are non-muscle invasive. Non-muscle invasive recurrences can be treated in the same fashion as non-muscle invasive cancer that is found at initial diagnosis (e.g. intravesical therapy). Radical cystectomy is recommended for muscle invasive recurrence. 15% of patients who undergo partial cystectomy will eventually require radical cystectomy.

7. 5-year cancer specific survival rate for all stages is approximately 68%.

8. Systemic chemotherapy (neoadjuvant or adjuvant) with partial cystectomy has not been well studied. However, its use with partial cystectomy is extrapolated from radical cystectomy data. Therefore, *neoadjuvant systemic chemotherapy is recommended before partial cystectomy.* Consider adjuvant chemotherapy when neoadjuvant chemotherapy was not given (especially for patients with a regional node metastasis). Partial cystectomy without chemotherapy can be utilized for patients not eligible for cisplatin based chemotherapy.

Partial Cystectomy for Non-urothelial Bladder Cancer

1. Partial cystectomy is the usually the treatment of choice for bladder pheochromocytoma.

2. Partial cystectomy may be used for urachal adenocarcinomas and non-urologic cancers that invade the bladder by local extension.

TURBT With Chemoradiation (Trimodality Therapy)

1. Trimodality therapy is used for urothelial carcinoma of the bladder (not for pure non-urothelial cancer).
2. TURBT with chemoradiation is often called trimodality therapy because it consists of 3 modes of treatment: maximal TURBT, chemotherapy, and external beam radiation. Maximal TURBT removes as much of the tumor as possible. Then, external beam radiation (XRT) is administered concomitantly with systemic radio-sensitizing chemotherapy. Radio-sensitizing chemotherapy is directly cytotoxic to cancer cells, but it also causes cancer cells to be more susceptible to radiation (resulting in greater cell kill than chemotherapy or radiation alone). For trimodality therapy, commonly used radiosensitizing chemotherapy regimens (which are administered systemically, not intravesically) include gemcitabine, 5-fluorouracil + mitomycin, and cisplatin based regimens (e.g. cisplatin alone, cisplatin + 5-fluorouracil, cisplatin + paclitaxel).
3. *Trimodality therapy is less effective for cancers that have any of the following characteristics: TURBT did not resect all grossly visible tumor, stage T3-T4, multifocal CIS, extensive CIS, or hydronephrosis caused by the cancer.* Patients with any of these characteristics have a low cure rate and a substantial risk of needing salvage cystectomy. Patients with a small bladder capacity are also poor candidates for this approach because the bladder may shrink after radiation. The ideal candidate would have all of the following characteristics.
   a. The bladder tumor does not cause hydronephrosis
   b. Absence of multifocal or extensive CIS
   c. Small and solitary bladder tumor
   d. Stage T2
   e. No regional or distant metastasis (N0M0)
   f. Ample bladder capacity before treatment
   g. Good bladder function before treatment
4. *Before chemoradiation, perform "maximal TURBT" and assess for CIS.*
   a. Maximal TURBT—this procedure removes the maximum possible amount of grossly visible tumor that can be resected safely, ideally without perforating the bladder. It includes re-resection of previous tumor sites and resection of any new tumor sites. *Maximal TURBT reduces the risk of persistent tumor and increases the chance of complete response to chemoradiation.* It may also improve disease free survival.
   b. Assessment for CIS—patients with multifocal or extensive CIS are not ideal candidates for trimodality therapy. To determine if CIS is present, biopsy areas that appear suspicious for CIS (using blue light or narrow band imaging can help identify these areas) and obtain random biopsies of normal appearing mucosa. Include biopsies of the prostatic urethra if indicated (for indications, see page 54).
5. After maximal TURBT, XRT is administered with concomitant systemic chemotherapy. Mid way through chemoradiation, perform cystoscopy, chest imaging, and abdominal/pelvic imaging (CT or MRI).
   a. If persistent or recurrent non-metastatic UC is found in the bladder, then cystectomy is recommended.
   b. If metastatic UC is found, then administer systemic chemotherapy.
   c. If no tumor is found (i.e. complete response), then additional chemoradiation is delivered to complete the treatment course.
6. This trimodality approach is more expensive than primary cystectomy and commits the patient to a long treatment regimen.

7. Recurrence in the bladder occurs in approximately 43% of patients; nearly two-thirds of these recurrences are non-muscle invasive. Non-muscle invasive recurrences can be treated in the same fashion as non-muscle invasive cancer that is found at initial diagnosis (e.g. intravesical therapy). Radical cystectomy is recommended for muscle invasive recurrence after trimodality therapy.

8. Approximately 25% of patients undergoing trimodality therapy will eventually require cystectomy, usually because of incomplete response to chemoradiation. The delay in cystectomy (compared to initial cystectomy) may increase the risk of disease progression (although this point is controversial). After incomplete response to chemoradiation, the patient may not be healthy enough to undergo cystectomy. Furthermore, cystectomy after radiation may have a higher complication rate and may limit the options for urinary diversion.

9. In appropriately selected patients, trimodality therapy can achieve a similar cancer specific survival and overall survival as radical cystectomy.

Comparison of Therapies for Muscle Invasive Bladder UC

	Mean (range)		
	Radical Cystectomy	**Partial Cystectomy**	**TURBT with Chemo & XRT**
5-Year cancer specific survival (all stages)	68% (55-79%)	68% (35-87%)	68% (47-82%)
Treatment related mortality	2-3%	< 5%	4%
Require cystectomy after therapy	—	15% (7-19%)	25% (8-46%)
Local recurrence rate†	≤ 12%	32%* (19-44%)	43%* (29-57%)

TURBT = transurethral resection of bladder tumor; XRT = external beam radiation
* Non-muscle invasive recurrences in the bladder can be treated by TURBT with or without intravesical therapy.
† Local recurrence after cystectomy is defined as pelvic recurrence. Local recurrence after partial cystectomy or trimodality therapy is defined as recurrence within the bladder.

Summary of Initial Treatment for Bladder Tumors

Histologic Type of Primary Bladder Tumor		Usual Initial Treatment for Non-metastatic Disease
Urothelial Carcinoma	Usual Type	Varies Depending on Tumor Stage
	Mixed Histology	Treated same as Usual Type
	Micropapillary, Plasmacytoid, or Sarcomatoid Variant	Radical Cystectomy*
Non-Urothelial Tumors	Squamous Cell Carcinoma	Radical Cystectomy*
	Adenocarcinoma	Radical Cystectomy*
	Urachal Carcinoma	Partial or Radical Cystectomy*
	Small Cell Carcinoma	Systemic Chemotherapy†
	Pheochromocytoma	Partial Cystectomy

* Radiation and systemic chemotherapy are generally ineffective.
† In patients who respond to chemotherapy, consolidation with radical cystectomy and/or pelvic radiation may be administered.

Systemic Therapy for Metastatic Urothelial Carcinoma

Example Treatment Paradigm
1. The preferred first-line treatment for metastatic urothelial carcinoma (UC) is cisplatin based systemic chemotherapy using either ddMVAC (dose dense methotrexate, vinblastine, adriamycin, cisplatin) or GC (gemcitabine and cisplatin).
2. If the patient progresses after platinum based chemotherapy, then the preferred second-line treatment is pembrolizumab, although other options include nivolumab, avelumab, or erdafitinib.
3. If the patient fails second-line treatment with a PD-1/PD-L1 pathway inhibitor, then the preferred third line treatment options are erdafitinib or enfortumab vedotin.

Systemic Chemotherapy
1. *Systemic chemotherapy for UC is not curative.*
2. *Cisplatin is the most effective systemic chemotherapy agent against UC.* Combination chemotherapy is more effective than a single agent.
3. The first line regimen for metastatic bladder UC is either ddMVAC (dose dense methotrexate, vinblastine, adriamycin, cisplatin) or GC (gemcitabine and cisplatin). The NCCN no longer recommends conventional MVAC (given on a 28 day cycle) because ddMVAC (given on a 14 day cycle) is more effective and better tolerated. GC and conventional MVAC achieve a similar survival, but GC is less toxic. GC has higher rate of anemia and thrombocytopenia, whereas MVAC has a higher rate of neutropenia, sepsis, mucositis, alopecia, and fatigue.
4. For patients with M1 disease who are not eligible for cisplatin, carboplatin may be used in place of carboplatin, but carboplatin based regimens appear to be less effective. For M0 patients undergoing radical cystectomy and who are not eligible for a cisplatin based perioperative regimen, a carboplatin based regimen should not be used instead.
5. Cisplatin kills cancer cells by cross linking DNA. Its dose limiting toxicity is nephrotoxicity. Other side effects include neurotoxicity, hearing loss, diminished cardiac function, nausea, and vomiting. Patients with hearing loss, neuropathy, poor performance status, or renal insufficiency may not be eligible for cisplatin based chemotherapy.

Targeted Systemic Therapies
1. There are many biochemical pathways that allow cancer to grow. Targeted therapy inhibits one or more of these specific pathways, which leads to reduced cancer growth. Cancer cells tend to be more dependant on these processes than normal cells; therefore, targeted therapy has the potential to treat the cancer while having less impact on normal tissue (which may lead to less side effects). In other words, targeted therapy acts upon a specific process used by cancer cells (and some normal cells), whereas chemotherapy acts upon all cells (whether they are cancerous or not). Examples of these targeted pathways include the PD-1/PD-L1 pathway, the FGFR/FGF pathway, and the nectin/microtubule pathway.
2. PD-1/PD-L1 pathway—the programmed death receptor-1 (PD-1) is located on lymphocytes. When certain proteins bind to PD-1, the immune system has a reduced capacity to attack normal tissues (decreasing auto-immune reactions) and a reduced capacity to attack malignant tissues (hindering the body's ability to kill cancer). PD-L1 (programmed death ligand 1) is a protein that binds to the PD-1 receptor. Many cancers evade the body's defenses by expressing a high level of PD-L1, which binds to PD-1 and inhibits the immune system's ability to kill cancer.

a. Medicines can block the binding of PD-L1 to PD-1 by attaching to PD-L1 (PD-L1 inhibitors) or by attaching to the PD-1 receptor (PD-1 inhibitors). However, both PD-1 and PD-L1 inhibitors achieve their anticancer effects by inhibiting the PD-1/PD-L1 pathway.

b. The increased immune activity from blocking the PD-1/PD-L1 pathway can also result in an attack on normal tissue (which leads to some of the side effects). Since all PD-1 inhibitors and PD-L1 inhibitors block the same pathway, they all tend to have similar side effects.

c. Medications that block the PD-1/PD-L1 pathway are often called immune check point inhibitors because they block an important regulatory component of the immune system.

3. FGFR/FGF pathway—fibroblast growth factor receptor (FGFR) is located on many types of cells. When fibroblast growth factor (FGF) binds to FGFR, many processes are stimulated, including cell division (i.e. mitosis), cell migration, and endothelial cell proliferation (leading to angiogenesis). In cancer cells, genetic alterations in the FGFR gene can lead to increased activation of the FGFR/FGF pathway, which stimulates mitosis (leading to cancer growth), cell migration (leading to cancer invading into surrounding tissue), and angiogenesis (leading to cancer survival and increased capacity for growth).

a. Medicines that block the binding of FGF to FGFR can inhibit cancer survival, cancer growth, and cancer invasion.

b. Medicines that block the FGFR/FGF pathway can impair growth, survival, and angiogenesis of normal tissue (which leads to some of the side effects).

c. FGFR is a member of the tyrosine kinase family of molecules. Therefore, medications that inhibit the FGFR/FGF pathway may be referred to as tyrosine kinase inhibitors. Since the FGFR/FGF pathway is also involved in angiogenesis, medications that block this pathway may be referred to as angiogenesis inhibitors.

4. Nectin/microtubule pathway—for details on how this pathway is utilized, see enfortumab vedotin, page 83.

5. Examples of targeted therapies
   a. PD-1 inhibitors—e.g. pembrolizumab, nivolumab.
   b. PD-L1 inhibitors—e.g. avelumab, atezolizumab.
   c. FGFR inhibitors—e.g. erdafitinib.
   d. Microtubule disrupter—e.g. enfortumab vedotin.

Pembrolizumab

1. Mechanism of action—pembrolizumab is a PD-1 inhibitor. It is an antibody that binds to PD-1 and blocks the binding of proteins to PD-1, which gives the immune system a greater capacity to attack cancer.

2. Intravenous pembrolizumab is FDA approved for the treatment of bladder cancer in the following clinical situations.

   a. Patients who have BCG unresponsive carcinoma in situ (with or without papillary tumors) who are not eligible for or have elected not to undergo cystectomy.

   b. In locally advanced or metastatic urothelial cancer, it is approved for
      i. Patients who are not eligible for cisplatin containing chemotherapy and whose tumors express PD-L1.
      ii. Patients who are not eligible for any platinum containing chemotherapy (regardless PD-L1 status).
      iii. Patients with cancer progression during or after platinum containing chemotherapy (regardless PD-L1 status), including those who progress within 12 months of receiving platinum based neoadjuvant or adjuvant chemotherapy.

3. Side effects
   a. Common—fatigue, musculoskeletal pain, decreased appetite, pruritus, diarrhea, nausea, rash, fever, cough, dyspnea, constipation, abdominal pain, peripheral edema, and infusion related reactions.
   b. Less common—*immune mediated side effects* (pneumonitis, colitis, hepatitis, thyroiditis, pituitary inflammation, nephritis, etc.)
4. Dose—pembrolizumab is administered intravenously. See the full prescribing information for dose and administration.
5. Monitoring during therapy—monitoring should include serum creatinine, electrolytes, glucose, liver function tests, and thyroid function tests.

Other Inhibitors of the PD-1/PDL-1 Pathway
1. These include PD-1 inhibitors (nivolumab) and PDL-1 inhibitors (atezolizumab and avelumab)
2. These medications are used for the treatment of locally advanced or metastatic urothelial bladder cancer in patients.
3. Side effects—similar to pembrolizumab, see above.

Erdafitinib
1. Mechanism of action—erdafitinib an FGFR inhibitor. It binds to FGFR types 1 through 4, which blocks the binding of FGF to these FGFRs.
2. Erdafitinib is FDA approved for the treatment of locally advanced and metastatic UC in patients whose cancers have susceptible FGFR2 or FGFR3 genetic mutations and who progress during or after platinum containing chemotherapy, including those who progress within 12 months of receiving platinum based neoadjuvant or adjuvant chemotherapy.
3. Side effects
   a. Abnormal blood tests—decreased hemoglobin, increased creatinine, decreased sodium, decreased magnesium, increased calcium, increased or decreased phosphate, decreased albumin, and elevated liver function tests.
   b. Common side effects—stomatitis (inflammation of the mouth), fatigue, dry mouth, dry skin, dry eye, diarrhea, constipation, abdominal pain, nausea, decreased appetite, dysgeusia (altered taste), musculoskeletal pain, and onycholysis (detachment of the fingernail or toenail from the nail bed).
   c. Serious side effects—hyperphosphatemia, ocular disorders (such as central serous retinopathy/retinal pigment epithelial detachment which can cause a visual field defect).
4. Dose—erdafitinib is administered *orally*. See the full prescribing information for dose and administration.
5. Monitoring during therapy—monitoring should include ophthalmological exams and serum phosphate measurements.

Enfortumab Vedotin
1. Mechanism of action—enfortumab vedotin is an antibody-drug conjugate (an antibody attached to a therapeutic drug). The antibody binds to the nectin-4 receptor on the surface of cells. The therapeutic drug, called monomethyl auristatin E (MMAE), is a microtubule inhibitor. The antibody-drug conjugate binds to the nectin-4 receptor, which causes the conjugate to be internalized into the cell. Inside the cell, MMAE is released from the antibody. Then, MMAE causes microtubule disruption, which leads to cell death. The gene for nectin-4 is frequently amplified in bladder cancer, leading to overexpression of Nectin-4 receptor. The overexpression of nectin-4 on bladder cancer allows Enfortumab vedotin to preferentially target cancer cells instead of normal cells.

2. Enfortumab vedotin is FDA approved for the treatment of locally advanced or metastatic urothelial cancer in patients who have previously received a platinum containing chemotherapy regimen and a PD-1/PD-L1 pathway inhibitor.
3. Side effects
    a. Abnormal blood tests—elevated glucose, decreased white blood cells, decreased hemoglobin, increased creatinine, and decreased phosphate.
    b. Common side effects—fatigue, peripheral neuropathy, decreased appetite, nausea, diarrhea, dysgeusia (altered taste), rash, alopecia, dry eye, dry skin, and pruritus.
    c. Serious side effects—hyperglycemia, ocular disorders, and peripheral neuropathy.
4. Dose—enfortumab vedotin is administered intravenously. See the full prescribing information for dose and administration.
5. Monitoring during therapy—monitoring should include serum glucose. Also consider ophthalmological exams.

Recurrence

Non-metastatic Recurrence in Patients with an Intact Bladder
1. If urine tumor marker is suspicious for malignancy, but cystoscopy shows no tumor, then perform the evaluation described on page 117.
2. Muscle invasive recurrence after intravesical therapy, trimodality therapy, or any other bladder sparing therapy—the preferred treatment is radical cystectomy.
3. Non-muscle invasive recurrence after intravesical chemotherapy—in patients with low grade stage Ta tumors that recur frequently despite intravesical chemotherapy, then intravesical BCG may be tried (the efficacy of BCG is not altered by prior intravesical chemotherapy).
4. Non-muscle invasive recurrence after intravesical BCG
    a. For patients who are tumor free after induction BCG and then recur during BCG maintenance with high risk cancer, radical cystectomy is the usually preferred management.
    b. For patients who are tumor free after completing BCG and then recur within 12 months of their last BCG dose with high risk cancer, radical cystectomy is the preferred management.
    c. For patients who are tumor free after completing BCG and then recur > 12 months after their last BCG dose with high risk cancer, treatment options include radical cystectomy or repeat BCG therapy (induction and maintenance). Repeating BCG is likely more favored in those with a longer time between the last BCG dose and recurrence.
5. Non-muscle invasive recurrence after trimodality therapy or after partial cystectomy—these recurrences can be treated similar to de novo non-muscle invasive bladder cancer (i.e. with intravesical therapy) or with radical cystectomy. Intravesical therapy may be favored for low risk recurrences, where radical cystectomy may be favored for high risk recurrences.

Statistics Regarding Recurrence
1. Factors that increase the risk of recurrence
    a. Larger tumor size (especially > 3 cm)
    b. Higher tumor stage
    c. Higher tumor grade or presence of CIS
    d. Multiple tumors
    e. Prior history of tumors

    f. Tumor aneuploidy

    g. Lymphovascular invasion

    h. Positive urine tumor marker after treatment

    i. Visible bladder tumor within 6 months after treatment

2. Bladder recurrence after TURBT

    a. CIS—80% will recur after TURBT, only 30% recur after BCG.

    b. Ta—50% will recur after TURBT alone, most within one year.

    c. T1—more than 70% recur after TURBT alone.

3. After Cystectomy

    a. The rate of pelvic recurrence after cystectomy is $\leq$ 12%. Patients with pelvic recurrence after cystectomy have a very poor prognosis.

    b. Recurrence usually occurs within 2 years after cystectomy.

    c. After cystectomy without urethrectomy, urethral recurrence occurs in up to 10% of cases and usually occurs within 2 years.

4. Upper tract recurrence

    a. *Patients with CIS in the bladder are more likely to have an upper tract recurrence than those without CIS.*

    b. Up to 4% of those with papillary bladder UC develop upper tract UC later in life. Up to 20% with bladder CIS develop upper tract UC.

    c. see History of Urothelial Carcinoma of the Bladder, page 93.

REFERENCES

General

AUA/SUO—Chang SS, et al: Diagnosis and treatment of non-muscle invasive bladder cancer: AUA/SUO guideline. AUA Education and Research, Inc., 2020. (www.auanet.org/guidelines).

AUA/ASCO/ASTRO/SUO—Chang SS, et al: Treatment of non-metastatic muscle invasive bladder cancer: AUA/ACSO/ASTRO/SUO guideline. AUA Education and Research, Inc., 2020. (www.auanet.org/guidelines).

Bladder Cancer: 2nd International Consultation on Bladder Cancer. Ed. M Soloway & S Khoury. Plymouth, United Kingdom: Health Publication Ltd., 2012.

EAU—Babjuk M, et al: Non-muscle invasive bladder cancer. European Association of Urology, 2021. (www.uroweb.org).

EAU—Witjes JA, et al: Muscle invasive and metastatic bladder cancer. European Association of Urology, 2021. (www.uroweb.org).

NCCN—National Comprehensive Cancer Network clinical practice guidelines in oncology: Bladder cancer. V.3.2021, 2021. (www.nccn.org).

Variant Histology & Non-urothelial Tumors

Beilan JA, et al: Pheochromocytoma of the urinary bladder: a systematic review of the contemporary literature. BMC Urology, 13: 22, 2013.

Black PC, et al: The impact of variant histology on the outcome of bladder cancer treated with curative intent. Urol Oncol, 27: 3, 2009.

Herr, HW, et al: Urachal carcinoma: contemporary surgical outcomes. J Urol, 178: 74, 2007.

Royce TJ, et al: Clinical characteristics and outcomes of non-urothelial cell carcinoma of the bladder: results from the National Cancer Data Base. Urol Oncol, 36(2): 78.e1, 2018.

Weiss RE, Fair WR: Urachal anomalies and urachal carcinoma. AUA Update Series, Vol. 17, Lesson 38, 1998.

Enhanced Visualization with Cystoscopy & TURBT (Blue Light & NBI)

Bach T, et al: Technical solutions to improve the management of non-muscle invasive transitional cell carcinoma: summary of a European Association of Urology Section for Uro-technology (ESUT) and Section for Uro-Oncology (ESOU) expert meeting and current and future perspectives. BJU Int, 115(1): 14, 2015.

Daneshmand S, et al: Efficacy and safety of blue light flexible cystoscopy with hexaminolevulinate in the surveillance of bladder cancer: a phase III, comparative, multicenter study. J Urol, 199(5): 1158, 2018.

Dragoescu PO, et al: Improved diagnosis and long term recurrence rate reduction for non-muscle invasive bladder cancer patients undergoing fluorescent hexylaminolevulinate photodynamic diagnosis. Rom J Morph Embryol, 58(4): 1279, 2017.

Kang W, et al: Narrow band imaging assisted transurethral resection reduces the recurrence risk of non-muscle invasive bladder cancer: a systematic review and met-analysis. Oncotarget, 8(14): 23880, 2017.

Kim SB, et al: Detection and recurrence rate of transurethral resection of bladder tumors by narrow band imaging: prospective, randomized comparison with white light cystoscopy. Investig Clin Urol, 59: 98, 2018.

Rolevich AI, et al: Results of a prospective randomized study assessing the efficacy of fluorescent cystoscopy assisted transurethral resection and single instillation of doxorubicin in patients with non-muscle invasive bladder cancer. World J Urol, 35(5): 745, 2017.

TURBT

Bolat D, et al: Comparing the short term outcomes and complications of monopolar and bipolar transurethral resection of bladder tumors in patients with coronary artery disease: a prospective randomized controlled study. Int Braz J Urol, 44: 717, 2018.

Cumberbatch MGK, et al: Repeat transurethral resection in non-muscle invasive bladder cancer: a systematic review. Eur Urol, 73(6): 925, 2018.

Divrik RF, et al: The effect of repeat transurethral resection on recurrence and progression rates in patients with T1 tumors of the bladder who received intravesical mitomycin: a prospective randomized clinical trial. J Urol, 175: 1641, 2006.

Herr HW: Role of repeat resection in non-muscle invasive bladder cancer. J Natl Compr Canc Netw, 13(8): 1041, 2015.

Mano R, et al: Resection of ureteral orifice during transurethral resection of bladder tumor. J Urol, 188(6, part 1): 2129, 2012.

Naselli A, et al: Role of restaging transurethral resection for T1 non-muscle invasive bladder cancer: a systematic review and meta-analysis. Eur Urol Focus, 4(4): 558, 2018.

Sharma G, et al: Safety and efficacy of bipolar versus monopolar transurethral resection of bladder tumor: a systematic review and meta-analysis. World J Urol, 39(2): 377, 2021.

Vianello A, et al: Repeated white light transurethral resection of the bladder in nonmuscle invasive urothelial bladder cancer: a systematic review and meta-analysis. J Endourol, 25(11): 1703, 2011.

TURP with TURBT

Dellabella M, et al: Oncological safety and quality of life in men undergoing simultaneous transurethral resection of bladder tumor and prostate: results from a randomized controlled trial. World J Urol, 36(10): 1629, 2018.

Ham WS, et al: Long term outcome of simultaneous transurethral resection of bladder tumor and prostate in patients with non-muscle invasive bladder tumor and bladder outlet obstruction. J Urol, 181(4): 1594, 2009.

Jaidaine M, et al: Tumor recurrence in prostatic urethra following simultaneous resection of bladder tumor and prostate. Urology, 75(6): 1392, 2010.

Laor E, et al: The influence of simultaneous resection of bladder tumors and prostate on the occurrence of prostatic urethral tumors. J Urol, 126:171,1981.

Ugurlu O, et al: Effects of simultaneous transurethral resection of prostate and solitary bladder tumors smaller than 3 cm on oncologic results. Urology, 70: 55, 2007.

Vicente J, et al: Tumor recurrence in prostatic urethra following simultaneous resection of bladder tumor and prostate. Eur Urol, 15: 40, 1988.

Urethra and Prostatic Urethra Involvement

Freeman JA, Esrig D, Stein JP, et al: Management of the patient with bladder cancer: urethral recurrence. Urol Clin North Am, 21: 645, 1994.

Hardeman SW, Soloway MS: Urethral recurrence following radical cystectomy. J Urol, 144: 666, 1990.

Lebret T, Herve JM, Barre P, et al: Urethral recurrence of transitional cell carcinoma of the bladder. Eur Urol, 33: 170, 1998.

Mungan MU, et al: Risk factors for mucosal prostatic urethral involvement in superficial transitional cell carcinoma of the bladder. Eur Urol, 48(5): 760, 2005.

Sakamoto N, et al: An adequate sampling of the prostate to identify prostatic involvement by urothelial carcinoma in bladder cancer patients. J Urol, 149: 318, 1993.

Stenzl A, Draxl H, Posch B, et al: The risk of urethral tumors in female bladder cancer: can the urethra be used for orthotopic reconstruction of the lower urinary tract? J Urol, 153: 950, 1995.

Intravesical Therapy

AUA/SUNA—Baumgartner R, et al: Intravesical administration of therapeutic medication for the treatment of bladder cancer. AUA Education and Research, Inc., 2020. (www.auanet.org).

Au JL, et al: Methods to improve efficacy of intravesical mitomycin C: results of a randomized phase III trial. J Natl Cancer Inst, 93: 597, 2001.

Bohle A, et al: Intravesical bacillus Calmette-Guerin versus mitomycin C for superficial bladder cancer: a formal meta-analysis of comparative studies on recurrence and toxicity. J Urol, 169: 90, 2003.

Bosschieter J, et al: Value of an immediate intravesical instillation of mitomycin C in patients with non-muscle invasive bladder cancer: a prospective multicenter randomized study in 2243 patients. Eur Urol, 73(2): 226, 2018.

Chen S, et al: Maintenance versus non-maintenance intravesical bacillus Calmette Guerin instillation for non-muscle invasive bladder cancer: a systematic review and meta-analysis of randomized clinical trials. Int J Surg, 52: 248, 2018.

Chou R, et al: Intravesical therapy for the treatment of nonmuscle invasive bladder cancer: systematic review & meta-analysis. J Urol, 197: 1189, 2017.

Han RF, et al: Can intravesical bacillus Calmette-Guerin reduce the risk of recurrence in patients with superficial bladder cancer? A meta-analysis of randomized trials. Urology, 67: 1216, 2006.

Lamm DL, et al: Maintenance bacillus Calmette-Guerin immunotherapy for recurrent Ta, T1 and carcinoma in situ transitional cell carcinoma of the bladder: a randomized SWOG study. J Urol, 163: 1124, 2000.

Oddens J, et al: Final results of an EORTC-GU cancers group randomized study of maintenance Bacillus Calmette Guerin in intermediate and high risk Ta, T1 papillary carcinoma of the urinary bladder. One third dose versus full dose and 1 year versus 3 years of maintenance. Eur Urol, 63(3): 462, 2013.

O'Donnell MA, et al: Interim results from a national multicenter phase II trial of combination with bacillus Calmette Guerin plus interferon alfa-2B for superficial bladder cancer. J Urol, 172: 888, 2004.

O'Donnell MA, et al: Salvage intravesical therapy with interferon-α2B plus low dose bacillus Calmette Guerin is effective in patients with superficial bladder cancer in whom bacillus Calmette Guerin alone previously failed. J Urol, 166: 1300, 2001.

Shelley MD, et al: A systematic review of intravesical bacillus Calmette-Guerin plus transurethral resection versus transurethral resection alone in Ta and T1 bladder cancer. BJU Int, 88: 209, 2001.

Shelley MD, et al: Intravesical bacillus Calmette-Guerin is superior to mitomycin C in reducing tumor recurrence in high risk superficial bladder cancer: a meta-analysis of randomized trials. BJU Int, 93: 485, 2004.

Shelley MD, et al: Intravesical gemcitabine therapy for non muscle invasive bladder cancer (NIMBC): a systematic review. BJU Int, 109: 496, 2012.

Skinner EC, et al: SWOG S0353: Phase II trial of intravesical gemcitabine in patients with non-muscle invasive bladder cancer and recurrence after 2 prior courses of intravesical bacillus Calmette Guerin. J Urol, 190(4): 1200, 2013.

Steinberg G, et al: Efficacy and safety of valrubicin for the treatment of bacillus Calmette Guerin refractory carcinoma in situ of the bladder. J Urol, 163: 761, 2000.

Sylvester RJ, et al: Long term efficacy results of EORTC genito-urinary group randomized phase 3 study 30911 comparing intravesical instillation of epirubicin, bacillus Calmette Guerin, and bacillus Calmette Guerin plus isoniazid in patients with intermediate and high risk stage Ta T1 urothelial carcinoma of the bladder. Eur Urol, 57(5): 766. 2010.

Sylvester RJ, et al: A single immediate postoperative instillation of chemotherapy decreases the risk of recurrence in patients with stage Ta T1 bladder cancer: a meta-analysis of published results of randomized clinical trials. J Urol, 171: 2186, 2004.

Sylvester RJ, et al: Intravesical bacillus Calmette-Guerin reduces the risk of progression in patients with superficial bladder cancer: a meta-analysis of the published results of randomized clinical trials. J Urol, 168: 1964, 2002.

Sylvester RJ, et al: Bacillus Calmette-Guerin versus chemotherapy for the intravesical treatment of patients with carcinoma in situ of the bladder: a meta-analysis of the published results of randomized clinical trials. J Urol, 174: 86, 2005.

Sylvester RJ, et al: The schedule and duration of intravesical chemotherapy in patients with non-muscle invasive bladder cancer: a systematic review of the published results of randomized clinical trials. Eur Urol, 53: 709, 2008.

Tabayoyong WB, et al: Systematic review on the utilization of maintenance intravesical chemotherapy in the management of non-muscle invasive bladder cancer. Eur Urol Focus, 4(4): 512, 2018.

Ye Z, et al: The efficacy and safety of intravesical gemcitabine vs bacillus Calmette Guerin for adjuvant treatment of non-muscle invasive bladder cancer: a meta-analysis. Onco Targets Ther, 11: 4641, 2018.

Prevention of BCG Side Effects

Colombel M, et al: The effect of ofloxacin on bacillus Calmette Guerin induced toxicity in patients with superficial bladder cancer: results of a randomized prospective double blind placebo controlled multicenter study. J Urol, 176: 935, 2006.

Damiano R, et al: Short term administration of prulifloxacin in patients with non-muscle invasive bladder cancer: an effective option for the prevention of bacillus Calmette Guerin induced toxicity. BJU Int, 104: 633, 2009.

Vegt P, et al: Does isoniazid reduce side effects of intravesical bacillus calmette-guerin therapy in superficial bladder cancer? J Urol, 157: 1246, 1997.

Radical Cystectomy

Abbas F, et al: Incidental prostatic adenocarcinoma in patients undergoing radical cystoprostatectomy for bladder cancer. Eur Urol, 30: 322, 1996.

Gschwend JE, et al: Radical cystectomy for invasive bladder cancer: contemporary results and remaining controversies. Eur Urol, 38: 121, 2000.

Herr HW, et al: Does early cystectomy improve the survival of patients with high risk superficial bladder tumors? J Urol, 166: 1296, 2001.

Klotz L: Prostate capsule sparing radical cystectomy: oncologic safety and clinical outcome. Ther Adv Urol, 1(1): 43, 2009.

Pederzoli F, et al: Surgical factors associated with male and female sexual dysfunction after radical cystectomy: what do we know and how can we improve outcomes? Sex Med Rev, 6: 469, 2018.

Sanchez-Ortiz RF, Huang WC, et al: An interval longer than 12 weeks between the diagnosis of muscle invasion and cystectomy is associated with worse outcome in bladder carcinoma. J Urol, 169: 110, 2003.

Schilling D, et al: Cystectomy in women. BJU Int, 102: 1289, 2008.

Smith ZL, Soloway MS: Prostate capsule sparing radical cystectomy - a safe procedure for few. Cent European J Urol, 69: 32, 2016.

Stein JP, et al: Radical cystectomy in the treatment of invasive bladder cancer: Long-term results in 1,054 patients. J Clin Oncol, 19(3): 666, 2001.

Partial Cystectomy

Capitanio U, et al: Partial cystectomy does not undermine cancer control in appropriately selected patients with urothelial carcinoma of the bladder. Urology, 74(4): 858, 2009.

Dandekar NP, et al: Partial cystectomy for invasive bladder cancer. J Surg Oncol, 60(1): 24, 1995.

Danzig MR, et al: Partial cystectomy for primary bladder tumors in contemporary patients with diverse tumor locations. Urology Practice, 3(1): 55, 2016.

Ebbing J, et al: Oncological outcomes, quality of life outcomes and complications of partial cystectomy for selected cases of muscle invasive bladder cancer. Sci Rep, 8(1): 8360, 2018.

Holzbeierlein JM, et al: Partial cystectomy: a contemporary review of the Memorial Sloan Kettering Cancer Center experience and recommendations for patient selection. J Urol, 172: 878, 2004.

Kassouf W, et al: Partial cystectomy for muscle invasive urothelial carcinoma of the bladder. J Urol, 175: 2058, 2006.

Knoedler JJ, et al: Does partial cystectomy compromise oncologic outcomes for patients with bladder cancer compared to radical cystectomy? A matched case control analysis. J Urol, 188(4): 1115, 2012.

Shao IH, et al: Outcomes and prognostic factors of simple partial cystectomy for localized bladder urothelial cell carcinoma. Kaohsiung J Med Sci, 32(4): 191, 2016.

Smaldone MC, et al: Long term results of selective partial cystectomy for invasive urothelial carcinoma. Urology, 72(3): 613, 2008.

Pelvic Lymph Node Dissection

Gschwend JE, et al: Extended versus limited lymph node dissection in bladder cancer patients undergoing radical cystectomy: survival results from a prospective randomized trial. Eur Urol, 75(4): 604, 2019.

Herr HW, et al: Surgical factors influence bladder cancer outcomes: a cooperative group report. J Clin Oncol, 22(14): 2781, 2004.

Konety BR, et al: Extent of pelvic lymphadenectomy and its impact on outcome in patients diagnosed with bladder cancer: analysis of data from the Surveillance Epidemiology and End Results program data base. J Urol, 169(3): 946, 2003.

Leissner J, et al: Lymphadenectomy in patients with transitional cell carcinoma of the urinary bladder; significance for staging and prognosis. BJU Int, 85(7): 817, 2000.

Wright JL, et al: The association between extent of lymphadenectomy and survival among patients with lymph node metastases undergoing radical cystectomy. Cancer, 112(11): 2401, 2008.

Neoadjuvant & Adjuvant Therapy with Cystectomy

Advanced Bladder Cancer (ABC) Meta-analysis Collaboration: Neoadjuvant chemotherapy in invasive bladder cancer: update of a systematic review and meta-analysis of individual patient data. Eur Urol, 48(2): 202, 2005.

Advanced Bladder Cancer (ABC) Meta-analysis Collaboration: Adjuvant chemotherapy for invasive bladder cancer: Cochrane Database Syst Rev, Issue 2: CD006018, 2006.

Bayoumi Y, et al: Survival benefit of adjuvant radiotherapy in stage III and IV bladder cancer: results of 170 patients. Cancer Manag Res, 6: 459, 2014.

Fischer-Valuck BW, et al: Effectiveness of postoperative radiotherapy after radical cystectomy for locally advance bladder cancer. Cancer Med, 8(8): 3698, 2019.

International Collaboration of Trialists: International phase III trial assessing neoadjuvant cisplatin, methotrexate, and vinblastine chemotherapy for muscle invasive bladder cancer. J Clin Oncol 29(16): 2171, 2011.

Iwata T, et al: The role of adjuvant radiotherapy after surgery for upper and lower urinary tract urothelial carcinoma: a systematic review. Urol Oncol, 37(10): 659, 2019.

Leow JJ, et al: Adjuvant chemotherapy for invasive bladder cancer: a 2013 updated systematic review and meta-analysis of randomized trials. Eur Urol, 66(1): 42, 2014.

Sherif A, et al: Neoadjuvant cisplatinum based chemotherapy in patients with invasive bladder cancer. Eur Urol, 45: 297, 2004.

Winquist E, et al: Neoadjuvant chemotherapy for transitional cell carcinoma of the bladder: a systematic review and meta-analysis. J Urol, 171(2): 561, 2004.

Zaghloul MS, et al: Randomized phase III trial of adjuvant sequential chemotherapy plus radiotherapy versus adjuvant radiotherapy alone for locally advanced bladder cancer after radical cystectomy: urothelial carcinoma subgroup analysis. J Clin Oncol, 37 (7, suppl): abstract 351, 2019 (https://doi.org/10.1200/JCO.2019.37.7_suppl.351)

Bladder Sparing With TURBT & Chemoradiation (Trimodality Therapy)

Arcangeli G, et al: Radical cystectomy versus organ sparing trimodality treatment in muscle invasive bladder cancer: a systematic review of clinical trials. Crit Rev Oncol Hematol, 95(3): 387, 2015.

Fahmy O, et al: A systematic review and meta-analysis on the oncological long term outcomes after trimodality therapy and radical cystectomy with or without neoadjuvant chemotherapy for muscle invasive bladder cancer. Urol Oncol, 36(2): 43, 2018.

Giacalone NJ, et al: Long term outcomes after bladder preserving trimodality therapy for patients with muscle invasive bladder cancer: an updated analysis of the Massachusetts General Hospital. Eur Urol, 71(6): 952, 2017.

Mak RH, et al: Long term outcomes in patients with muscle invasive bladder cancer after selective bladder preserving combined modality therapy: a pooled analysis of Radiation Therapy Oncology Group protocols 8802, 8903, 9506, 9706, 9906, 0233. J Clin Oncol, 32(34): 3801, 2014.

Ploussard G, et al: Critical analysis of bladder sparing with trimodal therapy in muscle invasive bladder cancer: a systematic review. Eur Urol, 66(1): 120, 2014.

Ray-Zack MD, et al: Comparing radical cystectomy with trimodal therapy for patients diagnosed with bladder cancer: critical assessment of statistical methodology and interpretation of observational data. J Clin Oncol, 37 (7, supplement): abstract 373, 2019.
(https://doi.org/10.1200/JCO.2019.37.7_suppl.373).

Russell CM, et al: The role of transurethral resection in trimodal therapy for muscle invasive bladder cancer. Bladder Cancer, 2(4): 381, 2016.

Sanchez A, et al: Incidence, clinicopathological risk factors, management and outcomes of nonmuscle invasive recurrence after complete response to trimodality therapy for muscle invasive bladder cancer. J Urol, 199(2): 407, 2018.

Shipley WU, et al: Selective bladder preservation by combined modality protocol treatment: long term outcomes of 190 patients with invasive bladder cancer. Urology, 60: 62, 2002.

Smith ZL, et al: Bladder preservation in the treatment of muscle invasive bladder cancer (MIBC): a review of the literature and a practical approach to therapy. BJU Int, 112: 12, 2013.

Vashistha V, et al: Radical cystectomy compared to combined modality treatment for muscle invasive bladder cancer: a systematic review and meta-analysis. Int J Radiat Oncol Biol Phys, 97(5): 1002, 2017.

Systemic Chemotherapy for Metastatic Disease

Sternberg CN, et al: Seven year update of an EORTC phase III trial of high dose intensity M-VAC chemotherapy and G-CSF versus classic M-VAC in advance urothelial tract tumors. Eur J Cancer, 42(1): 50, 2006 [update of J Clin Oncol, 19(10): 2638, 2001.

von der Maase H, et al: Long term survival results of a randomized trial comparing gemcitabine plus cisplatin with methotrexate, vinblastine, doxorubicin, plus cisplatin in patients with bladder cancer. J Clin Oncol, 23(21): 4602, 2005 [update of J Clin Oncol, 18(17): 3068, 2000].

UPPER URINARY TRACT UROTHELIAL CANCER

General Information

1. The ureter is conceptually divided into two regions.
   a. Pelvic ureter—the portion that is below the common iliac artery. This portion comprises the lower third of the ureter, and is often called "the lower ureter."
   b. Abdominal ureter—the portion of that is above the common iliac artery. This portion comprises the upper two-thirds of the ureter, and includes the mid ureter and upper ureter.
2. The upper urinary tract (also called the collecting system) is composed of the calyces, infundibula, renal pelvis, and ureters. Urothelium covers the entire inner surface of the upper urinary tract; therefore, upper tract urothelial cancer (UTUC) can arise anywhere in the collecting system.
3. The low incidence of UTUC has made it difficult to conduct randomized clinical trials. The diagnosis and management of UTUC is based mainly on expert opinion and retrospective series rather than on quality evidence.
4. *Approximately 90% of upper urinary tract cancers are urothelial cancer.* Pure squamous cell carcinoma of the upper urinary tract is often associated with chronic inflammation (mainly from infection or urolithiasis). UTUC of variant histology is usually high grade, more aggressive, and has a worse prognosis than pure urothelial carcinoma (see page 65).
5. Approximately 22-47% of patients with a UTUC subsequently develop urothelial carcinoma (UC) of the bladder.
6. After treatment of UTUC, the risk of recurrence in the contralateral upper urinary tract is 2-6% (i.e. bilateral UTUC develops in 2-6% of cases).

Risk Factors for UTUC

1. Tobacco smoking
2. Cyclophosphamide or ifosfamide chemotherapy (see page 49 for details).
3. Chronic phenacetin use—this analgesic has a chemical structure that is similar to aniline dye. Phenacetin has been taken off the market.
4. Chronic inflammation—chronic inflammation from infection or stones increases the risk upper tract cancer, particularly squamous cell carcinoma
5. Aristolochic acid—a toxin produced by the Aristolochia plant. Oral consumption increases the risk of renal insufficiency and UTUC. Patients with a specific genetic mutation are far more susceptible to the toxic effects of aristolochic acid. Aristolochia is used as a medicinal Chinese herb and has been found as a contaminant of wheat in the Balkan areas.
6. Balkan nephropathy (Danubian endemic nephropathy)—an interstitial nephritis that causes renal insufficiency in people endemic to the Balkan peninsula in southeastern Europe, especially along the Danube river and its tributaries (Croatia, Bosnia and Herzegovina, Serbia, Romania, Bulgaria). Balkan nephropathy is thought to arise from consumption of wheat that is contaminated with aristolochia. Patients with Balkan nephropathy have a 100-200 fold greater risk of UTUC than the general population and are more likely to develop bilateral UTUC.
7. Chemical exposure—chemicals that cause UTUC are similar to those that cause urothelial carcinoma of the bladder. See page 49.

8. Lynch syndrome (hereditary nonpolyposis colorectal cancer)—an autosomal dominant syndrome that increases the risk of developing multiple malignancies, including cancer of the prostate, upper urinary tract, colon, rectum, small bowel, stomach, biliary tract, pancreas, endometrium, ovary, and brain.
9. History of urothelial carcinoma of the bladder—15-50% of patients with UTUC have a history of bladder cancer. In patients with bladder cancer, each of the following characteristics increases the risk of UTUC.
   a. A history of CIS or high grade urothelial carcinoma of the bladder—in patients treated with bladder sparing therapy, UTUC occurs in up to 20% of patients with bladder CIS.
   b. A history of bladder cancer at the ureter orifice, trigone, or bladder neck.
   c. A history of multifocal bladder cancer.
   d. Vesicoureteral reflux (VUR) and a history of bladder cancer—these patients have a 15 to 22 fold higher risk of UTUC. Surveillance of the upper tracts should be performed more frequently in these patients.
   e. Placement of a ureteral stent immediately after transurethral resection of a bladder tumor increases the risk of UTUC by 3 fold.
   f. Urothelial cancer at the ureteral margin or in the distal ureter during cystectomy—after radical cystectomy, UTUC occurs in 2-6% of patients with cancer in the distal ureter or at the ureter margin.

Metastasis

1. Most common metastatic sites: lungs, liver, bones, regional lymph nodes.
2. Invasive renal pelvis UTUC may be less likely to metastasize than invasive ureteral UTUC because the renal parenchyma may serve as a barrier that prevents the spread of tumor.
3. Lymphatic metastases from tumors of the renal pelvis and upper ureter initially spread to the retroperitoneal lymph nodes, whereas distal ureteral tumors initially spread to the pelvic lymph nodes.

Presentation

1. The most common age of presentation is 50-70 years.
2. *The most common presenting symptom of UTUC is hematuria* (occurs in 75% of cases). Flank pain is present in up to 30% of patients and usually arises from ureteral obstruction that is caused by the tumor.
3. On pyelogram, UTUC may appear as a filling defect (50-70% of cases) and/or it may generate hydronephrosis or ureter obstruction (10-30% of cases). *When an UTUC causes hydronephrosis, the tumor is more likely to be invasive.*
4. At initial presentation, UTUC is more likely to be stage T2 or higher than bladder cancer (56% versus 25%).
5. *The most common location of UTUC is the renal pelvis.* When UTUC is in the ureter, it usually occurs in the distal ureter.
6. Most tumors are unifocal (solitary) at presentation.
7. Up to 17% of patients with UTUC present with concomitant bladder urothelial cancer. When a patient has tumors in the upper tract and in the bladder, the tumors are usually clonally related (i.e. genetically similar).
8. 5% of patients with UTUC have Lynch syndrome.

Work Up

1. Medical history—information obtained should include a personal history of cancer, smoking, use of oral herb therapies, recurrent upper tract urinary infections, urolithiasis, exposure to cyclophosphamide or ifosfamide, and residence in the Balkan peninsula of southeastern Europe. Family history should include inquiry for cancers associated with Lynch syndrome.

2. The following tests should be performed (except when contraindicated).
   a. Cystoscopy—cystoscopy is performed because of the high incidence of associated bladder tumors.
   b. Voided urine tumor marker (cytology, FISH, etc.)—although voided urine tumor markers perform poorly when used to detect UTUC, they are usually included in the evaluation.
   c. Upper urinary tract imaging—*CT urogram (CTU) is preferred because it is more specific and more sensitive than intravenous urogram (IVU) for detecting UTUC.* MR urogram is another option. *Hydronephrosis caused by the tumor suggests the presence of an advanced tumor stage.* If IVU, pyelogram, or ureteroscopy are used for upper tract imaging, then consider also performing abdominal pelvic cross sectional imaging (CT or MRI). For more details on upper tract imaging, see page 51.
   d. BUN, creatinine, liver function tests, and complete blood count.
3. Tests performed in select circumstances
   a. Retrograde pyelogram (RPG)—RPG may be necessary when poor renal function limits the utility of CT urogram, IVU, or MR urogram.
   b. Ureteroscopy—especially useful in patients who cannot undergo pyelogram because of iodine allergy, when other imaging is inconclusive, or when a benign diagnosis is suspected. Ureteroscopy can be performed with narrow band imaging to help detect cancer (see page 50).
      i. Some physicians confirm the presence of urothelial carcinoma using ureteroscopy before proceeding to surgical, whereas other urologists feel that diagnostic ureteroscopy is unnecessary when other testing is highly suggestive of UTUC.
      ii. For diagnostic ureteroscopy, visualize the entire upper urinary tract and obtain an upper urinary tract wash cytology using normal saline. Then, perform a biopsy using a brush, cold cup forceps, or basket.
      iii. Ureteroscopy and the risk of systemic spread of cancer— theoretically, ureteroscopy may increase the risk of spreading malignancy through pyelovenous or pyelolymphatic backflow. However, *several large retrospective series and meta-analyses in patients with UTUC reveal that ureteroscopy before nephroureterectomy does not increase the risk of developing metastasis and does not alter cancer specific survival nor overall survival.*
      iv. Ureteroscopy and the risk of recurrence in the bladder—although the data are conflicting, *most studies show an increased risk of developing bladder cancer after ureteroscopy for UTUC* (even in patients with no history of bladder cancer). Limited evidence suggests that using an immediate postoperative dose of intravesical chemotherapy can reduce the risk of intravesical recurrence after ureteroscopy.
   c. Upper urinary tract wash cytology (barbotage cytology)—the accuracy of wash cytology for detecting UTUC has not been well defined. False negatives and false positives can occur. At least one study showed that barbotage (wash) cytology can detect most UTUCs. *Upper tract wash cytology should be obtained before pyelography* because contrast exposure can reduce the quality of the cytology specimen.
   d. Renal scan—in select cases, renal scan may help predict whether the patient will require dialysis after nephroureterectomy or whether the ipsilateral kidney functions enough to make renal sparing worth while.

e. Metastatic evaluation—metastatic evaluation is recommended for cases where high grade or invasive UTUC is present or suspected.
   i. If IVU was obtained rather than CTU or MR urogram, then perform abdominal and pelvic cross section imaging (CT or MRI).
   ii. If CTU and MR urogram are contraindicated, then use FDG-PET/CT.
   iii. Chest imaging—chest CT is usually preferred over chest x-ray.
   iv. Bone imaging—bone imaging is recommended for patients with bone pain, elevated alkaline phosphatase, or at high risk for bone metastasis (e.g. multiple soft tissue metastasis). Bone scan is usually the initial test. MRI or FDG-PET/CT may also be used.
   v. Brain imaging—brain MRI (with and without gadolinium) is recommended for patients with symptoms suggestive of a central nervous system metastasis or in patients at higher risk of brain metastasis (e.g. small cell carcinoma or multiple metastasis outside the central nervous system). CT scan with intravenous contrast may be used if MRI with gadolinium is contraindicated.
f. Germline genetic testing for Lynch syndrome—5% of patients with UTUC have Lynch syndrome. Genetic testing is an option for all patients with UTUC, but is highly recommended in patients with any of the following characteristics.
   i. UTUC diagnosed at age < 60 (especially when there is no previous history of bladder cancer).
   ii. Personal history of other cancers associated with Lynch syndrome (e.g. prostate, colon, rectum, small bowel, stomach, biliary tract, pancreas, endometrium, ovary, or brain).
   iii. Family history of UTUC (especially in a first degree relative)
   iv. Family history of other cancers associated with lynch syndrome (especially a first or second degree relative diagnosed with cancer before age 50, or multiple first or second degree relatives diagnosed with cancer at any age).
   v. Known family history of Lynch syndrome.

Stage, Grade, and Prognosis

Predictors of Prognosis
The following factors increase the recurrence rate and reduce the cancer specific survival.
   a. Tumor in the ureter (rather than tumor in the renal pelvis or calyces)
   b. Multifocal tumor
   c. Higher pathological stage
   d. Higher tumor grade
   e. Lymphovascular invasion
   f. Extensive tumor necrosis (> 10%)
   g. Lymph node metastasis or distant metastasis
   h. Extranodal extension
   i. Variant histology
   j. Positive surgical margins during surgical excision

Grade
High grade lesions are usually high stage. Higher grade lesions progress more often, recur more often, and have a worse prognosis. Low grade is often abbreviated as "LG", and high grade is often abbreviated as "HG". For example, T1HG is a stage T1 high grade tumor.

Grade	Histologic Description
Low Grade	Well differentiated
High Grade	Poorly differentiated or undifferentiated

Stage (AJCC 2017)
This classification refers to clinical and pathological staging. Higher stage lesions progress more often, recur more often, and have a worse prognosis.

Primary Tumor (T)

Tx	Primary tumor cannot be assessed
T0	No evidence of primary tumor
Ta	Papillary noninvasive carcinoma
Tis	Carcinoma in situ
T1	Tumor invades subepithelial connective tissue
T2	Tumor invades muscularis
T3	For renal pelvis only: tumor invades beyond muscularis into peripelvic fat or into the renal parenchyma.
	For ureter only: tumor invades beyond muscularis into periureteric fat.
T4	Tumor invades adjacent organs, or through the kidney into the perinephric fat.

Regional Lymph Nodes (N)
Laterality does not affect the N classification.

Nx	Regional lymph nodes cannot be assessed
N0	No regional lymph node metastasis
N1	Metastasis ≤ 2 cm in greatest dimension, in a single lymph node.
N2	Metastasis > 2 cm in a single lymph node; or multiple lymph nodes

Distant Metastasis (M)

M0	No distant metastasis
M1	Distant metastasis

Used with the permission of the American College of Surgeons. Amin, M.B., Edge, S.B., Greene, F.L., et al. (Eds.) AJCC Cancer Staging Manual, 8th Ed. Springer New York, 2017.

Risk Stratification
1. Low risk for recurrence and progression—low risk requires all of the following criteria.
    a. Low grade tumor on biopsy
    b. Cytology (voided or upper tract wash) shows no high grade cells
    c. Papillary tumor (not sessile)
    d. Tumor size < 1.5 cm
    e. Solitary tumor (not multifocal)
    f. Imaging does not suggest an invasive tumor.
    g. Pure urothelial carcinoma (no variant histology)—variant histology has a worse prognosis than pure urothelial carcinoma (see page 65); therefore, more aggressive treatment may be favored.
    h. The cancer does not cause hydronephrosis—*Hydronephrosis caused by the tumor suggests the presence of an advanced tumor stage.*
    i. No history of cystectomy for high grade urothelial cancer of the bladder
2. High risk for recurrence and progression—any tumor that does not qualify as low risk.

Treatment

General Concepts

1. *The most important prognostic factor is tumor stage.* Tumors that are high grade, large, broad base, sessile, or variant histology are more likely to be high stage. *Tumor stage is difficult to determine from imaging and from endoscopic resection, whereas tumor grade can easily be determined by cytology or biopsy. Therefore, treatment decisions are often based on tumor grade rather than tumor stage.*

2. When imaging or cytology suggest the presence of UTUC, performing ureteroscopy to confirm the diagnosis before treatment is optional. Endoscopy should be considered when a benign diagnosis is suspected (to confirm that there is no cancer).

3. The standard treatment of UTUC is en bloc nephroureterectomy with removal of the entire ureter (including the intramural ureter) with a cuff of bladder. For high grade or high stage UTUC, radical nephroureterectomy (RNU) achieves better cancer control than endoscopic management. *For low grade UTUC, retrospective data shows that disease specific survival is similar in patients who undergo antegrade endoscopic treatment, retrograde endoscopic treatment, or nephroureterectomy.*

4. For patients with a positive upper tract urine tumor marker but with an otherwise normal evaluation (imaging, endoscopy, and biopsies are all normal), management options include close surveillance, upper tract intracavitary therapy, or nephroureterectomy.

   a. Close surveillance is probably the most commonly used option (with repeat ureteroscopy, upper tract urine wash cytology, and biopsy).

   b. These patients may have CIS of the upper urinary tract that is not prominent enough to be seen during ureteroscopy. Using narrow band imaging during ureteroscopy may help find CIS that does not show up when using white light.

Renal Sparing Therapies (Nephron Preserving Therapies)

1. These therapies preserve all or part of the ipsilateral kidney and its collecting system. *Renal sparing therapy is the preferred approach for patients with low risk cancer.*

2. Renal sparing therapy is usually restricted to low grade, low stage tumors, except in the following circumstances

   a. Distal ureter tumor of any stage and grade—these tumors can be treated with distal ureterectomy and ureteral reimplant.

   b. An imperative indication for renal sparing therapy is present—renal sparing is an option regardless of stage and grade when any of the following characteristics are present.
      i. Absent or poorly functioning contralateral kidney
      ii. Poor overall renal function
      iii. Bilateral UTUC
      iv. At risk for bilateral UTUC (e.g. Lynch syndrome, Balkan nephropathy, Chinese herb abuse, phenacetin abuse)
      vi. Patients who are not candidates for more aggressive treatment.

3. Renal sparing therapies include endoscopic management, intracavitary therapy, ureterectomy, and partial nephrectomy.

4. *Recurrences after renal sparing therapy almost always occur distal to the location of the original tumor.*

Endoscopic Management (Resection and/or Fulguration)
1. Endoscopic treatment can be accomplished antegrade (percutaneously) or retrograde (through the bladder). The antegrade approach is often restricted to tumors in the upper third of the collecting system. The retrograde approach is preferred in most cases because it avoids the risk of seeding tumor along a percutaneous tract.
2. Endoscopic management is usually restricted to patients with any of the following characteristics: low risk cancer, an imperative indication for renal preservation, or when the morbidity of surgical excision is unacceptable.
3. *For low grade UTUC, disease specific survival is similar in patients who undergo antegrade endoscopic treatment, retrograde endoscopic treatment, or nephroureterectomy. For high grade UTUC, disease specific survival is lower with endoscopic treatment than with nephroureterectomy.*
4. Tumors can be treated by loop resection (using a ureteral resectoscope), snaring (using a basket or other grasping device to ensnare the tumor and pluck it off at the stalk), or fulguration (using electrocautery or laser ablation). In each case, tumor tissue should be obtained for pathologic analysis.
   a. Snaring—snaring can be accomplished with a cold cup biopsy forceps (for small lesions) or with a stone basket (for larger papillary lesions that have a relatively narrow stalk). To extract the specimen, remove the ureteroscope from the patient. Avoid pulling the specimen through the working channel of the ureteroscope. The base of the tumor may be biopsied with cold cup forceps and then fulgurated with electrocautery or laser energy.
   b. Fulguration—if fulguration is performed, a biopsy should be obtained first so that the tumor type and grade can be determined. The holmium:YAG laser is particularly well suited for fulguration in the upper tract because its depth of penetration is less than 0.5 mm. The depth of penetration for the neodymium:YAG laser is 5-6 mm; thus, it is more likely to cause perforation. For UTUC fulguration, a commonly used setting for the holmium:YAG laser is 0.6-1.0 joules at 10 Hz.
   c. *Only treat the intraluminal tumor. Do not attempt to resect or ablate deep into the wall of the upper urinary tract because this increases the risk of perforation.* Perforation may allow tumor cells to spread outside the urinary system and may increase the risk of complications.
5. After endoscopic treatment, a ureteral stent is usually left in place for several weeks to facilitate healing.
6. Risks of endoscopic treatment include ureter perforation, ureteral stricture, gross hematuria, and infection.
   a. Ureteral stricture has been reported in 5-25% of cases and appears to be more likely when fulguration is done with electrocautery rather than with a laser. Ureter stricture may indicate UTUC recurrence; therefore, the ureter stricture should be biopsied. If it is benign, then balloon dilation or stricture incision may be attempted.
   b. Collecting system perforation is uncommon. When perforation occurs, the procedure should be terminated and a ureteral stent should be placed. The stent is left in place for several weeks. Another attempt at endoscopic management may be tried when the perforation has healed.
7. In patients with low grade tumors, recurrence in the ipsilateral upper urinary tract is approximately 30-50% at 5 years.
8. Approximately 20-30% of patients treated endoscopically will eventually require delayed nephroureterectomy.

Intracavitary Therapy: General Information

1. Intracavitary therapy is treatment that is administered within a body cavity. For the bladder, intracavitary therapy is called intravesical therapy. For the upper urinary tract, intracavitary therapy is instillation of medicine into the collecting system so that it will contact the upper tract urothelial surface.

2. The benefit of intracavitary therapy for UTUC has not been proven in large randomized trials.

3. Intracavitary therapy is used only to treat non-metastatic UTUC that is stage Ta, T1, or CIS. Indications for UTUC intracavitary therapy include

   a. To treat upper tract CIS—intracavitary therapy for UTUC appears to be more effective for CIS than for papillary UC.

   b. To treat residual pathologic stage Ta or T1 UTUC.

   c. As prophylaxis to prevent recurrence after complete endoscopic treatment of pathologic stage Ta or T1 UTUC.

4. BCG—this is the most studied and most commonly used agent for intracavitary treatment of UTUC. The concentration of BCG (typically 0.5-2.4 mg/cc) and the volume infused (typically 40-250 cc) are highly variable. Reported contact time ranges from 10 minutes to 4 hours; thus, it seems reasonable to attempt a contact time of at least 1-2 hours.

   a. Induction therapy—the usual induction course is one instillation per week for 6 weeks. When there is an inadequate response, another 6-week course may be administered. If there is recurrent or persist tumor after 6-12 instillations, then surgical extirpation is recommended.

   b. Maintenance therapy can be administered using schedules similar to those used for bladder cancer.

   c. Upper urinary tract intracavitary BCG can be administered in patients with a urinary diversion. In patients with a neobladder or continent cutaneous diversion, a catheter is temporarily placed to drain BCG from the diversion.

5. Intracavitary chemotherapy—the more commonly used agents include mitomycin C, gemcitabine, and epirubicin. For UTUC, intracavitary chemotherapy is not used for an immediate postoperative instillation. However, it is used for induction therapy (starting 3-4 weeks after tumor excision/fulguration) and for maintenance therapy. *The FDA approved mitomycin semi-solid gel for the treatment of low grade UTUC* (see page 101 for more information, including dose and administration).

   a. Induction and maintenance therapy can be given using a schedule similar to the schedule used for bladder cancer. For details on chemotherapy agents and their induction dose schedule, see page 66.

   b. Thiotepa should be avoided for treatment of UTUC because it frequently causes myelosuppression.

Intracavitary Therapy: Instillation of Non-gel Non-viscous Agents

1. The following protocol should not be used for gel formulations.

2. Intracavitary upper tract therapy is initiated only when all of the following criteria are met.

   a. At least 4-6 weeks have passed after open urinary surgery and 3-4 weeks have passed after endoscopic urinary surgery.

   b. Absence of extravasation from the urinary tract.

   c. Absence of urinary obstruction.

   d. Absence of urinary infection.

   e. Absence of gross hematuria.

3. Before each treatment
   a. A urinalysis should be performed before each treatment. Do not give intracavitary therapy when there is urinary infection or gross hematuria.
   b. When using a nephrostomy tube or ureteral catheter, consider performing a nephrostogram before each instillation to rule out obstruction and extravasation.
4. The intracavitary agent can be administered by one of the following routes:
   a. Irrigation through a nephrostomy tube.
   b. Irrigation through a ureteral catheter.
   c. Instillation into the bladder in the presence of vesicoureteral reflux.
5. Intravesical instillation
   a. Intravesical instillation to treat UTUC is only effective when vesicoureteral reflux (VUR) reaches the tumor site. VUR can usually be achieved temporarily by placing a ureteral stent. VUR will be present in 75-80% of cases when a ureteral stent has been in place for at least one week (the rate of VUR is lower within 7 days after stent placement). At least one week after stent placement, a cystogram is performed (in the supine or Trendelenburg position) to determine: 1) if VUR is present, 2) the bladder volume at which VUR occurs, and 3) if VUR goes high enough to reach the tumor site. For VUR to reach the calyces, a bladder volume of 120-240 ml is typically required.
   b. After instillation, the patient remains in the supine or Trendelenburg position for at least 15-30 minutes. The patient often voids (or is catheterized if necessary) by 2 hours after instillation.
   c. Disadvantages of this approach include that it may not be as efficient as ureter irrigation at distributing the solution across the entire surface of the upper tract urothelium. Advantages include the ability to treat concomitant superficial bladder tumors.
6. Irrigation through a nephrostomy tube
   a. There is no simple way hold a non-viscous agent in the upper urinary tract because it will promptly drain down the ureter. For non-viscous liquids, a slow continuous irrigation is required so that the agent remains in contact with the urothelium for the required period of time.
   b. The patient is placed in the supine position. The therapeutic agent is placed 15 cm above the kidney and instilled over 2 hours. Consider using a pressure vent (prevents the pressure from rising above a set limit). Higher infusion pressures (up to 40 cm water) have been used, but pressures < 15 cm water may be safer. The pressure must be kept low enough to prevent pyelovenous backflow, pyelolymphatic backflow, and collecting system rupture.
   c. Consider performing a nephrostogram before each irrigation to rule out extravasation and obstruction. Ideally, nephrostogram should show complete filling of the upper tract collecting system at the planned infusion pressure.
   d. Disadvantages of this approach include rare seeding of tumor along the nephrostomy tract.
7. Irrigation through a ureteral catheter
   a. A ureteral catheter is placed through the urethra and bladder, up the ureter, and into the renal pelvis. A retrograde pyelogram is performed to determine if the contrast will flow adequately around the catheter.
   b. Some urologists advocate using a ureteral catheter that is ≤ 5 French to allow enough space for the agent to drain around the ureteral catheter.
   c. The pressure must be kept low enough to prevent pyelovenous backflow, pyelolymphatic backflow, and collecting system rupture.
   d. Disadvantages of this approach include the need to place a ureteral catheter for each treatment.

8. Monitoring during therapy
   a. Stop the infusion for pain, fevers, bleeding, or extravasation.
   b. For patients with high grade cancers, some urologists have suggested performing abdominal/pelvic imaging (CT or MRI) and chest x-ray to check for metastatic progression at 1 month after starting intracavitary therapy and then every 3 months thereafter.
9. Side effects
   a. BCG—common side effects include voiding symptoms, hematuria, low grade fever. Rare side effects include sepsis, severe gross hematuria, renal granulomas, and ureteral stricture. Renal function is rarely affected. For more details on BCG side effects, see page 69.
   b. Side effects of other agents—mitomycin C (see page 68), thiotepa (see page 68), interferon (see page 72).
   c. Voiding symptoms—can occur when the irrigant contacts the bladder.
   d. Pyelovenous backflow, pyelolymphatic backflow, collecting system rupture, extravasation—these events may cause systemic absorption of the irrigant. You can minimize the risk of these events by confirming the absence of urinary obstruction and extravasation on pretreatment imaging and by avoiding high infusion pressures during irrigation.

Intracavitary Therapy: Mitomycin Gel

1. Mitomycin gel (U.S. brand name Jelmyto) is the only medication that is FDA approved for upper tract UTUC. FDA approval was based on the preliminary results from the OLYMPUS trial. Jelmyto is approved for pyelocalyceal administration in the treatment of patients with unresected or incompletely resected low grade UTUC.
2. Mechanism of action—mitomycin is an alkylating agent (which causes cell death by inhibiting DNA synthesis). After instillation, Jelmyto turns into a semi-solid gel that fills the pyelocalyceal cavity and exposes the adjacent urothelium to mitomycin for several hours.
3. OLYMPUS trial (based on data reported in the prescribing information)
   a. 71 patients were studied. Patients met all of the following criteria.
      i. No current or previous CIS of the urinary tract.
      ii. No concomitant untreated urothelial cancer in the ureter, bladder, or urethra.
      iii. At least one papillary UTUC that was still present when treatment was begun. The tumor could be untreated (no resection attempted) or incompletely resected, but it had to be low grade, located above the ureteropelvic junction, and 5-15 mm in size. Tumors larger than 15 mm could undergo debulking to meet the size criterion.
   b. Jelmyto was instilled by ureteral catheter or nephrostomy tube into the renal pelvis. Treatment consisted of a 6-week induction course (one dose each week for 6 weeks). Patients who had a complete response at 3 months were allowed to undergo maintenance therapy of one dose per month (up to a maximum of 11 maintenance doses after the 6 week induction course).
   c. Complete response was defined as negative urine cytology and absence of grossly visible tumor on ureteroscopy.
   d. 58% of patients achieved a complete response at 3 months after starting therapy. Of the patients that had a complete response at 3 months, 46% had a sustained complete response at 12 months.
   e. Temporary dose interruption was required in 34% of patients, mainly because of renal dysfunction, ureter obstruction, urinary infection, or flank pain. Jelmyto was permanently discontinued in 23% of patients.

4. Jelmyto should only be administered when all of the following criteria are met.

   a. At least 3-4 weeks have passed after endoscopic treatment of the tumor.

   b. Absence of extravasation from the urinary tract.

   c. Absence of urinary obstruction.

   d. Absence of urinary infection.

   e. Absence of gross hematuria.

5. Before administration

   a. Before instilling Jelmyto, it is prudent to wait at least 4-6 weeks after open urinary surgery and at least 3-4 weeks after endoscopic urinary surgery. *Jelmyto is contraindicated when there is perforation anywhere in the urinary tract.* Consider performing pyelogram prior to treatment to rule out extravasation.

   b. The volume of the Jelmyto dose is determined from a pyelogram. Perform a pyelogram with dilute (50%) contrast, and measure the volume of injection at the time point when the entire renal pelvis and calyces are visualized and contrast flows below the ureteropelvic junction. This volume measurement should be determined at low pressure and in the absence of pyelovenous backflow, pyelolymphatic backflow, collecting system rupture, and extravasation. Repeat this measurement 3 times and record the average of the 3 measurements. The volume of the instilled dose will be either the average of the 3 measurements or 15 ml (whichever is less).

   c. Check a complete blood count before each instillation.

   d. The patient should take 1.3 grams of sodium bicarbonate orally the evening prior to instillation and the morning before instillation. If the patient is not undergoing general anesthesia for the instillation, then an additional 1.3 gram oral dose of sodium bicarbonate is taken 30 minutes before the instillation. Sodium bicarbonate is administered because studies for bladder cancer show that intravesical mitomycin C is more effective when urine is alkaline (urine pH > 6).

   e. Consider withholding diuretics starting one day prior to instillation, and resume the diuretic 4 hours after instillation.

6. Instillation

   a. Dose—the concentration of Jelmyto is 4 mg/ml. The volume for each instillation is based on pyelogram (with a maximum volume of 15 ml per dose). Jelmyto is instilled into the renal pelvis through a ureteral catheter or nephrostomy tube. General anesthesia may be required to place a ureteral catheter (the ureter catheter is typically removed after each instillation).

   b. Jelmyto must be instilled as a chilled solution at 27° F to 41° F (at this temperature, it becomes a viscous liquid that can be injected through a catheter). Once inside the renal pelvis, Jelmyto is warmed by body heat to > 66° F, which causes the Jelmyto to become a semi-solid gel. When instilling Jelmyto, the syringe must be emptied within one minute (otherwise Jelmyto may become a gel prematurely, preventing complete instillation). Normal urine flow dissolves the semi-solid gel, slowly releasing the mitomycin gel in the urine over 4 to 6 hours. Since adequate urine flow is require to dissolve Jelmyto, it should not be used in patients with glomerular filtration rate < 30 ml/min.

7. After instillation—monitor the patient for signs and symptoms of infection and urinary tract obstruction (e.g. flank pain, fever, nausea, vomiting, or an increase in creatinine).

8. Side effects include
   a. *Ureter obstruction*—occurred in 58% of patients, most of whom required placement of a ureter stent. The obstruction may be caused by the gel itself, ureter inflammation, sloughed tumor tissue, or stenosis. In patients who had ureter obstruction, one third required balloon dilation of the ureter (although it is unclear if the stenosis occurred because of endoscopic procedures or because of mitomycin).
   b. Bone marrow suppression (myelosuppression)—systemic absorption of mitomycin can cause myelosuppression, particularly thrombocytopenia and neutropenia. However, myelosuppression is severe in only 3% of cases. *Systemic absorption through an intact urothelium is rare because mitomycin has a high molecular weight.* However, mitomycin is more likely to enter the systemic circulation when there is pyelovenous backflow, pyelolymphatic backflow, perforation of the collecting system, or urine extravasation.
   c. *Contact dermatitis*—mitomycin can cause a rash when it comes into contact with the skin. Skin irritation can be minimized by avoiding contact with urine (especially urine that is produced within 6 hours after instillation) by siting on the toilet to urinate, flushing the toilet several times after use, washing the hands and genitals with soap and water after voiding, immediately washing skin with soap and water when it has come in contact with urine (such as from urine incontinence or nephrostomy leakage), and immediately removing and washing clothes soiled by urine (wash them separately from clothes that have no urine contamination).
   d. Other side effects that were common (but rarely severe) include flank pain (39%), abdominal pain (23%), hematuria (32%), renal dysfunction (25%), nausea/vomiting (24%), fatigue (24%), dysuria (21%), and urinary infection (34%).

Radical Nephroureterectomy (RNU)

1. En bloc RNU with removal of a cuff of bladder around the ureteral orifice is considered the gold standard for treating non-metastatic high risk UTUC because of the following findings.
   a. When the ureter distal to the tumor is not completely excised, there is a high risk of recurrence in the ureteral tissue that is left behind (16-58%).
   b. The risk of multifocal ipsilateral urothelial carcinoma is high (15-44%).
   c. The risk of developing a contralateral upper tract tumor is low (< 8%).
2. RNU consists of en bloc removal of the kidney, renal pelvis, and the entire ureter. Transection of the ureter (not removing it en bloc) is discouraged because it may increase the risk of tumor spillage.
3. Removal of cuff of tissue around the ureteral orifice
   a. Various techniques have been described to help simplify removal of the distal ureter. No study has shown convincing data that these techniques are as oncologically effective as excision of the ureter en bloc with a cuff of bladder.
   b. *Excision of a cuff of tissue around the ureteral orifice during RNU is recommended by the EAU and NCCN guidelines.*
   c. For patients with their native bladder, remove the intramural ureter, the ureteral orifice, and a cuff of bladder around the ureteral orifice.
   d. For patients with a urinary diversion or neobladder, remove the ureteral anastomosis and a cuff of bowel.
4. A regional lymph node dissection (LND) should be performed for high grade or invasive cancers. See Regional Lymph Node Dissection, page 105.

5. Prospective randomized data and retrospective data suggests that open RNU and minimally invasive (laparoscopic/robotic) RNU achieve similar cancer control for N0M0 patients with stage $\leq$ T1. *The EAU 2021 guideline states that minimally invasive RNU is contraindicated in the presence of invasive or large UTUC (stage T3 T4 and or N+) because cancer control is worse compared to the open approach.* Also, patients undergoing laparoscopic RNU generally do not undergo sufficient lymphadenectomy. Port site metastases have been reported with laparoscopic RNU, but are rare.

6. *An immediate postoperative single dose of intravesical chemotherapy is strongly recommended (if not contraindicated) because randomized trials show that it decreases intravesical recurrence after RNU.* The instillation is usually given within 2-10 days after RNU. A postoperative cystogram can be performed before instillation to verify the absence of extravasation. The most commonly used agent for this indication is mitomycin C. For contraindications of intravesical chemotherapy, see page 67. For other details on intravesical chemotherapy, see page 65.

7. Neoadjuvant or adjuvant therapy may be considered in patients with high grade or high stage disease. See page 106.

8. Survival—disease specific survival after RNU can be predicted by nomogram [see J Urol, 189(5): 1662, 2013].

Survival After Radical Nephroureterectomy for Upper Tract Urothelial Cancer		
Pathologic Stage* (AJCC 2017)	5 Year Disease Specific Survival	10 Year Disease Specific Survival
Ta	93-100%	90%
CIS	82-100%	90%
T1	91-95%	85%
T2	70-75%	70%
T3	40-54%	45%
T4	12-14%	6%

* Nearly 60% of patients did not undergo lymphadenectomy (Nx). Of those patients who underwent lymphadenectomy, only 1 out of 10 were N+.

Partial Nephrectomy

Partial nephrectomy is rarely performed, and is usually restricted to patients with all of the following characteristics.

1. Preservation of renal function is imperative.
2. Low grade, low stage tumor that is located in the intrarenal collecting system (renal calyces or infundibula) and can be completely removed by partial nephrectomy.
3. The tumor cannot be sufficiently eradicated with endoscopic management and intracavitary therapy.

Segmental Ureterectomy with Ureteroureterostomy (SU)

1. SU is usually restricted to patients with all of the following characteristics.
   a. Preservation of renal function is imperative.
   b. Low grade, low stage tumor that is confined to one segment of the ureter.
   c. No tumor in the renal pelvis or intrarenal collecting system.
   d. The tumor cannot be sufficiently eradicated with endoscopic management and intracavitary therapy.
2. Segmental resection of the proximal or mid ureter is associated with a higher risk of recurrence than segmental resection of the distal ureter (distal ureterectomy).

Total Ureterectomy With Creation of an Ileal Ureter (TU)

1. TU is usually restricted to patients with all of the following characteristics.
   a. Preservation of renal function is imperative.
   b. Low grade, low stage tumor in the ureter that is not amenable to segmental ureterectomy (e.g. tumors in multiple ureter segments).
   c. No tumor in the renal pelvis or intrarenal collecting system.
   d. The tumor cannot be sufficiently eradicated with endoscopic management and intracavitary therapy.
2. Complications from an ileal ureter can be significant; thus, TU is typically used as a last resort for renal sparing when other options are not feasible.

Distal Ureter Resection With Ureteral Reimplant (DU)

1. DU is utilized to remove tumor in the distal third of the ureter (the pelvic ureter) and may be used for UTUC of any grade or T stage.
2. Remove the entire distal ureter. For patients with their native bladder, remove the intramural ureter, the ureteral orifice, and a cuff of bladder around the ureteral orifice. For patients with a urinary diversion or neobladder, remove the ureteral anastomosis and a cuff of bowel. The remaining ureter is reimplanted into the bladder (or urinary diversion).
   a. It is unknown whether a refluxing or non-refluxing ureteral reimplant is best. However, a non-refluxing reimplant may decrease the risk of infection and the risk of upper tract seeding from bladder cancer.
   b. The gap between the bladder and ureter can be bridged using a psoas hitch and/or Boari flap (see Ureteral Reimplant, page 607).
3. Regional lymph node dissection should be performed for high risk cancers.
4. When the tumor is confined to the intramural ureter, the tumor can be treated with transurethral resection of the intramural ureter and the ureteral orifice, followed by intravesical therapy in the presence of reflux up the ipsilateral ureter (a ureteral stent may be necessary).

Regional Lymph Node Dissection (LND)

1. Lymphatic metastases from tumors of the renal pelvis and upper ureter initially spread to the retroperitoneal lymph nodes, whereas distal ureteral tumors initially spread to the pelvic lymph nodes.
2. The template for the LND depends on the location of the UTUC. There is no universally accepted LND template, but some urologists utilize the following templates based on tumor location. *Removal of all the lymph nodes in the template (as opposed to sampling only some nodes) reduces the risk of local recurrence and may improve cancer specific survival.*
   a. Pelvic ureter—remove the ipsilateral pelvic lymph nodes (common iliac, external iliac, internal iliac, and obturator).
   b. Left abdominal ureter or left renal pelvis—remove left renal hilar, paraaortic, and interaortocaval nodes. The superior limit of dissection is the renal hilum. The inferior limit is the aortic bifurcation. For tumors of the mid ureter (especially the distal mid ureter), remove the nodes listed for the pelvic ureter.
   c. Right abdominal ureter or right renal pelvis—remove right renal hilar, paracaval, retrocaval, and interaortocaval nodes. The superior limit of dissection is the renal hilum. The inferior limit is the bifurcation of the inferior vena cava. For tumors of the mid ureter (especially the distal mid ureter), remove the nodes listed for the pelvic ureter.
3. *In patients who are undergoing extirpative surgery, regional LND should be performed for cancer that is high grade, high risk, or suspected of being invasive. Several retrospective studies suggest that LND improves cancer specific survival in men with pathologic stage ≥ T2 UTUC*, although the curative potential of LND is still controversial.

4. LND can be considered even in patients with low grade tumor because preoperative tumor staging is inaccurate. Thus, if there is a suspicion that the tumor may be invasive despite being low grade, perform a LND.
5. Side effects from retroperitoneal LND for UTUC are similar to the side effects seen with retroperitoneal LND for testis cancer (including impaired ejaculation; see page 148). Side effects from pelvic LND for UTUC are similar to the side effects seen with pelvic LND for prostate and bladder cancer (see page 220).

Neoadjuvant or Adjuvant Therapy with Surgical Extirpation

1. Neoadjuvant and/or adjuvant therapy may be utilized with extirpative surgery for high risk UTUC.
2. Neoadjuvant therapy
   a. Neoadjuvant systemic chemotherapy has not been well studied in UTUC, but its use for UTUC is based on its efficacy for treating urothelial carcinoma of the bladder. *Retrospective data shows that neoadjuvant systemic chemotherapy for UTUC lowers the risk of recurrence, improves cancer specific survival, and improves overall survival.*
   b. When the expected decline in renal function from nephroureterectomy will preclude the use of adjuvant chemotherapy, then neoadjuvant chemotherapy should be considered.
   c. Neoadjuvant radiation is not recommended.
3. Adjuvant therapy
   a. Adjuvant systemic chemotherapy—in the POUT trial, 261 M0 patients with stage pT2-pT4 or N1-N3 were randomized to no adjuvant therapy or to adjuvant chemotherapy using cisplatin and gemcitabine in patients with glomerular filtration rate (GFR) $\geq$ 50 ml/min or carboplatin and gemcitabine in patients with GFR < 50 ml/min. At a median follow up of 30 months, *adjuvant chemotherapy significantly improved disease free survival.* Retrospective data shows that adjuvant systemic chemotherapy improves cancer specific and overall survival.
   b. Adjuvant radiation—the role of adjuvant radiation for UTUC is poorly defined. Limited data suggests that adjuvant external beam radiation to the renal fossa or ureteral bed after nephroureterectomy may reduce local recurrence, but it does not prevent metastases or improve survival.
4. Based on data from treating urothelial carcinoma of the bladder, the preferred perioperative chemotherapy regimen (neoadjuvant or adjuvant) is either ddMVAC (dose dense methotrexate, vinblastine, adriamycin, cisplatin) or GC (gemcitabine and cisplatin). Substituting carboplatin for cisplatin in perioperative may reduce the response rate and survival.

Treatment of Metastatic UTUC (N1-3 or M1)

1. The most common metastatic sites are lungs, liver, bones, and regional lymph nodes.
2. Metastatic UTUC (N1-3 or M1) is usually treated with systemic chemotherapy. If the patient is stage N1-N3 and M0, is treated initially with systemic chemotherapy, and if chemotherapy sufficiently downstages the disease, then RNU may be an option for select patients.
3. Systemic agents used to treat UTUC are the same as those used for urothelial carcinoma of the bladder (see page 81).
4. When the local tumor is causing problematic symptoms (such as significant gross hematuria), then external beam radiation may be utilized for local tumor control.

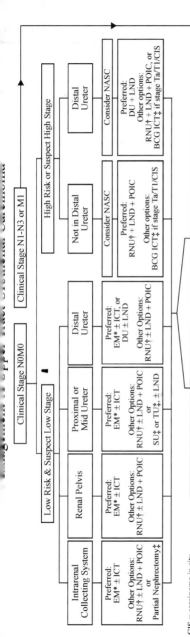

Management of Upper Tract Urothelial Carcinoma

Clinical Stage N0M0 | **Clinical Stage N1-N3 or M1**

Low Risk & Suspect Low Stage | **High Risk or Suspect High Stage**

Low Risk & Suspect Low Stage:

Intrarenal Collecting System
Preferred: EM* ± ICT
Other Options: RNU† ± LND + POIC or Partial Nephrectomy‡

Renal Pelvis
Preferred: EM* ± ICT
Other Options: RNU† ± LND + POIC

Proximal or Mid Ureter
Preferred: EM* ± ICT
Other Options: RNU† ± LND + POIC or SU‡ or TU‡, ± LND

Distal Ureter
Preferred: EM* ± ICT, or DU ± LND
Other Options: RNU† ± LND + POIC

High Risk or Suspect High Stage:

Not in Distal Ureter
Consider NASC
Preferred: RNU† ± LND + POIC
Other options: BCG ICT‡ if stage Ta/T1/CIS

Distal Ureter
Consider NASC
Preferred: DU + LND
Other options: RNU† ± LND + POIC, or BCG ICT‡ if stage Ta/T1/CIS

N0 & Low T stage (pT0, pTa, pTis, or pT1) → Surveillance

N1-N3 or High T stage (pT2-T4) → Systemic Chemotherapy ± Radiation

Clinical Stage N1-N3 or M1 → Systemic Chemotherapy ± Radiation

CIS = carcinoma in situ
EM = endoscopic management
chemo = chemotherapy
ICT = intracavitary therapy (induction with or without maintenance)

RNU = radical nephroureterectomy; LND = regional lymph node dissection; POIC = postoperative intravesical chemo (single dose); NASC = neoadjuvant systemic chemo; DU = distal ureterectomy with ureteral re-implant; SU = segmental ureterectomy; TU = total ureterectomy with ileal ureter; BCG = Bacillus Calmette Guerin;

* Endoscopic management (EM) includes resection and/or fulguration, and may be accomplished using an antegrade or retrograde approach. Renal sparing approaches are most successful for tumors with all of the following characteristics: low grade, solitary, papillary, size < 1.5 cm, and no suspicion of invasion on imaging.

† Renal sparing is preferred for patients at low risk or with any imperative indication (poor overall renal function, absent or poorly functioning contralateral kidney, risk for or presence of bilateral upper tract tumor, or unable to tolerate therapy that is more invasive. LND may be done for low grade tumor because preoperative T staging is inaccurate.

‡ These options are typically used only when preservation of renal function is imperative (see †) and the tumor burden is too large for endoscopic management.

Follow Up And Recurrence

1. Approximately 22-47% of patients with a UTUC subsequently develop urothelial carcinoma (UC) of the bladder. Therefore, surveillance of the bladder is recommended after treatment of UTUC. ✓

2. After treatment of UTUC, the risk of recurrence in the contralateral upper urinary tract is 2-6%. Monitoring of the contralateral collecting system is usually recommended.

3. The following example follow up regimens are adapted from multiple clinical guidelines.

4. Low grade and low stage (Ta-T1, N0) treated with renal sparing surgery
   a. Cystoscopy (to detect metachronous bladder tumors) every 3 months for 1 year, then less often.
   b. Routine use of urinary tumors markers is usually not recommended, but may be considered in select cases.
   c. Upper tract imaging (preferably with CTU) every 3-6 months for 1 year, then less often. If IVU or retrograde pyelogram are used for upper tract imaging, consider performing abdominal and pelvic cross sectional imaging (CT or MRI) each time the upper tract is imaged.
   d. Ureteroscopy of the treated side—strongly consider performing a ureteroscopy at 3 months post-treatment in all patients. Thereafter, ureteroscopy should be considered every 3-12 months for 1 year and then less often, especially in patients with a higher risk of recurrence (e.g. large, multifocal, and/or recurrent tumors). Ureteroscopy should be done in addition to the upper tract radiographic imaging that is recommended in "c" above.

5. Low grade and low stage (Ta-T1, N0) treated with RNU
   a. Cystoscopy (to detect metachronous bladder tumors) every 3 months for 1 year, then less often.
   b. Routine use of urinary tumors markers is usually not recommended, but may be considered in select cases.
   c. Routine upper tract imaging and abdominal pelvic cross sectional imaging are usually not recommended.

6. High grade (including CIS) or high stage (T2-T4 or N1-N3) treated with either renal sparing surgery or with RNU
   a. Cystoscopy and urine cytology—every 3 months for 1-2 years, then less often.
   b. Upper tract imaging—every 3-6 months (preferably with CTU) for 2 years, then annually. If IVU or retrograde pyelogram are used for upper tract imaging, then perform abdominal and pelvic cross sectional imaging (CT or MRI) each time the upper tract is imaged.
   c. Chest imaging (preferably with chest CT)—every 3-6 months for 2 years, then annually.
   d. If renal sparing treatment was utilized—perform ureteroscopy and upper tract wash cytology of the treated side at 3 month and 6 months post-treatment, then consider performing these tests less often thereafter. Using narrow band imaging in addition to white light may help detect recurrent tumor.
   e. After nephroureterectomy, monitor renal function periodically.

REFERENCES

General

EAU—**Roupret M, et al: Upper urinary tract urothelial call carcinoma. European Association of Urology, 2021. (www.uroweb.org).**

NCCN—**National Comprehensive Cancer Network clinical practice guidelines in oncology: Bladder cancer. V.3.2021, 2021. (www.nccn.org).**

Wang LJ, et al: Multidetector computerized tomography urography is more accurate than excretory urography for diagnosing transitional cell carcinoma of the upper urinary tract in adults with hematuria. J Urol, 183(1): 48, 2010.

Risk Factors for UTUC (Including Genetic Predisposition)

Audenet F, et al: A proportion of hereditary upper urinary tract urothelial carcinomas are mis-classified as sporadic according to a multi-institutional database analysis proposal of patient specific risk identification tool. BJU Int, 110: E583, 2012.

Chen, CH, et al: Aristolochic acid associated urothelial cancer in Taiwan. Proc Natl Acad Sci USA, 109(21): 8241, 2012.

Crockett DG, et al: Upper urinary tract carcinoma in Lynch syndrome cases. J Urol, 185(5): 1627, 2011.

Grollman AP, et al: Aristolochic acid and the etiology of endemic (Balkan) nephropathy. Proc Natl Acad Sci USA, 104(29): 12129, 2007.

Hurle R, et al: Upper urinary tract tumors developing after treatment of superficial bladder cancer: 7 year follow up of 591 consecutive patients. Urology, 53: 1144, 1999.

Jelakovic B, et al: Aristolactam-DNA adducts are a biomarker of environmental exposure to aristolochic acid. Kidney Int, 81: 559, 2012.

Picozzi S, et al: Upper urinary tract recurrence following radical cystectomy for bladder cancer: a meta-analysis on 13,185 patients. J Urol, 188: 2046, 2012.

Ross RK, et al: Analgesics, cigarette smoking, and other risk factors for cancer of the renal pelvis and ureter. Cancer Research, 49: 1045, 1989.

Sountoulides P, et al: Does ureteral stenting increase the risk of metachronous upper urinary tract urothelial carcinoma in patients with bladder tumors? A systematic review and meta-analysis. J Urol, 205(4): 956, 2021.

Tollefson MK, et al: Significance of distal ureteral margin at radical cystectomy for urothelial carcinoma. J Urol, 183(1): 81, 2010.

Volkmer BG, et al: Upper urinary tract recurrence after radical cystectomy for bladder cancer - who is at risk? J Urol, 182(6): 2632, 2009.

Wright JL, et al: Predictors of upper tract urothelial cell carcinoma after primary bladder cancer: a population based analysis. J Urol, 181(3): 1035, 2009.

Variant Histology

Chung HS, et al: Effects of variant histology on the oncologic outcomes of patients with upper urinary tract carcinoma after radical nephroureterectomy: a propensity score matched analysis. Clin Genitourin Cancer, 17(3): e394, 2019.

Mori K, et al: Prognostic value of variant histology in upper tract urothelial carcinoma treated with nephroureterectomy: a systematic review and meta-analysis. J Urol, 203(6): 1075, 2020.

Zamboni S, et al: Incidence and survival outcomes in patients with upper urinary tract urothelial carcinoma diagnosed with variant histology and treated with nephroureterectomy. BJU Int, 124(5): 738, 2019.

Upper Urinary Tract Cytology

Malm C, et al: Diagnostic accuracy of upper tract urothelial carcinoma: how samples are collected matters. Scand J Urol, 51(2): 137, 2017.

Sadek S, et al: The value of upper tract cytology after transurethral resection of bladder tumor. J Urol, 161(1): 77, 1999.

Smith AK, et al: Is there a role for cytology in the diagnosis of upper tract urothelial cancer. J Urol, 181(4, suppl): 132 (abstract 368), 2009.

Influence of Ureteroscopy Before Nephroureterectomy: Recurrence & Survival

Baboudjian M, et al: Diagnostic ureteroscopy prior to nephroureterectomy for urothelial carcinoma is associated with a high risk of bladder recurrence despite technical precautions to avoid tumor spillage. World J Urol, 38(1): 159, 2020.

Boorjian S, et al: Impact of delay to nephroureterectomy for patients undergoing ureteroscopic biopsy and tumor ablation of upper tract transitional cell carcinoma. Urology, 66(2): 283, 2005.

Capitanio U, et al: Comparison of oncologic outcomes for open and laparoscopic nephroureterectomy: a multi-institutional analysis of 1249 cases. Eur Urol, 56: 1, 2009.

Chung Y, et al: Impact of diagnostic ureteroscopy before radical nephroureterectomy on intravesical recurrence in patients with upper tract urothelial cancer. Invest Clin Urol, 61: 158, 2020.

Guo RQ, et al: Impact of ureteroscopy before radical nephroureterectomy for upper tract urothelial carcinomas on oncological outcomes: a meta-analysis. BJU Int, 121: 184, 2018.

Gurbuz C, et al: The impact of previous ureteroscopic tumor ablation on oncologic outcomes after radical nephroureterectomy for upper tract urothelial carcinoma. J Endourol, 25(5): 775, 2011.

Hendin BN, et al: Impact of diagnostic ureteroscopy on long term survival in patients with upper tract transitional cell carcinoma. J Urol, 161: 783, 1999.

Lee HS, et al: The diagnostic ureteroscopy before radical nephroureterectomy in upper urinary tract urothelial carcinoma is not associated with higher intravesical recurrence. World J Surg Oncol, 16(1): 135, 2018.

Liu Z, et al: Oncologic outcomes of patients undergoing diagnostic ureteroscopy before radical nephrectomy for upper urinary tract urothelial carcinomas: a systematic review and meta-analysis. J Laparoendosc Adv Surg Tech A, 28(11): 1316, 2018.

Margulis V, et al: Outcomes of radical nephroureterectomy: a series from the upper tract urothelial carcinoma collaboration. Cancer, 115: 1224, 2009.

Endoscopic Management

Chen GL, Bagley DH: Ureteroscopic surgery for upper tract transitional cell carcinoma: complications and management. J Endourol, 15(4): 399, 2001.

Cutress ML, et al: Endoscopic versus laparoscopic management of noninvasive upper tract urothelial carcinoma: 20 year single center experience. J Urol, 189(6): 2054, 2013.

Gadzinski AJ, et al: Long term outcomes of immediate versus delayed nephroureterectomy for upper tract urothelial carcinoma. J Endourol, 26(5): 566, 2012.

Gadzinski AJ, et al: Long term outcomes of nephroureterectomy versus endoscopic management of upper tract urothelial carcinoma. J Urol, 183(6): 2148, 2010.

Grasso M, et al: Ureteroscopic and extirpative treatment of upper urinary tract urothelial carcinoma: a 15 year comprehensive review of 160 consecutive patients. BJU Int, 110: 1618, 2012.

Lee BR, et al: 13-year survival comparison of percutaneous and open nephroureterectomy approaches for management of transitional cell carcinoma of renal collecting system. J Endourol, 13(4): 289, 1999.

Lucas SM, et al: Conservative management in selected patients with upper tract urothelial carcinoma compares favorably with early radical surgery. BJU Int, 102(2): 172, 2008.

Raymundo EM, et al: Third prize: the role of endoscopic nephron sparing surgery in the management of upper tract urothelial carcinoma. J Endourol, 25(3): 377, 2011.

Roupret M, et al: Comparison of open nephroureterectomy and ureteroscopic and percutaneous management of upper urinary tract transitional cell carcinoma. Urology, 67(6): 1181, 2005.

Upfill-Brown A, et al: Treatment utilization and overall survival inpatients receiving radical nephroureterectomy versus endoscopic management for upper tract urothelial carcinoma: evaluation of updated treatment guidelines. World J Urol, 37(6): 1157, 2019.

Villa L, et al: Which patients with upper urinary tract urothelial carcinoma can be safely treated with flexible ureteroscopy with Holmium:YAG laser photoablation? Long term results from a high volume institution. J Urol, 199(1): 66, 2018.

Intracavitary Therapy

Bassi P, et al: Intracavitary therapy of noninvasive transitional cell carcinomas of the upper urinary tract. Urol Int, 67: 189, 2001.

Bohle A: Editorial comment. Eur Urol, 38: 705, 2000.

Foerster B, et al: Endocavitary treatment for upper tract urothelial carcinoma: a meta-analysis of the current literature. Urol Oncol, 37(7): 430, 2019.

Gallioli A, et al: Adjuvant single dose upper urinary tract instillation of mitomycin C after therapeutic ureteroscopy for upper tract urothelial carcinoma: a single center prospective non-randomized trial. J Endourol, 34(5): 573, 2020.

Nishino Y, et al: Bacillus Calmette Guerin instillation treatment for carcinoma in situ of the upper urinary tract. BJU Int, 85: 799, 2000.

Nissenkorn I, et al: Long term intravesical thiotepa treatment in patients with superficial bladder tumors and vesicoureteral reflux. J Urol, 133: 198, 1985.

Nonomura N, et al: Bacillus Calmette Guerin perfusion therapy for treatment of transitional cell carcinoma in situ of the upper tract. Eur Urol, 38: 701, 2000.

Rastinehad AR, et al: a 20 year experience with percutaneous resection of upper tract transitional carcinoma: is there an oncologic benefit with adjuvant Bacillus Calmette Guerin therapy? Urology, 73(1): 27, 2009.

Rastinehad AR, Smith AD: Bacillus Calmette-Guérin for upper tract urothelial cancer: is there a role? J Endourol, 23(4): 563, 2009.

Thalmann GN, et al: Long term experience with Bacillus Calmette Guerin therapy of upper urinary tract transitional cell carcinoma in patients not eligible for surgery. J Urol, 168: 1381, 2002.

Yokogi H, et al: Bacillus Calmette Guerin perfusion therapy for carcinoma in situ of the upper urinary tract. Br J Urol, 77: 676, 1996.

Reflux Through a Ureteral Stent for Intracavitary Therapy

Hubner WA, et al: The double-J ureteral stent: in vivo and in vitro flow studies. J Urol, 148: 278, 1992.

Irie A, et al: Intravesical instillation of Bacille Calmette Guerin for carcinoma in situ of the urothelium involving the upper urinary tract using vesicoureteral reflux created by a double pigtail catheter. Urology, 59: 53, 2002.

Korkes F, et al: Is a ureter stent an effective way to deliver drugs such as bacillus Calmette Guerin to the upper urinary tract? An experimental study. Ther Adv Urol, 11:1, 2019.

Yossepowitch O, et al: Assessment of vesicoureteral reflux in patients with self retaining ureteral stents: implications for upper urinary tract instillation. J Urol, 173(3): 890, 2005.

Partial Nephrectomy

Goel MC, et al. Partial nephrectomy for renal urothelial tumors: clinical update. Urology, 67(3): 490, 2006.

Distal Ureterectomy and Segmental Ureterectomy

Abrate A, et al: Segmental resection of distal ureter with termino-terminal ureteric anastomosis vs bladder cuff removal and ureteric re-implantation for upper tract urothelial carcinoma: results of a multicenter study. BJU Int, 124(1): 116, 2019.

Abrate A, et al: Segmental ureterectomy vs radical nephroureterectomy for ureteral carcinoma in patients with a preoperative glomerular filtration rate less than 90 ml/min/1.73 m^2: a multicenter study. Urol Oncol, 38(6): 601.e11, 2020.

Bagrodia A, et al: Comparative analysis of oncologic outcomes of partial ureterectomy vs radical nephroureterectomy in upper tract urothelial carcinoma. Urology, 81(5): 972, 2013.

Colin P, et al: Comparison of oncological outcomes after segmental ureterectomy or radical nephroureterectomy in urothelial carcinomas of the upper urinary tract: results from large French multicentre study. BJU Int, 110: 1134, 2012.

Jeldres C, et al: Segmental ureterectomy can safely be performed in patients with transitional cell carcinoma of the ureter J Urol, 183(4): 1324, 2010.

Jia Z, et al: Segmental ureterectomy can be performed safely in patients with urothelial carcinoma of the distal ureter. Can Urol Assoc J, 13(7): e202, 2019.

Lughezzani G, et al: Nephroureterectomy and segmental ureterectomy in the treatment of invasive upper tract urothelial carcinoma: a population based study of 2299 patients. Eur J Cancer, 45(18): 3291, 2009.

Pohar, KS and Sheinfeld J: When is partial ureterectomy acceptable for transitional cell carcinoma of the ureter? J Endourol, 15(4): 405, 2001.

Seisen T, et al: Oncologic outcomes of kidney sparing surgery versus radical nephroureterectomy for upper tract urothelial carcinoma: a systematic review by the EAU non-muscle invasive bladder cancer guidelines panel. Eur Urol, 70(6): 1052, 2016.

Simonato A, et al: Elective segmental ureterectomy for transitional cell carcinoma of the ureter: long term follow up in a series of 73 patients. BJU Int, 110: E744, 2012.

Veccia A, et al: Segmental ureterectomy for upper tract urothelial carcinoma: a systematic review of comparative studies. Clin Genitourin Cancer, 18(1): e10, 2020.

Nephroureterectomy

Capitanio U, et al: Comparison of oncologic outcomes for open and laparoscopic nephroureterectomy: a multi-institutional analysis of 1249 cases. Eur Urol, 56: 1, 2009.

Karam JA, et al: Carcinoma in situ of the upper urinary tract treated with radical nephroureterectomy - results from a multicenter study. Eur Urol, 54: 961, 2008.

Manabe D, et al: Comparative study of oncologic outcome of laparoscopic nephroureterectomy and standard nephroureterectomy for upper tract transitional cell carcinoma. Urology, 69: 457, 2007.

Margulis V, et al: Outcomes of radical nephroureterectomy: a series from the Upper Tract Urothelial Carcinoma Collaboration. Cancer, 115(6): 1224, 2009.

Roupret M, et al: Oncologic control after open or laparoscopic nephroureterectomy for upper urinary tract transitional cell carcinoma. Urology, 69: 656, 2007.

Roupret M, et al: Prediction of cancer specific survival after radical nephroureterectomy for upper tract urothelial carcinoma. J Urol, 189(5): 1662, 2013.

Sakamoto N, et al: Prophylactic intravesical installation of mitomycin C and cytosine arabinoside for prevention of recurrent bladder tumors following surgery for upper urinary tract tumors: a prospective randomized study. Int J Urol, 8: 212, 2001.

Waldert M, et al: The oncological results of laparoscopic nephroureterectomy for upper urinary tract transitional cell cancer are equal to those of open nephroureterectomy. BJU Int, 103: 66, 2008.

Yuasa T, et al: Radical nephroureterectomy as initial treatment for carcinoma in situ of upper urinary tract. Urology, 68: 972, 2006.

Bladder Cuff Excision with Nephroureterectomy & Method of Cuff Excision

Capitanio U, et al: Comparison of oncologic outcomes for open and laparoscopic nephroureterectomy: a multi-institutional analysis of 1249 cases. Eur Urol, 56: 1, 2009.

Gkougkousis EG, et al: Management of the distal ureter during nephroureterectomy for upper tract transitional cell carcinoma: a review. Urol Int, 85:249, 2010.

Laguna MP, et al: The endoscopic approach to the distal ureter in nephroureterectomy for upper urinary tract tumor. J Urol, 166: 2017, 2001.

Lai S, et al: Assessing the impact of different distal ureter management techniques during radical nephrectomy for primary upper urinary tract urothelial carcinoma on oncological outcomes: a systematic review and meta-analysis. Int J Surg, 75: 165, 2020.

Lee SM, et al: Distal ureter management during nephroureterectomy: evidence from a systematic review and cumulative analysis. J Endourol, 33(4): 263, 2019.

Li WM, et al: Oncologic outcomes following three different approaches to the distal ureter and bladder cuff in nephroureterectomy for primary upper urinary tract urothelial carcinoma. Eur Urol, 57: 963, 2010.

Lughezzani G, et al: Nephroureterectomy and segmental ureterectomy in the treatment of invasive upper tract urothelial carcinoma: a population based study of 2299 patients. Eur J Cancer, 45(18): 3291, 2009.

Lughezzani G, et al: Should bladder cuff excision remain the standard of care at nephroureterectomy in patients with urothelial carcinoma of the renal pelvis? A population based study. Eur Urol, 57: 956, 2010.

Phe V, et al: Does the surgical technique for management of the distal ureter influence the outcome after nephroureterectomy? BJU Int, 108: 130: 2010.

Walton TJ, et al: Comparative outcomes following endoscopic ureteral detachment and formal bladder cuff excision in open nephroureterectomy for upper urinary tract transitional cell carcinoma. J Urol, 181(2): 532, 2009.

Regional Lymphadenectomy

Brausi MA, et al: Retroperitoneal lymph node dissection in conjunction with nephroureterectomy in the treatment of infiltrative transitional cell carcinoma of the upper urinary tract. Eur Urol, 52(2): 1414, 2007.

Dominguez-Escrig JL, et al: Potential benefit of lymph node dissection during radical nephroureterectomy for upper tract urothelial carcinoma: a systematic review by the European Association of Urology Guidelines Panel on non-muscle invasive bladder cancer. Eur Urol Focus, 5(2): 224, 2019.

Dong F, et al: Lymph node dissection could bring survival benefits to patients diagnosed with clinical node negative upper urinary tract urothelial cancer: a population based propensity score matched study. Int J Clin Oncol, 24(3): 296, 2019.

Grimes N, et al: Lymph node dissection during nephroureterectomy: establishing the existing evidence based on a review of the literature. Arab J Urol, 17(3): 167, 2019.

Kondo T, et al: Impact of the extent of regional lymphadenectomy on the survival of patients with urothelial carcinoma of the upper urinary tract. J Urol, 178 (4, part 1): 1212, 2007.

Roscigno W, et al: Impact of lymph node dissection on cancer specific survival in patients with upper tract urothelial carcinoma treated with radical nephroureterectomy. J Urol, 181: 2482, 2009.

Tamhankar AS, et al: Current status of lymphadenectomy during radical nephroureterectomy for upper tract urothelial cancer - yes, no or maybe? Ind J Surg Oncol, 9(3): 418, 2018.

Zhai, TS, et al: Effect of lymph node dissection on stage specific survival in patients with upper urinary tract urothelial carcinoma treated with nephroureterectomy. BNC Cancer, 19: 1207, 2019.

Prognosis and Survival after Nephroureterectomy

Bolenz C, et al: Lymphovascular invasion and pathologic tumor stage are significant outcome predictors for patients with upper tract urothelial carcinoma. Urology, 72: 364, 2008.

Kikuchi E, et al: Lymphovascular invasion predicts clinical outcomes in patients with node-negative upper tract urothelial carcinoma. J Clin Oncol, 27: 612, 2008.

Margulis V, et al: Outcomes of radical nephroureterectomy: a series from the upper tract urothelial carcinoma collaboration. Cancer, 115: 1224, 2009.

Intravesical Chemotherapy Instillation After Nephroureterectomy

Harraz AM, et al: Single versus maintenance intravesical chemotherapy for the prevention of bladder recurrence after radical nephroureterectomy for upper tract urothelial carcinoma: a randomized clinical trial. Clin Genotourin Cancer, 17(6): e1108, 2019.

Hwang EC, et al: Single dose intravesical chemotherapy after nephroureterectomy for upper tract urothelial carcinoma. Cochrane Database Syst Rev, 5: CD013160, 2019.

Yoo SH, et al: Intravesical chemotherapy after radical nephroureterectomy for primary upper tract urothelial carcinoma: a systematic review and network meta-analysis. J Clin Med, 8: 1059, 2019.

Neoadjuvant and Adjuvant Therapy with Nephroureterectomy

Cozad S, et al: Adjuvant radiotherapy in high stage transitional cell carcinoma of the renal pelvis and ureter. Int J Radiat Oncol Biol Phys, 24: 743, 1992.

Foerster B, et al: Efficacy of preoperative chemotherapy for high risk upper tract urothelial carcinoma. J Urol, 203(6): 1101, 2020.

Hellenthal NJ, et al: Adjuvant chemotherapy for high risk upper tract urothelial carcinoma: results from the Upper Tract Urothelial Carcinoma Collaboration. J Urol, 182(3): 900, 2009.

Iwata T, et al: The role of adjuvant radiotherapy after surgery for upper and lower urinary tract urothelial carcinoma: a systematic review. Urol Oncol, 37(10): 659, 2019.

Kang M, et al: Role of adjuvant chemotherapy in advanced stage upper urinary tract urothelial carcinoma after radical nephroureterectomy: competing risk analysis after propensity score matching. J Cancer, 10(27): 6896, 2019.

Kim DK, et al: Effect of neoadjuvant chemotherapy on locally advanced upper tract urothelial carcinoma: a systematic review and meta-analysis. Crit Rev Oncol Hematol, 135: 59, 2019.

Li K, et al: Impact of neoadjuvant chemotherapy on survival prognosis and pathological downstaging in patients presenting with high risk upper tract urothelial carcinoma. Medicine, 99: 18, 2020.

Margulis V, et al: Phase II trial of neoadjuvant systemic chemotherapy followed by extirpative surgery in patients with high grade upper tract urothelial carcinoma. J Urol, 203: 690, 2020.

Martini A, et al: Neoadjuvant versus adjuvant chemotherapy for upper tract urothelial carcinoma. Urol Oncol, 38(8): 684.e9, 2020.

Matsunaga T, et al: Adjuvant chemotherapy improves overall survival in patients with localized upper tract urothelial carcinoma harboring pathologic vascular invasion: a propensity score matched analysis of multi-institutional cohort. World J Urol, 38: 3183, 2020.

POUT—Birtle A, et al: Adjuvant chemotherapy in upper tract urothelial carcinoma (the POUT trial): a phase 3, open label randomized controlled trial. Lancet, 395: 1268, 2020.

Quhal F, et al: Efficacy of neoadjuvant and adjuvant chemotherapy for localized and locally advanced upper tract urothelial carcinoma: a systematic review and meta-analysis. Int J Clin Oncol, 25: 1037, 2020.

Zhai TS, et al: Perioperative chemotherapy on survival in patients with upper urinary tract urothelial carcinoma undergoing nephroureterectomy: a population based study. Front Oncol, 10: 481, 2020.

TUMOR MARKERS FOR UROTHELIAL CANCER

Indications for Performing Urinary Tumor Markers
1. Irritative voiding symptoms (dysuria, frequency, etc.).
2. Hematuria (microscopic or gross)
3. Preoperative evaluation of urothelial tumors
4. Post-treatment surveillance of urothelial tumors
   a. After endoscopic resection
   b. After cystectomy
      i. From the urinary diversion.
      ii. Lavage cytology of urethral stump (see Urethrectomy, page 74).
5. Screening in high risk groups. For conditions that increase risk of urothelial tumors, see Risk Factors for Bladder Cancer on page 49 and Risk factors for UTUC on page 92.

Urine Cytology
1. Urine cytology detects abnormal appearing exfoliated urothelial cells.
2. Poorly differentiated tumors have less cohesive cells. Thus, the higher the tumor grade, the more likely urine cytology will detect the tumor (i.e. the sensitivity of urine cytology is greater for high grade tumors).

Urothelial Carcinoma Grade	Approximate Sensitivity of Urine Cytology
Low Grade	< 50%
High Grade (including CIS)	> 90%

3. The diagnostic yield of urine cytology is increased when at least 3 urine samples are analyzed.
4. For bladder cancers, bladder washings provide a better diagnostic yield than voided urine.
5. Urine cytology can remain positive for up to 3 months after BCG therapy.
6. The inflammation from intravesical therapy can hinder the accuracy of cytology.

Other Tumor Markers
1. Bladder cancer detection is highest when urine cytology is combined with another tumor marker.
2. Most markers have a higher sensitivity and lower specificity than cytology.
3. When urine cytology is atypical or inconclusive, other urine tumor markers may help determine the risk that urothelial malignancy is present.
4. BTA (bladder tumor antigen)—detects a complement factor H-related protein in the urine.
   a. BTA TRAK®—a quantitative test performed in a lab.
   b. BTA stat®—a qualitative test performed in the office.
   c. False positive results are more common in patients with gross hematuria, genitourinary inflammation (e.g. infection, recent intravesical therapy), urolithiasis, urinary foreign bodies (e.g. stents, nephrostomy tubes), bowel interposition (e.g. conduit, neobladder), non-urothelial genitourinary cancer, and recent urinary tract instrumentation.

5. NMP22®—detects nuclear matrix protein in the urine.
   a. NMP22® test—a quantitative test performed in a lab.
   b. NMP22® bladderchek®—a qualitative test performed in the office.
   c. False positives are more common in patients with genitourinary inflammation, urolithiasis, urinary foreign bodies, bowel interposition, non-urothelial genitourinary cancer, and recent urinary tract instrumentation.
6. ImmunoCyt™—detects two antigens (carcinoembryonic antigen and mucin glycoprotein) in exfoliated urothelial cells. For low grade tumors, ImmunoCyt™ has a higher sensitivity than cytology and FISH (i.e. it is better at detecting low grade tumors). ImmunoCyt™ is performed in a lab.
7. Urovysion™—uses fluorescence in situ hybridization (FISH) to detect chromosomal abnormalities in exfoliated urothelial cells. FISH is performed in a lab.
   a. Urovysion™ detects extra copies of chromosome 3, 7, and 17 and the loss of the 9p21 locus.
   b. FISH and urine cytology have a higher specificity than ImmunoCyt™, NMP22®, and BTA (i.e. FISH and cytology are more reliable at predicting the absence of cancer when the test is negative).
   c. FISH has a low rate of false positive results during urinary infection and inflammation. *FISH results are rarely affected by recent intravesical therapy* (whereas the inflammation generated by recent intravesical therapy can often hinder the accuracy of cytology).
   d. *The presence of a persistently abnormal FISH after induction BCG is associated with a higher likelihood of recurrence and progression. Therefore, FISH can be used to identify patients at risk for early failure after induction BCG.*

Positive Urine Tumor Marker Without Visible Tumor In the Bladder

1. Urothelial tumor markers can be positive before a grossly visible tumor develops (microscopic cancer). The source of the positive urinary tumor marker may be the upper tracts, bladder, prostate, or urethra. Also, false positive results can occur.
2. For patients with positive urine cytology within 6 months of treatment for bladder cancer, the source of the positive cytology rarely arises from the prostatic urethra or upper tracts (they almost always recur in the bladder). For patients that have a positive urine cytology and no history of urothelial carcinoma (UC), the source of the positive cytology is usually the bladder, but a significant number also arise from the prostatic urethra and upper tracts.

History of the Patient when the Positive Urine Cytology Develops	Approximate % that Develop UC	Location UC Develops (%)		
		Bladder	Prostatic Urethra	Upper Tract
No history of UC (asymptomatic)	94%	74%	7%	5%
No history of UC (symptomatic)*	70%	77%	9%	5%
< 6 months after TURBT	84-100%	100%	-	-
< 6 months after intravesical therapy	58-88%	100%	-	-

UC = urothelial carcinoma; TURBT = Transurethral resection of bladder tumor
* Symptoms include hematuria and voiding symptoms.

3. Example evaluation for patients who develop positive cytology within 6 months of TURBT or intravesical induction therapy—most of these patients will eventually have a recurrence in the bladder.
    a. If a urine tumor marker is positive, but there is no visible tumor in the bladder during white light cystoscopy, then perform upper tract imaging if not done recently (ideally CT urogram).
    b. If enhanced cystoscopy technologies are available, perform cystoscopy with blue light or with narrow band imaging (see page 50) and biopsy suspicious lesions.
    c. Consider performing random bladder biopsies and prostatic urethra biopsies (even in the absence of visible abnormalities).
    d. If the source of the positive marker is not found and it is within 3-6 months of when the positive marker first appeared, then repeat the above process (starting at step "a") in 3 months. If the source of the positive marker is not found and it is longer than 6-12 months from when the positive marker first appeared, then consider performing the evaluation suggested in #4 below.
4. Example evaluation in patients with no history of bladder cancer or a history of bladder cancer treated > 6 months prior.
    a. If a urine tumor marker is positive, but there is no visible tumor in the bladder during white light cystoscopy, then perform upper tract imaging if not done recently (ideally CT urogram). Also, if enhanced cystoscopy technologies are available, perform cystoscopy with blue light or with narrow band imaging (see page 50) and biopsy suspicious lesions.
    b. If step "a" above fails to reveal the source of the positive tumor marker, then perform cystoscopy, bladder wash cytology, random bladder biopsies, and prostatic urethra biopsy (see Prostatic Urethra Biopsies, page 54).
    c. If step "b" above fails to reveal the source of the positive tumor marker, then perform cystoscopy, bladder wash cytology, differential ureteral wash cytology, and repeat random bladder biopsies.
    d. If step "c" above fails to reveal the source of the positive tumor marker then perform bilateral ureteroscopy (ideally with both white light and with narrow band imaging) and bilateral ureter wash cytology. Biopsy suspicious lesions.
    e. If step "d" above fails to reveal the source of the positive tumor marker then consider evaluating the gastrointestinal tract and female reproductive organs.
    f. If step "e" above fails to reveal the source of the positive tumor marker, then perform cystoscopy (consider using blue light or narrow band imaging) and urine tumor marker in 3 months.
    g. If step "f" above fails to reveal the source of the positive tumor marker, consider repeating the above process (starting at step "a") in 3 months.

REFERENCES

Bladder Cancer: 2nd International Consultation on Bladder Cancer. Ed. M Soloway & S Khoury. Plymouth, United Kingdom: Health Publication Ltd., 2012.

Friedrich MG, et al: Comparison of multitarget fluorescence in situ hybridization in urine with other non-invasive tests for detecting bladder cancer. BJU Int, 92(9), 911, 2003.

Schwalb DM, et al: The management of positive urinary cytology in the absence of visible disease. AUA Update Series, Vol. 13, Lesson 36, 1994.

Sharma S, et al: Exclusion criteria enhance the specificity and positive predictive value of NMP22 and BTA stat. J Urol, 162(1): 53, 1999.

PENILE TUMORS

Benign Penile Lesions

Papilloma (Pearly Penile Papules, Hirsute Papilloma)
1. These benign lesions consist of rows of 1 to 2 mm white/yellow papules on the corona of the glans.
2. These lesions do not contain human papilloma virus (HPV).
3. Treatment is usually unnecessary. Laser ablation has been reported.

Condyloma Acuminatum (Genital Warts)
1. Nontender wart-like lesions or papillary frondular lesions.
2. Condyloma acuminatum is a sexually transmitted disease caused by HPV.
3. HPV rarely leads to cervical carcinoma, penile carcinoma, and anal cancer.
4. For details, see Condyloma Acuminatum, page 690.

Zoon's (Plasma Cell) Balanitis
1. Zoon's balanitis is seen on the glans or prepuce of uncircumcised men.
2. Exam reveals an asymptomatic, well-circumscribed, red, flat lesion that contains pinpoint darker red spots ("cayenne pepper spots"). It may look similar to carcinoma in situ. Diagnosis requires biopsy. Histology shows plasma cells in the dermis.
3. Treatment—options include surveillance, topical steroids, circumcision, or CO_2 laser ablation.

Premalignant Penile Lesions

Buschke-Lowenstein Tumor (Giant Condyloma)
1. An exophytic cauliflower-like mass in the genital or anorectal region.
2. It is usually benign (i.e. it does not metastasize), but it can be *locally invasive*. There are rare reports of progression to invasive carcinoma.
3. HPV has been found in these tumors (especially HPV 6 and HPV 11).
4. Treatment—complete excision (it tends to recur after inadequate excision).

Bowenoid Papulosis
1. Presentation—red-brown papules on the glans or shaft. The average age of diagnosis is 20-30 and it usually occurs in circumcised men.
2. HPV is usually identified in these lesions (especially HPV 16).
3. Bowenoid papulosis is generally considered to be benign. However, there have been rare reports of Bowenoid papulosis progressing to invasive cancer (especially in immunosuppressed men); therefore, observation is prudent.
4. Its histologic appearance is similar to carcinoma in situ (CIS).
5. Treatment—options include surveillance, topical 5-fluorouracil (for dose see Carcinoma in Situ, page 120), topical imiquimod 5% cream, excision, and ablation (laser, cryotherapy, cautery).

Characteristic	Bowenoid Papulosis	CIS
Usual Age at diagnosis	20-30	50-60
Usual foreskin status	Circumcised	Uncircumcised
HPV has been detected	Yes	Yes
Risk of Developing SCC	Rare	10%

Carcinoma in Situ (Erythroplasia of Queyrat, Bowen's disease, PIN)
1. Carcinoma in situ (CIS) of the penile shaft is called Bowen's disease, whereas CIS of the foreskin or glans is called Erythroplasia of Queyrat. CIS is also called penile intraepithelial neoplasia (PIN).
2. 10% of men with CIS eventually develop invasive SCC of the penis.
3. HPV has been detected in CIS, especially HPV types 16 and 18.
4. Presentation—asymptomatic red, velvety, well-marginated skin plaques, usually in uncircumcised men age 50-60 years. Rare in circumcised men.
5. Evaluation—biopsy.
6. Treatment options
   a. Topical therapy with 5% 5-fluorouracil (5-FU) or 5% imiquimod—eradicates CIS in ~ 50% of cases. These therapies can cause dermatitis, which may simulate worsening of CIS. If topical therapy fails, it should not be repeated. Doses: 5% 5-fluorouracil topically BID for 2-6 weeks [5% Cream: 25 grams]; Imiquimod 5% cream topically three times per week at night for 4-16 weeks [5% cream: 250 mg single use packets].
   b. Wide local excision—circumcision may be used for lesions confined to the foreskin. Mohs' surgery is best utilized for lesions < 1 cm in size.
   c. Ablation (such as laser or cryotherapy)
   d. Glans resurfacing for lesions confined to the glans.
7. Long-term yearly follow up is required because of the risk of malignancy.

Lichen Sclerosus (Balanitis Xerotica Obliterans)
1. Lichen sclerosus (LS) is now the preferred term for this condition.
2. LS arises from chronic infection, trauma, or inflammation.
3. 2-9% of men with LS develop penile cancer. The mean time from diagnosis of LS to development of penile cancer is 12 years.
4. Presentation—flat white patches (often a mosaic pattern) on the glans and prepuce, sometimes extending to the meatus or fossa navicularis.
   a. Occurs in males (circumcised and uncircumcised) and females.
   b. LS is usually *asymptomatic*. Symptoms may include pruritus, burning, painful erections in males, and dyspareunia in females.
   c. *20% of men with LS have associated meatal and or urethral strictures.*
5. Evaluation—if LS is atypical or progresses rapidly, perform a biopsy to rule out malignancy. Men with obstructive voiding symptoms or LS near the meatus should be evaluated for urethral strictures.
6. Treatment
   a. Asymptomatic LS—no therapy required.
   b. Symptomatic LS—topical steroids relieve itching and burning (e.g. 0.1% triamcinolone acetonide BID topically for up to 2 weeks).
   c. Avoid excision of LS (recurrence rate is high). Phimosis may be treated with circumcision. Treat urethral or meatal strictures accordingly.
7. Long-term yearly follow up is required because of the risk of malignancy.

Leukoplakia
1. Leukoplakia is usually associated with chronic irritation or inflammation.
2. Malignant transformation occurs in 10-20% of cases.
3. Presentation—sharply marginated white scaly plaques, often involving the meatus. Symptoms are irritative in nature.
4. Evaluation—biopsy.
5. Treatment—complete excision and long-term follow up.

Cutaneous Horn
1. A cutaneous horn is a mound of hyperkeratosis, usually on the glans.
2. The cutaneous horn is benign, but up to 33% of these horns arise from underlying malignancy (i.e. SCC is at the base of the horn).
3. Treatment—complete excision with long-term follow up.

Squamous Cell Carcinoma (SCC)

General Information
1. Squamous cell carcinoma (SCC) accounts for $\geq$ 95% of penile cancers.
2. SCC of the penis is rare in the United States. In some regions of Asia and Africa, penile cancer is the most common malignant tumor in men.
3. Female sexual partners of patients with penile cancer do not have a higher risk of cervical cancer.

Risk Factors for Penile Cancer
1. Uncircumcised—*presence of the foreskin is the most important risk factor for penile SCC.* Circumcision in a newborn virtually eliminates the risk of penile cancer. Circumcision before puberty may lower the risk of penile SCC. Men circumcised after puberty have the same risk of penile SCC as uncircumcised men. *Circumcision does not protect against CIS.*
2. Premalignant lesions (see Premalignant Penile Lesions, page 119)
3. Chronic inflammation of the penile skin
4. Phimosis—phimosis may contribute to chronic inflammation, which may increase the risk of penile cancer.
5. Psoralen and ultra violet light type A (PUVA), which is used to treat psoriasis, increases the risk of penile SCC when the penis is not shielded.
6. Tobacco use (includes smoking and chewing tobacco)
7. Human papilloma virus (HPV) infection—*especially types 16 and 18.*
8. The following agents do not increase the risk of penile SCC.
   a. Carcinogens (topical contact)—these increase the risk of scrotal cancer.
   b. Sexually transmitted diseases other than HPV.
   c. Smegma—smegma is not a carcinogen.

Presentation
1. Mean age of presentation = 55-60, but it can occur at any age.
2. The presence of the penile lesion is usually the reason for presentation. The lesion is usually *not* painful, but may have a discharge or foul odor.
3. The lesion may be nodular, ulcerative, fungating, or obscured by phimosis.
4. The common presenting locations (from most to least common) are: glans, prepuce, and shaft. In 30% of cases, multiple penile sites may be involved.
5. Most penile cancers are superficial and low grade.
6. Paraneoplastic syndromes may be present, most commonly *hypercalcemia.*
7. 50% of men present with palpable inguinal lymph nodes (see Inguinal Lymph Node Dissection, page 125).
8. Less than 10% of men present with distant metastasis.
9. Delay in seeking treatment is common. Men often wait longer than a year.

Metastasis
1. The most common site of metastasis is the inguinal lymph nodes (ILNs).
2. Metastatic spread occurs in a stepwise fashion: from the penis to the sentinel node, to other superficial inguinal nodes, to deep inguinal nodes, to pelvic nodes, and then to distant sites.
   a. *The sentinel node is the first lymph node to which the cancer metastasizes. It is usually located in the superior-medial zone of the superficial inguinal node group; however, its position is variable.*
   b. Penis lymphatics do not drain directly to the pelvic nodes. Metastases must travel through the ILN to reach the ipsilateral pelvic nodes. Metastases do not spread from the ILN to the contralateral pelvic nodes.
3. *Penile cancer can spread bilaterally to the inguinal lymph nodes (ILNs) because the penile lymphatics drain to both sides.*
4. Distant metastasis—most to least common: lung, liver, bone, brain. Less than 10% of men present with distant metastasis.

Work Up

1. History and physical exam (especially genitals and inguinal lymph nodes). If the inguinal nodes are difficult to assess on physical exam (e.g. obese patient), then obtain an inguinal and pelvic CT or MRI with IV contrast.
2. Biopsy of the primary lesion—perform a biopsy before treatment (excisional, incisional, or core biopsy).
3. When organ sparing therapy is being considered and invasion of the corpus cavernosum is suspected, penile ultrasound or MRI with gadolinium (with or without an artificial erection) may help determine if invasion is present.
4. For details on evaluation and treatment, see page 128.
5. Biopsy of non-palpable inguinal lymph nodes
   a. Non-dynamic sentinel node biopsy—the biopsy is directed at *the usual anatomic location of the sentinel node (the superior-medial region of the superficial inguinal node group)*. This technique depends on the assumption that the sentinel node resides in the usual location. Since the position of the sentinel node is variable, non-dynamic biopsy frequently misses nodal metastases. In fact, some men have developed extensive metastatic disease despite having a negative non-dynamic sentinel node biopsy. Therefore, *non-dynamic sentinel node biopsy is not recommended because it has a high false negative rate (up to 50%)*.
   b. Dynamic sentinel node biopsy (DSNB)—the biopsy is directed based on functional information that identifies the true location of the sentinel node(s). Technetium-99m labeled nanocolloid and blue dye are injected intradermal around the penile tumor (if it was not excised) or around the scar (if the tumor was excised) 1 day prior to inguinal node dissection. The injected material travels from the tumor, through the lymphatic channels, to the sentinel node(s). Preoperative lymphoscintigraphy, intraoperative hand held gamma ray detection, and intraoperative identification of blue stained lymph tissue helps identify the sentinel nodes, which are excised. When performed correctly, the false negative rate for DSNB is < 15%. This technique should only be performed by centers that have extensive experience (e.g. > 20 procedures per year). *DSNB is an option for men with non-palpable ILNs, but should not be performed in men with palpable ILNs nodes.*
6. Biopsy of palpable inguinal lymph nodes—if the clinician elects to assess the ILNs before node dissection, percutaneous needle biopsy of the palpable node(s) is the preferred initial approach (if necessary, this biopsy can be performed with ultrasound or CT guidance). If the percutaneous needle biopsy is benign, then perform an excisional biopsy of the palpable node (because needle biopsy has a substantial false negative rate).
7. Metastatic evaluation should be performed in patients who have palpable inguinal lymph nodes, who are risk for cancer in the inguinal lymph nodes, or who have proven cancer in the inguinal lymph nodes.
   a. Cross sectional imaging of the chest, abdomen, and pelvis (using CT, MRI, or PET/CT). Chest x-ray is an alternative for imaging the chest.
   b. Blood tests including serum calcium (check for paraneoplastic syndrome) and liver function tests (check for liver metastasis).
8. Obtain a bone scan when the patient has bone pain, elevated calcium, or elevated alkaline phosphatase.

Stage (AJCC 2017)

Primary Tumor (T)

Tx	Primary tumor cannot be assessed
T0	No evidence of primary tumor
Tis	Carcinoma in situ (penile intraepithelial neoplasia)
Ta	Noninvasive localized squamous cell carcinoma
T1	Glans: Tumor invades lamina propria
	Foreskin: Tumor invades dermis, lamina propria, or dartos fascia
	Shaft: Tumor invades connective tissue between epidermis and corpora, regardless of location
T1a	Tumor is without lymphovascular invasion or perineural invasion and is not high grade (i.e. not grade 3 or sarcomatoid)
T1b	Tumor exhibits lymphovascular invasion and/or perineural invasion or is high grade (i.e. Grade 3 or sarcomatoid)
T2	Tumor invades into corpus spongiosum (either glans or ventral shaft) with or without urethral invasion.
T3	Tumor invades into corpora cavernosum (including tunica albuginea) with or without urethral invasion
T4	Tumor invades into adjacent structures (i.e scrotum, prostate, pubic bone)

Regional Lymph Nodes (N) - Clinical Stage

cNx	Regional lymph nodes cannot be assessed
cN0	No palpable or visibly enlarged inguinal lymph nodes
cN1	Palpable mobile unilateral inguinal lymph node
cN2	Palpable mobile ≥ 2 unilateral inguinal nodes or bilateral inguinal lymph nodes
cN3	Palpable fixed inguinal nodal mass or pelvic lymphadenopathy unilateral or bilateral

Regional Lymph Nodes (N) - Pathologic Stage

Pathologic stage is based on biopsy or surgical specimen.

pNx	Lymph node metastasis cannot be assessed
pN0	No lymph node metastasis
pN1	≤ 2 unilateral inguinal metastases, no extranodal extension
pN2	≥ 3 unilateral inguinal metastases or bilateral metastases, no extranodal extension
pN3	Extranodal extension of lymph node metastasis or pelvic lymph node metastases

Distant Metastasis (M)

M0	No distant metastasis
M1	Distant metastasis present

Used with the permission of the American College of Surgeons. Amin, M.B., Edge, S.B., Greene, F.L., et al. (Eds.) AJCC Cancer Staging Manual, 8th Ed. Springer New York, 2017.

Grade

Higher grade implies worse prognosis.

Descriptive Grade	Numerical Grade	Histologic Description
Low grade	Grade 1	Well differentiated
Intermediate Grade	Grade 2	Moderately differentiated
High Grade	Grade 3	Poorly differentiated, undifferentiated, or sarcomatoid

Pathologic Variants of Penile SCC
1. Classic (usual)—the most common variant.
2. Verrucous—this tumor can be locally invasive, but it does not metastasize. Therefore, it has an excellent prognosis.
3. HPV is commonly found in the basaloid and warty variants, but is uncommon in the verrucous and papillary variants.
4. Sarcomatoid—*very aggressive and has a poor prognosis. Most men die within 1 year of diagnosis.*
5. Other variants include warty (condylomatous), papillary, basaloid, and adenosquamous.

Type of Penile SCC	Cancer Specific Mortality	Risk of ILN Metastasis at Initial Presentation
Verrucous	Very low	None
Papillary	Low	Low
Warty (Condylomatous)	Low	Low
Adenosquamous	Low	Intermediate to High
Classic (usual)	Intermediate	Low to Intermediate
Basaloid	Intermediate	Intermediate
Sarcomatoid	Very High	High

SCC = squamous cell carcinoma; ILN = Inguinal lymph node

Treatment of Penile SCC

For details on evaluation and treatment, see page 128.

Size of Negative Surgical Margin
1. For excision of the primary tumor, a 2 cm tumor-free margin was recommended in the past, but a 5 mm tumor-free margin is now considered safe.
2. For cases of high grade or high T stage, the clinician may consider increasing the size of the margin to 8 to 10 mm.

Penectomy
1. Partial penectomy
   a. Partial penectomy is indicated for tumors confined to the glans, prepuce, or distal shaft.
   b. Partial penectomy removes the distal penis, including the glans, the distal corpora, and the distal urethra. Try to leave 2-3 cm of penile length because this permits the patient to
      • Maintain some degree of sexual function.
      • Void in a standing position ("upright voiding").
   c. The urethral stump is used to create a new meatus at the end of the penis
   d. Local recurrence after partial penectomy is 4%.
2. Total penectomy
   a. Total penectomy is indicated for invasive tumors of the proximal shaft.
   b. Total penectomy removes all of the penis distal to the pubic bone.
   c. The urethral stump is diverted to the perineum (perineal urethrostomy) so the patient must void in a sitting position.
3. Advanced disease may require more extensive resection including removal of the scrotum, perineum, or entire corpus cavernosum.
4. Stenosis of the new meatus occurs in up to 10% of cases, but the stenosis rate can be minimized by spatulating the urethra.
5. Intraoperative frozen sections are recommended to achieve negative margins.

Glansectomy

1. Glansectomy removes all or some of the glans while leaving the corpora intact (whereas partial penectomy removes the distal corpora). Partial or complete glansectomy may be performed based on the tumor size and location.
2. Compared to partial penectomy, glansectomy is more likely to maintain upright voiding and more likely to preserve sexual function.
3. Glansectomy is typically utilized in men with Ta, T1, or T2 tumors that are confined to the glans.

Penile Sparing Therapy

1. Penile sparing therapies may be indicated in men who have any of the following characteristics.
   a. Men who refuse or who are unfit for penectomy or glansectomy.
   b. Men who want to preserve sexual function and penile anatomy.
   c. Men who have carcinoma in situ (Tis) or low grade Ta or T1 tumors.
2. *Penile sparing therapy has a higher local recurrence rate than partial penectomy, but these therapies appear to achieve comparable cancer specific survival in appropriately selected patients.*
3. Before penile sparing therapy, biopsy of the primary tumor is mandatory to confirm the presence of cancer.
4. Penile sparing therapies include
   a. Circumcision—reserved for lesions confined to the foreskin.
   b. Wedge resection—if tension free closure is not possible, use a skin graft.
   c. Mohs' surgery—removal of tumor layer by layer under microscopic control until negative margins are obtained. This is best utilized for lesions < 1 cm in diameter. Local recurrence rate is 30%.
   d. Laser ablation or laser excision—the neodymium:YAG, carbon dioxide, or KTP lasers are typically used. Local recurrence rate is 20%.
   e. Glans resurfacing—abrasive removal of the glans epithelium followed by a split thickness skin graft or buccal graft to cover the glans.
   f. Topical therapy (5-FU or imiquimod)—used mainly for CIS or stage Ta (see page 120). Local recurrence rate is 50%.
   g. Radiation—mainly used for men with stage T1 or T3 tumors < 4 cm in greatest dimension.
      i. Radiation has a higher local recurrence rate than partial or total penectomy.
      ii. Recurrence rate after radiation is higher when the cancer is ≥ 4 cm in size (i.e radiation is less effective for tumors ≥ 4 cm in size).
      iii. For stage T1 or T2 tumors that are < 4 cm in size, treatment options include brachytherapy alone, external beam radiation (XRT) alone, or XRT with systemic chemotherapy.
      iv. For tumors ≥ 4 cm in size or stage T3, XRT is administered with systemic chemotherapy.
      v. Side effects of radiation therapy include meatal or urethral stenosis (20-35%), glans necrosis (10-20%), and corporal fibrosis.
      vi. *Circumcision should be performed before radiation therapy to prevent radiation induced phimosis.*

Inguinal Lymph Node Dissection (ILND)

1. Men with non-palpable inguinal lymph nodes (ILNs) at presentation—25% will have ILN metastases. *ILND when men have non-palpable nodes ("early ILND") achieves longer survival than delaying ILND until men have recurrence with palpable nodes ("late ILND").* Thus, "early ILND" is recommended in men who have non-palpable inguinal nodes and risk factors for ILN metastases.

2. Primary tumor characteristics that are risk factors for ILN metastasis:
   a. Stage T1b or greater
   b. High grade (especially when the tumor is > 50% poorly differentiated)
   c. Lymphovascular invasion
3. Men with palpable inguinal nodes at presentation—50% have adenopathy from inflammation and 50% have adenopathy from metastasis. In the past, these men were given 6 weeks of antibiotics to differentiate inflammatory adenopathy from malignant adenopathy (node metastases were likely if adenopathy persisted after antibiotics). However, *immediate biopsy of the palpable inguinal nodes (preferably by percutaneous needle biopsy) is now the favored diagnostic approach.*
4. After treatment of the primary cancer, the development of palpable inguinal lymph nodes during follow up is usually caused by cancer.
5. For patients unwilling or unable to undergo ILND, external beam radiation can be delivered to the inguinal nodes.
6. Inguinal anatomy
   a. *The femoral vessels and the deep inguinal lymph nodes are found in the femoral triangle*, which is bounded by the sartorius laterally, the inguinal ligament superiorly, and the adductor longus medially. Progressing lateral to medial (toward the navel), structures in the femoral triangle are represented by "N(AVEL)". N = femoral Nerve; A = femoral Artery; V = femoral Vein; E = Empty space; L = deep inguinal Lymph nodes; structures in parenthesis are within the femoral sheath. The anterior surface of the femoral triangle is covered by fascia lata.
   b. *The fascia lata separates the superficial and deep inguinal lymph nodes.*
   c. Superficial inguinal lymph nodes—these nodes are superficial to the fascia lata and are divided into 5 zones (see diagram below).
   d. Deep inguinal lymph nodes—the deep inguinal nodes are deep to the fascia lata and are located medial to the femoral vein in the femoral triangle [see "N(AVEL)" description above]. The node of Cloquet is the most cephalad node in the deep inguinal region.
   e. The saphenous vein branches from the femoral vein in the deep inguinal region. Then, it passes anteriorly through an oval opening in the fascia lata (the fossa ovalis) and continues into the superficial inguinal region.
7. During ILND, inguinal skin flaps are developed *deep to Scarpa's fascia.* Some surgeons recommend that lymphatic vessels be ligated rather than cauterized or clipped. Gentle tissue handling helps prevent skin necrosis.
8. Complications of ILND include lymphocele, wound infection, skin flap necrosis, and lower extremity edema. Postoperative compression stockings and prophylactic antibiotics may help prevent complications.

Zonal Anatomy of the Superficial Inguinal Lymph Nodes (Daseler's Zones)

SL = superior lateral zone
SM = superior medial zone*
C   = central zone
IL   = inferior lateral zone
IM = inferior medial zone

* The sentinel lymph node
  is usually found in the
  superior medial zone.

- Femoral Artery
- Femoral Vein
- Inguinal Ligament
- Saphenous Vein

Standard Template ILND (Radical ILND or Full Template ILND)

1. Superficial node dissection—*nodes in all 5 superficial zones are removed.*
   The limits of the superficial dissection are
   a. Superior limit = external oblique fascia at level of spermatic cord.
   b. Lateral limit = a sagittal plane through the anterior superior iliac spine (ASIS).
   c. Medial limit = a sagittal plane through the ipsilateral pubic tubercle.
   d. Inferior limit = a transverse plane 20 cm inferior to the ASIS.
2. Deep node dissection—the deep inguinal nodes are removed from the femoral triangle, avoiding dissection lateral to the femoral artery (which avoids injury to the femoral nerve and profunda femoris artery).
3. During radical ILND, the saphenous vein is ligated where is arises from the femoral vein and where it passes through the fossa ovalis. Then, the vein segment between the ligatures is removed.
4. *A sartorius muscle flap is utilized to cover the femoral vessels after radical ILND because it reduces the incidence of hemorrhage from the femoral vessels.* The origin of the sartorius is mobilized from the anterior superior iliac spine, moved medial to cover the femoral vessels, and then sutured to the ilioinguinal ligament.

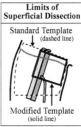

Limits of Superficial Dissection

Standard Template (dashed line)

Modified Template (solid line)

Modified Template ILND

1. Compared to the standard ILND, the modified ILND consists of
   a. A shorter skin incision.
   b. The area of the superficial dissection is smaller (the lateral and inferior limits are different from the standard template).
   c. Preservation of the saphenous vein.
   d. No sartorius muscle flap to cover the femoral vessels.
2. Superficial node dissection—*nodes in the central zone, superior medial zone, and the medial portion of the superior lateral zone are removed, but nodes in the inferior zones (which are inferior to the fossa ovalis) are not removed.* The limits of the superficial dissection are
   • Lateral limit = lateral edge of femoral artery.
   • Inferior limit = the fossa ovalis where the saphenous vein penetrates the fascia lata (no dissection of the inferior zones).
   • Superior limit and medial limit = same as for standard template ILND.
3. Deep node dissection—the deep inguinal nodes are removed from the femoral triangle, avoiding dissection lateral to the femoral artery.
4. Some urologists perform a "superficial" modified template ILND, which omits removal of the deep inguinal nodes because studies have shown that metastases to the deep inguinal nodes are unlikely if there is no cancer in the superficial nodes. However, the original modified ILND described by Catalona in 1988 includes removal of the deep inguinal nodes.
5. *Compared to standard ILND, modified ILND removes fewer inguinal nodes and has a higher false negative rate (0% versus $\leq 5.5\%$).*
6. *Modified ILND has a lower complication rate than standard ILND.*
7. *The modified ILND is utilized in men whose inguinal nodes are not palpable.* When cancer is found in the inguinal nodes during modified ILND, convert to a standard (radical) ILND.

Management of Squamous Cell Carcinoma of the Penis

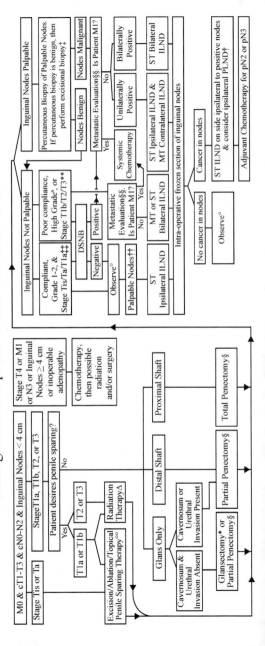

DSNB = Dynamic Sentinel Node Biopsy; MT = Modified Template; ST = Standard Template (radical); ILND = Inguinal Lymph Node Dissection; PLND = Pelvic Lymph Node Dissection; LVI = Lymphovascular Invasion; XRT = External Beam Radiation

a High grade includes grade 3 and sarcomatoid.

* Partial glansectomy may be considered in patients with stage T1a cancer.

† Consider ipsilateral PLND when cancer in the inguinal nodes has any of the following: ≥ 2 positive nodes, high grade, extranodal extension, or positive node of Cloquet.

§ For penectomy, a negative margin of 5 mm appears to be safe.

‡ If percutaneous biopsy is negative, then excisional biopsy of the palpable node is performed. If the percutaneous or excisional biopsy shows cancer, then perform ILND.

†† Lymph node metastases that appear after treatment of the primary tumor usually develop within 2-3 years postoperatively. Percutaneous or excisional biopsy can be performed to confirm the presence of cancer before proceeding to ILND.

‡‡ The risk of inguinal lymph node metastasis is < 10% in men with *all* of the following criteria: lower stage (Tis, Ta, or T1a), low grade, and LVI absent.

** The risk of inguinal lymph node metastasis is > 50% in men with *any* of the following criteria: higher stage (T2 or T3), high grade, or LVI present (T1b).

§§ Metastatic evaluation includes cross sectional imaging of the chest, abdomen, & pelvis using CT, MRI, or PET/CT. For chest imaging, chest x-ray may be used instead.

Δ Radiation has a higher risk of local recurrence than partial or total penectomy. For stage T1 or T2 tumors that are < 4 cm in size, treatment options include brachytherapy alone, external beam radiation (XRT) alone, or XRT with systemic chemotherapy. For tumors ≥ 4 cm in size or stage T3, the preferred treatment is XRT with systemic chemotherapy. Perform circumcision before radiation therapy to prevent radiation induced phimosis.

○ Follow with genital examination and inguinal node examination every 1-2 months for at least 2 years, then less often thereafter.

○○ When utilizing penile sparing therapy, pathological assessment of the lesion is mandatory, preferably by excisional biopsy. When excisional biopsy is performed, deep and radial surgical margins should be assessed. See the table below for penile sparing treatment options.

Penile sparing options for stage Tis and Ta	Penile sparing options for stage T1a	Penile sparing options for stage T1a	Penile sparing options for stage T1b
• Topical 5-fluorouracil (see page 120) or 5% imiquimod (see page 692).	• Radiation—see Δ above.	• Radiation—see Δ above.	• Radiation—see Δ above.
• Wide local excision—circumcision alone may be used for lesions confined to the foreskin.	• Wide local excision—circumcision alone may be used for lesions confined to the foreskin.	• Wide local excision—circumcision alone may be used for lesions confined to the foreskin.	• Wide local excision—circumcision alone may be used for lesions confined to the foreskin.
• Mohs' surgery—mainly for lesions < 1 cm in size.	• Mohs' surgery—mainly for lesions < 1 cm in size.	• Mohs' surgery—mainly for lesions < 1 cm in size.	• Glansectomy—for lesions confined to the glans.
• Laser excision/ablation	• Laser excision/ablation	• Laser excision/ablation	
• Glans resurfacing—for lesions confined to the glans.	• Glans resurfacing—for lesions confined to the glans.	• Glans resurfacing—for lesions confined to the glans.	
• Glansectomy—for lesions confined to the glans.	• Glansectomy—for lesions confined to the glans.	• Glansectomy—for lesions confined to the glans.	

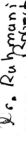

Pelvic Lymph Node Dissection (PLND)
1. Penis lymphatics do not drain directly to the pelvic nodes. Inguinal lymph node (ILN) metastases must be present before cancer can reach the pelvic nodes. It appears that metastases are unlikely to spread from the ILNs to the contralateral pelvic lymph nodes. However, one study suggested ≥ 4 inguinal lymph node metastases may support performing bilateral PLND.
2. Consider performing ipsilateral PLND in men any of the following characteristics: ≥ 2 inguinal ipsilateral node metastases, metastasis in the ipsilateral node of Cloquet, tumor extension through the capsule of the inguinal lymph nodes (pN3), presence of high grade tumor in the involved nodes, or imaging suggests suspicious pelvic nodes.
3. If metastasis are present in ≥ 4 inguinal nodes (total among both sides), consider performing bilateral PLND.

Systemic Chemotherapy
1. In men with ≥ 3 positive lymph node found at ILND (e.g. pN2 or pN3), adjuvant chemotherapy improves survival.
2. Chemotherapy may be used when the primary tumor or inguinal node metastases are unresectable: e.g. stage T4 or fixed inguinal nodes (cN3). Chemotherapy may shrink the tumor enough to permit excision.
3. *Chemotherapy regimens should include cisplatin.* Regimens include:
   a. Paclitaxel, ifosfamide, and cisplatin (TIP)—this is the preferred regimen for neoadjuvant treatment before node dissection, adjuvant treatment after node dissection, and for distant metastatic disease.
   b. 5-FU and cisplatin.
4. Bleomycin based regimens are no longer recommended because of unacceptable toxicity.

Follow Up and Survival for Penile SCC

Follow Up
1. Most recurrences occur within 2 years of treatment; therefore, intensive follow up is conducted for the first 2 years after therapy, with less intensive follow up thereafter.
2. Follow up should include
   a. Patient self examination of the penis and inguinal nodes.
   b. Examination by a physician, including penis and inguinal nodes.
   c. After ILND, perform chest imaging and abdominal/pelvic CT or MRI.

Prognosis and Survival
1. *Men with invasion of the corpus spongiosum (pT2) have a better prognosis than men with invasion of the corpus cavernosum (pT3).*
2. The following tumor characteristics are indicators of poor prognosis.
   a. Higher primary tumor stage
   b. Higher tumor grade
   c. Perineural invasion
   d. Basaloid or sarcomatoid histology
   e. More extensive lymph node involvement—*the most important determinant of survival in men with penile SCC is the extent of lymph node metastasis.*
3. Prognosis is significantly worse when the lymph node metastases have any of the following characteristics.
   a. More than 2 inguinal lymph node metastases.
   b. Bilateral inguinal node metastases.
   c. Pelvic lymph node metastasis.
   d. Extension of tumor through the capsule of a lymph node.

2017 AJCC Node Stage	Mean 5-year Overall Survival (range)	
pN0	80%	(74-100%)
pN1 with only 1 node metastasis (superficial inguinal)	81%	(75-82%)
pN2 (superficial inguinal)	50%	(17-80%)
pN2 (deep inguinal)	29%	(17-40%)
pN3 (pelvic)	< 10%%	(0-38%)

REFERENCES

Djajadiningrat RS, et al: Penile sparing surgery for penile cancer–does it affect survival? J Urol, 192(1): 120, 2014.

EAU—Hakenberg OW, et al: Guidelines on penile cancer. European Association of Urology, 2020. (www.uroweb.org).

ICUD—International Consultation on Urologic Diseases: 1st ICUD-SIU consultation on penile cancer. Ed. A Pompeo. Urology, 76(2A), 2010.

Leijte JA, et al: Recurrence patterns of squamous cell carcinoma of the penis: recommendations for follow up based on a two center analysis of 700 patients. Eur Urol, 54: 161, 2008.

NCCN—National Comprehensive Cancer Network clinical practice guidelines in oncology: Penile Cancer. V.1.2021, 2021. (www.nccn.org).

Types of SCC

Bezerra AL, et al: Clinicopathological features and human papillomavirus NDA prevalence of warty and squamous cell carcinoma of the penis. Am J Surg Pathol, 25(5): 673, 2001.

Cubilla AL, et al: Histologic classification of penile carcinoma and its relation to outcome in 61 patients with primary resection. Int J Surg Pathol, 9: 111, 2001.

Dai B, et al: Predicting regional lymph node metastasis in Chinese patients with penile squamous cell carcinoma: the role of histopathological classification, tumor stage, and depth of invasion. J Urol, 176(4, part 1): 1431, 2006.

Guimaraes G, et al: Penile squamous cell carcinoma clinicopathological features, nodal metastasis and outcome in 333 cases. J Urol, 182(2): 528, 2009.

Lymph Node Dissection

Catalona, WJ: Modified inguinal lymphadenectomy for carcinoma of the penis with preservation of the saphenous veins: technique and preliminary results. J Urol, 140(2): 306, 1988.

Ficarra V, et al: Nomogram predictive of pathological inguinal lymph node involvement in patients with squamous cell carcinoma of the penis. J Urol, 175(5); 1700, 2006.

Lont, AP, et al: Pelvic lymph node dissection for penile carcinoma: extent of inguinal lymph node involvement as an indicator for pelvic lymph node involvement and survival. J Urol, 177(3): 947, 2007.

Pettaway CA, Pagliaro L: Penile squamous carcinoma: Part II - contemporary management of the inguinal region. AUA Update Series, Vol. 31, Lesson 16, 2012.

Protzel C, et al: Lymphadenectomy in the surgical management of penile cancer. Eur Urol, 55: 1075, 2009.

Srinivas V, Morse MJ, Herr HW, et al: Penile cancer: relation of extent of nodal metastasis to survival. J Urol, 137: 880, 1987.

TESTICULAR TUMORS

General Information

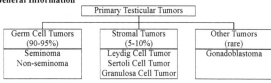

1. Typical (classic) seminoma is
   a. The most common testis tumor in adults. ✔
   b. The most common tumor in an undescended testis. ✔
2. Malignant lymphoma is
   a. The most common *bilateral* testis tumor (when primary and metastatic tumors are included).
   b. *The most common metastatic tumor of the testis.*
   c. The most common testis tumor in men > 50 years old.
3. Yolk sac tumor—the most common testis cancer in infants and children.
4. Leydig cell tumor—the most common non-germ cell tumor.
5. Gonadoblastoma—the most common testis tumor in patients with intersex.
6. Mixed tumors are more common than pure tumors.
7. Only 1% of testis tumors in adults are benign.

Risk Factors for Testis Cancer

1. Cryptorchidism—the higher the testis location, the higher the risk of cancer. The highest risk occurs with an intra-abdominal testes. *Cryptorchidism is more common on the right; thus, testis tumors are more common on the right.* In males with unilateral cryptorchidism, the contralateral descended testis has a slight increased risk of tumor.
2. HIV infection—increases the risk of developing testis cancer.
3. Gonadal dysgenesis with Y chromosome (testicular dysgenesis)—20-30% develop testicular tumors (usually gonadoblastomas). These patients should undergo prophylactic gonadectomy.
4. Testicular feminization > 30 years of age—the testes are removed after secondary sexual characteristics develop.
5. Presence of intratubular germ cell neoplasia.
6. Family history of testis cancer in a father or brother.
7. Personal history of testis cancer—*the cumulative risk of malignancy in the remaining testicle is 2-5% by 15 years after orchiectomy.*
8. Infertility—men with infertility are 2.8 times more likely to develop testis cancer than the general male population.
9. Klinefelter's syndrome—the patient's have an increased risk of extra-gonadal (mediastinal) germ cell cancer.
10. CHEK2 mutation—men with this mutation appear to be 4 times more likely to develop testis cancer.
11. Conditions that do not increase the risk of testicular cancer.
    a. Testis atrophy
    b. Trauma is *not* a cause of tumor, but often prompts medical evaluation.
    c. Testicular microlithiasis in the absence of a solid mass and in the absence other risk factors for testis cancer (see page 133).

Testicular Microlithiasis

1. In the past, there was concern that testicular microlithiasis may increase the risk of testis cancer. However, more recent data indicates that testicular microlithiasis does not increase the risk of testis cancer when there is no solid testis mass and no other risk factors for testis cancer (for risk factors see page 132).
2. Testicular microlithiasis without a concomitant solid testis mass
   a. The AUA 2019 guidelines states that testicular microlithiasis in men with no solid testis mass and no risk factors for testis cancer does not require further evaluation.
   b. For men with testicular microlithiasis (but no solid testis mass) and at least one risk for testis cancer, the AUA 2019 guideline recommends counselling the patient about the potential increased risk of testis cancer, and monitoring the patient with periodic self testis examination and follow up with a medical professional. The AUA did not specify what the medical follow up should consist of; however, it should include a testis exam. Follow up testicular ultrasound may be considered.
3. Testicular microlithiasis with a concomitant solid testis mass—these patients are assumed to have testis malignancy.

Presentation

1. Testis tumors are more common on the right because cryptorchidism is more common on the right.
2. *Most tumors present with a painless mass or swelling in the testis.* Exam typically reveals a firm, non-tender testis mass. Testicular pain occurs in only 10% of men with testis tumors and is probably caused by hemorrhage or infarction of the tumor.

Type of Testicular Tumor	Usual Age of Onset
Yolk sac tumor	0-10
Choriocarcinoma	20-30
Embryonal & teratoma	25-35
Classic Seminoma	30-40
Malignant lymphoma	> 50

3. 5-10% of testis cancers present with a hydrocele, which may obscure the tumor.
4. Gynecomastia occurs in 5% of men with germ cell cancers and in 30-50% of men with Sertoli or Leydig tumors.
5. Back pain or abdominal mass can occur with bulky retroperitoneal metastases. The presence of a metastasis at diagnosis is more likely with nonseminoma than with pure seminoma.
6. Bilateral testis tumors
   a. 1-3% of tumors are bilateral (including synchronous and metachronous).
   b. Lymphoma is the most common cause of bilateral testis tumors.

Metastasis From Testis Tumors

1. Testis tumors usually metastasize by lymphatic spread. Choriocarcinoma and yolk sac tumor may also metastasize hematogenously.
2. *Retroperitoneal lymph nodes are the most common site of metastasis.* The retroperitoneal nodes that are used to determine N stage (i.e. the regional nodes) include pre-aortic, para-aortic, retro-aortic, interaortocaval, pre-caval, para-caval, retro-caval, and nodes along the spermatic vein. Pelvic and inguinal nodes are not considered regional unless there was scrotal violation.
3. When the normal lymphatic flow from the testicle has *not* been altered, lymphatic spread occurs in a predictable and stepwise pattern.
   a. Right testis tumors spread to the *interaortocaval* retroperitoneal nodes.
   b. Left testis tumors spread to the *left para-aortic* retroperitoneal nodes.
   c. *Lymphatic metastases often spread from the right to the left retroperitoneum, but they usually do not spread from left to right.*

4. When the normal lymphatic flow from the testicle has been altered, lymphatic metastases may not follow the usual pattern.
   a. Metastasis to the inguinal nodes may occur when
      i. The tumor invades through the tunica vaginalis or into the scrotum.
      ii. There was previous scrotal or inguinal surgery (e.g. inguinal hernia repair, orchiopexy, trans-scrotal orchiectomy, trans-scrotal biopsy).
   b. Metastasis to the pelvic nodes may occur when the tumor invades into the epididymis or spermatic cord.
5. Distant non-node metastasis (most to least common)—lung, liver, brain, bone, kidney, adrenal, gastrointestinal tract, and spleen.
6. Spermatocytic seminoma has a very low metastatic potential.
7. Choriocarcinoma can present with distant metastasis in the presence of a small (sometimes clinically inapparent) primary testis tumor.

Work Up
1. History and physical exam including genitals, lymph nodes, abdomen, neurological, and breasts (check for gynecomastia).
2. Scrotal ultrasound with Doppler—both testes should be visualized with grey scale images and with Doppler.
   a. Most testis tumors are solid, heterogeneous, and hypoechoic on grey scale images and are vascular on Doppler images.
   b. *An intra-testicular lesion with solid elements is highly suspicious for testis cancer. All solid testis masses should be managed as malignancy unless further evaluation confirms a benign process.*
3. When malignancy is suspected, obtain the following tests before treatment: serum tumor markers (AFP, quantitative B-HCG, LDH), liver function tests (check for liver metastasis and hepatic causes of elevated AFP), CBC, and creatinine.
4. If the serum tumor markers are normal, but the testicular ultrasound and/or physical exam are inconclusive for solid tumor, then the scrotal ultrasound and physical exam should be repeated in 6 to 8 weeks. When repeat ultrasound is still inconclusive for tumor or when there is suspicion of a benign lesion, then multiparametric testicle MRI with Gadolinium may be helpful. However, testicle MRI should not be used routinely for evaluation.
5. See Initial Management of a Testicular Mass, page 155.

Stage for Germ Cell Tumors

TNM Staging System (AJCC 2017)
Primary Tumor (T) - Clinical Stage—clinical stage is based on biopsy for pTis and based on imaging and/or physical exam for cT4.
   cTx Primary tumor cannot be assessed
   cT0 No evidence of primary tumor
   cTis Germ cell neoplasia in situ
   cT4 Tumor invades scrotum with or without vascular/lymphatic invasion

<u>Primary Tumor (T) - Pathologic Stage</u>—pathological stage is based on radical orchiectomy.

pTx Primary tumor cannot be assessed

pT0 No evidence of primary tumor

pTis Germ cell neoplasia in situ

pT1 Tumor limited to the testis (including rete testis invasion) without lymphovascular invasion

Subclassification of pT1 applies only to pure seminoma:

T1a Tumor smaller than 3 cm in size

T1b Tumor 3 cm or larger in size

pT2 Tumor limited to the testis (including rete testis invasion) with lymphovascular invasion;

Tumor invading hilar soft tissue or epididymis or penetrating visceral mesothelial layer covering the external surface of the tunica albuginea with or without lymphovascular invasion

pT3 Tumor directly invades spermatic cord soft tissue with or without lymphovascular invasion

pT4 Tumor invades scrotum with or without lymphovascular invasion

<u>Regional Lymph Nodes (N) - Clinical Stage</u>

Nx Regional lymph nodes cannot be assessed

N0 No regional lymph node metastasis

N1 Metastasis with a lymph node mass 2 cm or smaller in greatest dimension; or

Multiple lymph nodes, none larger than 2 cm in greatest dimension

N2 Metastasis with a lymph node mass larger than 2 cm but not larger than 5 cm in greatest dimension; or

Multiple lymph nodes, any one mass larger than 2 cm but not larger than 5 cm in greatest dimension

N3 Metastasis with a lymph node mass larger than 5 cm in greatest dimension

<u>Regional Lymph Nodes (N) - Pathologic Stage</u>

pNx Regional lymph nodes cannot be assessed

pN0 No regional lymph node metastasis

pN1 Metastasis with a lymph node mass 2 cm or smaller in greatest dimension and less than or equal to 5 nodes positive, none larger than 2 cm in greatest dimension

pN2 Metastasis with a lymph node mass larger than 2 cm but not larger than 5 cm in greatest dimension; or more than 5 nodes positive, none larger than 5 cm; or evidence of extranodal extension of tumor

pN3 Metastasis with a lymph node mass larger than 5 cm in greatest dimension

<u>Distant Metastasis (M)</u>

M0 No distant metastases

M1 Distant metastases

M1a Non-retroperitoneal nodal or pulmonary metastases

M1b Non-pulmonary visceral metastases

> Used with the permission of the American College of Surgeons. Amin, M.B., Edge, S.B., Greene, F.L., et al. (Eds.) AJCC Cancer Staging Manual, 8th Ed. Springer New York, 2017.

<u>Serum Tumor Markers (S)</u> - *S stage is determined using the nadir value of the post-orchiectomy tumor markers.* N = upper limit of normal for LDH.

	LDH		HCG (mIu/ml)		AFP (ng/ml)
S0	Normal	&	Normal	&	Normal
S1	< 1.5 x N	&	< 5,000	&	< 1,000
S2	1.5-10 x N	or	5,000-50,000	or	1,000-10,000
S3	> 10 x N	or	> 50,000	or	> 10,000
Sx	Marker studies not available or not performed				

Stage Grouping

Stage 0	pTis	N0	M0	S0
Stage I	pT1-4	N0	M0	Sx
IA	pT1	N0	M0	S0
IB	pT2	N0	M0	S0
	pT3	N0	M0	S0
	pT4	N0	M0	S0
IS	Any pT/Tx	N0	M0	S1-3
Stage II	Any pT/Tx	N1-3	M0	Sx
IIA	Any pT/Tx	N1	M0	S0
	Any pT/Tx	N1	M0	S1
IIB	Any pT/Tx	N2	M0	S0
	Any pT/Tx	N2	M0	S1
IIC	Any pT/Tx	N3	M0	S0
	Any pT/Tx	N3	M0	S1
Stage III	Any pT/Tx	Any N	M1	Sx
IIIA	Any pT/Tx	Any N	M1a	S0
	Any pT/Tx	Any N	M1a	S1
IIIB	Any pT/Tx	N1-3	M0	S2
	Any pT/Tx	Any N	M1a	S2
IIIC	Any pT/Tx	N1-3	M0	S3
	Any pT/Tx	Any N	M1a	S3
	Any pT/Tx	Any N	M1b	Any S

Used with the permission of the American College of Surgeons. Amin, M.B., Edge, S.B., Greene, F.L., et al. (Eds.) AJCC Cancer Staging Manual, 8th Ed. Springer New York, 2017.

IGCCCG Risk Categories for Stage IIC and Stage III Germ Cell Tumors

Risk Status	Nonseminoma	Seminoma
Good Risk	All of the following: • Testicular or retroperitoneal primary tumor • M0 or M1a • S0 or S1*	All of the following: • Any primary site • M0 or M1a • Normal AFP
Intermediate Risk	All of the following: • Testicular or retroperitoneal primary tumor • M0 or M1a • S2*	All of the following: • Any primary site • M1b • Normal AFP
Poor Risk	Any of the following: • Mediastinal primary tumor • M1b • S3*	No patients are classified as poor risk

From J Clin Oncol, 15(2): 594, 1997 (the International Germ Cell Consensus Collaborative Group). For survival based on these risk groups, see page 153.
* For IGCCCG risk, S stage is determined on the first day of chemotherapy.

CT Scan of Abdomen and Pelvis
1. CT cannot differentiate between cancer, teratoma, necrosis, or fibrosis.
2. Abdominal CT has a 30% false negative rate (i.e. up to 30% of men with a normal abdominal CT will have tumor in the retroperitoneal nodes). Therefore, CT accurately stages approximately 70% of patients.
3. For initial staging, CT of the abdomen and pelvis should be performed with oral and intravenous contrast (if no contraindication exists).
4. If the abdominal CT shows tumor, obtain a chest CT.

Serum Tumor Markers

1. Tumor markers are measured before and after orchiectomy; however, *S stage is determined using the nadir value of the post-orchiectomy tumor markers.*

Tumor Marker	Half-life (days)
B-HCG	1-3
AFP	5-7
LDH-1	4.0-4.5

2. Beta-human chorionic gonadotropin (B-HCG)
   a. B-HCG is produced by syncytiotrophoblasts.
   b. *B-HCG is always elevated when choriocarcinoma is present.*
   c. Elevation of B-HCG can also occur with
      i. Marijuana use.
      ii. Hypergonadotropic hypogonadism (see page 538)—high levels of LH can cross react with some assays for HCG, resulting in a falsely high B-HCG.
      iii. Other cancers—liver, biliary, pancreatic, gastric, lung cancer, etc.
      iv. Hyperthyroidism
      v. Antibodies that interfere with an HCG assay (heterophile antibodies).
3. Alpha-fetoprotein (AFP)
   a. *AFP is never elevated in pure choriocarcinoma or in pure seminoma.*
   b. Elevation of AFP can also occur with
      i. Infants < 1 year old—it is normal for newborns to have elevated AFP, which usually declines to the low adult levels by one year of age.
      ii. Liver dysfunction—hepatitis, cirrhosis, etc.
      iii. Other cancers—liver, biliary, pancreatic, gastric, and lung cancer.
      iv. A portion of the male population has AFP levels up to 25 ng/ml in the absence of an abnormality (normal AFP is usually less than 8 ng/ml). *When AFP level is above the normal cut off, but is less than 25 ng/ml and relatively stable, this finding is usually not from testis cancer.*
      v. Other rare causes—ataxia telangiectasia, hereditary tyrosinemia, hereditary persistence of AFP, and antibodies that interfere with the AFP assay (heterophile antibodies).
4. Lactate dehydrogenase (LDH)
   a. The predominant LDH isoenzyme in testis cancer is LDH-1, but total LDH is usually measured because the other isoenzymes are negligible.
   b. LDH may be elevated in seminoma or nonseminoma.
   c. The magnitude of LDH elevation correlates with the volume of cancer.
   d. Elevation of LDH can occur with many other conditions, including liver disease, heart disease, kidney disease, other cancers, certain types of anemia, certain infections, skeletal muscle injury, etc.
   e. LDH is a less specific marker for testis cancer than B-HCG and AFP; therefore, *treatment decisions should not be made based on a mild elevation of LDH (e.g. < 3 times the upper limit of normal) when the B-HCG and AFP are normal.*

Gonadal Stromal Tumors

Granulosa Cell Tumors

1. Granulosa cell tumor is a rare benign tumor that usually occurs in the neonatal period. 75% are diagnosed within 1 month of birth.
2. Orchiectomy is curative.

Sertoli Cell Tumors

1. 10% of Sertoli cell tumors are malignant. The only reliable indicator of malignancy is the presence of metastasis.
2. Sertoli cell tumors may secrete estrogen or testosterone.
3. Presentation–painless testis mass. Virilization or gynecomastia may occur.
4. Treatment—non-metastatic Sertoli cell tumors are treated with orchiectomy followed by surveillance.

Leydig Cell Tumors
1. 10% of Leydig cell tumors are malignant. The only reliable indicator of malignancy is the presence of metastasis.
2. Histology—eosinophilic cells, extracellular *Reinke's crystals* (cigar shaped or lobular shaped red crystals).
3. Leydig cell tumors may produce testosterone and 17-ketosteroid.
4. Presentation—children usually present with precocious puberty (e.g. virilizing features such as pubic hair, masculine voice, and prominent external genitals). Adults often present with impotence, low libido, and feminizing features such as gynecomastia. Klinefelter's syndrome, adrenal cancer, and congenital adrenal hyperplasia may cause similar symptoms.
5. Treatment—non-metastatic Leydig cell tumors are treated with orchiectomy followed by surveillance. The persistence of virilizing or feminizing features after orchiectomy is not necessarily an indication of residual tumor because these changes can be irreversible. Metastatic tumors are often resistant to chemotherapy and radiation.

Germ Cell Neoplasia In Situ (GCNIS)

General Information
1. Previously used names for GCNIS include intratubular germ cell neoplasia and carcinoma in situ.
2. GCNIS is a non-invasive precursor of germ cell cancer (i.e. it is pre-malignant).
3. Risk factors for GCNIS—risk factors for GCNIS include: history of germ cell cancer (gonadal or extragonadal), atrophic testicle (< 12 cc), cryptorchidism, intersex, infertility, and age < 40 years old.
   a. When a testicular germ cell tumor is present, the surrounding parenchyma of the ipsilateral testis contains GCNIS in over 80% of cases and the parenchyma of the contralateral testicle contains GCNIS in 5% of cases.
   b. In men with multiple risk factors (e.g. a male with testis cancer and atrophy of contralateral testicle), the risk of GCNIS in the contralateral testis increases to at least 33%.
4. For patients with testicular germ cell cancer, some clinicians advocate for biopsy of the contralateral testicle if it is undescended or markedly atrophic (because these testes have a high risk of having GCNIS).
5. *When GCNIS is untreated, approximately 50% of men will develop a germ cell cancer in the involved testis within 5 years.*
6. GCNIS does not elevate serum tumor markers. *Testicle biopsy is the only way to diagnose GCNIS.* Testicle biopsy is done through inguinal exploration (the approach should not be trans-scrotal).
   a. Two separate testis sites should be biopsied. 3 cubic mm of tissue is removed at each site and preserved in Bouin's solution (not formalin).
   b. In adult males with germ cell testis tumors, biopsy of the contralateral testicle (at the time of orchiectomy) may be offered when the risk of GCNIS is high (i.e. multiple risk factors for GCNIS are present).
   c. In prepubertal males with germ cell tumors, biopsy of the contralateral testis is unnecessary because *children rarely have GCNIS.*
   d. History of cryptorchidism is a risk factor for GCNIS in adults; however, testis biopsy at the time of prepubertal orchiopexy is not recommended because the natural history of GCNIS in children is not well characterized.

Treatment

1. *Controversy exists regarding whether it is necessary to diagnose and treat GCNIS.* It is unclear if treating GCNIS improves survival compared to treating a germ cell cancer if it develops. Since the cure rate of germ cell cancers is high, some experts advocate not diagnosing or treating GCNIS unless it turns into a germ cell cancer.
2. Management options for GCNIS include surveillance, radical inguinal orchiectomy, testis radiation, or systemic chemotherapy.
   a. Treatment with radiation, chemotherapy, or orchiectomy can cause hypogonadism and infertility.
   b. Radiation is less likely to cause hypogonadism than orchiectomy, but both treatments eliminate sperm production from the treated testicle.
   c. Orchiectomy or radiation will cure almost all cases of GCNIS, but chemotherapy cures only 66% of cases.
   d. If a patient wishes to preserve fertility and/or testosterone production, then surveillance is the best option. If neither fertility nor testosterone production are a concern, then orchiectomy is the preferred treatment. Radiation is an option, but it can impair fertility and 50% develop hypogonadism. In most cases, chemotherapy is not recommended for the treatment of GCNIS because of its inferior cure rate.
3. Surveillance—in men with a solitary testicle or men who wish preserve fertility and/or testicular testosterone production, surveillance is usually recommended because other treatments can cause infertility and hypogonadism. Follow up is performed on a regular schedule and includes scrotal ultrasound, physical exam by a doctor, and physical exam by the patient (self testis exams).
4. Orchiectomy—achieves 100% cure in the treated testicle, but has the highest risk of hypogonadism among the management options.
5. External beam radiation to the testicle—achieves > 97% cure in the treated testicle, but 50% of patients will require testosterone replacement for post-radiation hypogonadism. The treatment dose is 18-20 Gy.
6. Chemotherapy—eradicates GCNIS in approximately 66% of cases.
   a. In most cases, chemotherapy is not recommended for treating GCNIS because of its systemic side effects and its lower cure rate. However, it is an excellent option for men who will already be undergoing chemotherapy for a germ cell cancer.
   b. Since the cure rate is only 66% after chemotherapy, post-chemotherapy biopsy of the testis can be performed to confirm resolution of GCNIS. However, the biopsy should be performed > 2 years after chemotherapy.

Seminoma

Types of Seminoma

1. Classic or typical seminoma (95% of seminomas)
   a. Gross pathology—lobulated and pale color.
   b. Histology—*large uniform cells with clear cytoplasm and distinct cell borders*. The nucleus may have 2 nucleoli or a single eccentric nucleolus (which makes the nucleus look like a "fried egg").
      i. Syncytiotrophoblasts (which produce B-HCG) are present in 10% of cases; thus, 10% of seminomas produce B-HCG.
      ii. Lymphocytic infiltrate is present in 20% of cases.

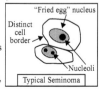

    c. Anaplastic seminoma—this term is of historical interest and is no longer used. It referred to classic seminoma with high mitotic activity. It became evident that mitotic activity did not impact prognosis; therefore, this designation was not useful and it was abandoned.
  2. Spermatocytic seminoma (5% of seminomas)
    a. Histology—cells of *varying size* that resemble maturing spermatogonia.
    b. Most spermatocytic seminomas are pure (i.e. they are not mixed with other germ cell cancers).
    c. Cryptorchidism does not increase the risk of spermatocytic seminoma (i.e. it does not occur more frequently in the undescended testicle).
    d. Spermatocytic seminoma presents at an older age than typical seminoma (usual presenting age > 50 versus 30-40 years, respectively).
    e. Spermatocytic seminoma rarely metastasizes.
    f. Spermatocytic seminoma is usually treated with radical inguinal orchiectomy and surveillance because of its *low metastatic potential.*

General Information on Seminoma
  1. *The diagnosis of pure seminoma requires a normal AFP and orchiectomy histology demonstrating only seminoma (no nonseminoma elements).*
  2. *Seminoma is the most common germ cell tumor* (65% of germ cell tumors).
  3. Age of presentation—spermatocytic seminoma presents at an older age than classic seminoma (peak age > 50 versus 30-40 years, respectively).
  4. At presentation, most cases of pure seminoma are confined to the testis (i.e. not metastatic). Metastases usually occur in the retroperitoneal lymph nodes. See Metastasis from Testis, page 133.
  5. *Pure seminoma never secretes AFP,* but it secretes B-HCG in 10% of cases.
  6. *Seminoma is radiosensitive and chemosensitive.*
  7. If histology shows only seminoma, but AFP is elevated, then the patient is assumed to have a unidentified non-seminoma elements, and is treated as a mixed germ cell tumor.

Nonseminoma

Mixed Germ Cell Tumor
  1. Mixed germ cell tumors are a mixture of seminoma and nonseminoma.
  2. Mixed germ cell tumors are treated using the protocol for non-seminoma.

Embryonal Carcinoma
  1. Usual presenting age = 25-35 years old.
  2. Gross pathology—a grey/white fleshy mass with poorly defined capsule. Necrosis and hemorrhage are often present.
  3. Histology—epithelial-like cells that form *papillary projections.*
  4. Tumor markers—may secrete AFP and/or B-HCG.
  5. Of the nonseminoma tumors, embryonal carcinoma is the most undifferentiated tumor. It has the capability to differentiate into any of other type of nonseminoma.

Yolk Sac Tumor
  1. Usual presenting age = children < 10 years old. Most present at age < 2.
  2. Gross pathology—a yellow or pale grey mass.
  3. Histology—epithelial-like cells that form cystic spaces. *Schiller-Duvall bodies,* embryoid bodies, and hyaline globules may be seen.
  4. Tumor markers—may secrete AFP and/or B-HCG.
  5. Metastasis—often metastasizes hematogenously, especially to the chest.

Choriocarcinoma

1. Usual presenting age = 20-30 years old.
2. Gross pathology—a grey white mass that tends to be peripheral in testis, and often has a central region of hemorrhage.
3. Histology—*syncytiotrophoblasts* (multiple nuclei, eosinophilic cytoplasm, secrete B-HCG) and *cytotrophoblasts* (single nucleus, clear cytoplasm).
4. Tumor markers—*never* secretes AFP and *always* secretes B-HCG.
5. Metastasis—early hematogenous spread, especially to the lungs. There may be a small primary testis tumor, but a large volume of metastasis.
6. Choriocarcinoma has the worst prognosis of all testis tumors.

Teratoma

1. Usual presenting age = 25-35 years old.
2. Gross pathology—teratoma is often cystic (the cyst lining stains positive for CEA). Gross appearance depends on the type of tissue that is present.
3. Histology—*multiple germ cell layers in different stages of maturation*: endoderm (gastrointestinal, respiratory tissue), mesoderm (bone, cartilage, muscle), or ectoderm (squamous epithelium, neural tissue). Teratoma is sometimes classified as having mature or immature elements, but this classification is of unknown significance and does not alter management.
4. Tumor markers—teratoma may secrete AFP.
5. *Teratoma is resistant to chemotherapy and radiation; therefore, it requires surgical resection.*
6. Although teratoma usually grows slowly, sometimes teratoma demonstrates rapid growth that encases or invades nearby structures ("teratoma growth syndrome").
7. *Rarely, teratoma can de-differentiate into somatic (non-germ cell) malignancies, such as sarcoma or adenocarcinoma. This condition is called teratoma with somatic type malignancy.* The previously used term "teratoma with malignant transformation" is no longer recommended.
8. *Prepubertal teratoma usually behaves in a benign fashion* (i.e. it does not metastasize or degenerate into somatic malignancy). Although post pubertal teratoma appears histologically benign, it has the potential to behave in a malignant fashion: it can de-differentiate into somatic malignancy and it can grow and invade local structures.

Tumor	Usual Age of Onset	Markers Secreted		Response to Therapy		Common Pathology Findings
		AFP	B-HCG	Radiation	Chemo	
Yolk Sac	< 10	Maybe	Maybe	Resistant	Sensitive	Schiller-Duvall bodies, embryoid bodies, hyaline globules
Chorio-carcinoma	20-30	Never	Always	Resistant	Sensitive	Syncytiotrophoblasts, cytotrophoblasts, central hemorrhage
Embryonal	25-35	Maybe	Maybe	Resistant	Sensitive	Papillary projections
Teratoma	25-35	Maybe	Never	Resistant	Resistant	Multiple germ cell layers, often cystic
Typical Seminoma	30-40	Never	Maybe	Sensitive	Sensitive	Clear cytoplasm, distinct cell borders, "fried egg" nucleus

Gonadoblastoma

1. Gonadoblastoma is a rare benign tumor that occurs almost exclusively in patients with gonadal dysgenesis from an intersex disorder.
2. Although gonadoblastoma is benign, 60% undergo transformation into a malignant germ cell tumor. Thus, bilateral gonadectomy is recommended.
3. Gonadoblastoma usually presents during or after puberty in phenotypic females with virilization or in males with hypospadias and cryptorchidism.

Treatment

Before Treatment

1. Obtain serum tumor markers (AFP, B-HCG, and LDH), liver function tests, complete blood count, and creatinine.
2. Counsel the patient regarding the potential side effects of surgical excision of the mass, including infertility and hypogonadism.
3. Discuss the option of placing a testicular prosthesis.
4. In patients of reproductive age, offer sperm banking prior to cancer treatment (ideally, the patient should preserve sperm before orchiectomy).

Surgical Excision of the Testis Mass

1. Avoid trans-scrotal biopsy and trans-scrotal surgery.
2. In adults at high risk for GCNIS (i.e. multiple risk factors present; see page 138), consider biopsy of the contralateral testicle during tumor excision. In prepubertal males, biopsy of the contralateral testis is unnecessary because *children rarely have GCNIS.*
3. Radical inguinal orchiectomy—when malignancy is suspected, *radical inguinal orchiectomy is the preferred treatment for men with a normal contralateral testicle.* Through an inguinal incision, the testis and its surrounding tunica vaginalis are excised en bloc with the ipsilateral spermatic cord up to the internal inguinal ring.
4. Testis sparing excision
   a. The rational for testis sparing is to preserve as much gonadal function as possible (i.e. preserve fertility and testosterone production). In adults, testis sparing is often done only when serum testosterone is adequate and preservation of fertility is desired (the testis may as well be removed if fertility is irrelevant and hypogonadism is already present).
   b. Testis masses that are non-palpable and < 2 cm in size are benign in at least 50% of cases. The AUA 2019 guideline states that testis sparing surgery should be offered to patients with testis masses < 2 cm, whereas the EAU 2021 guidelines did not specify a size cut-off, stating that the mass should be "suitable for enucleation."
   c. *Testis sparing is reasonable when the patient wishes to preserve gonadal function and any of the following conditions are present.*
      i. Tumor in a solitary testicle
      ii. The contralateral testicle is poorly functioning (i.e. it contributes minimally to fertility and/or testosterone production).
      iii. Synchronous bilateral testis tumors.
      iv. Tumor that is likely benign—e.g. when the serum tumor markers are normal and tumor size is < 2 cm in greatest dimension.
   d. *Testis sparing surgery has a higher local recurrence rate than radical orchiectomy (11% versus 0%).* The risk of local recurrence is higher for seminoma than for non-seminoma. Options for adjuvant treatment to reduce local recurrence include radiation to the ipsilateral testicle (for seminoma) or chemotherapy (for seminoma or non-seminoma).

e. Before testis sparing surgery, counsel the patient about the risk of infertility, hypogonadism (requires testosterone replacement in 7%), ipsilateral testis atrophy (3%), intraoperative radical orchiectomy, local recurrence, and need for adjuvant therapy to reduce local recurrence.

f. For testis sparing, mobilize the testis and spermatic cord *through an inguinal incision.* Occlude the spermatic cord and excise the mass. Frozen sections determine if the mass is benign and if surgical margins are negative. If it takes a long time to obtain the results of the frozen sections, then cool the testis to reduce ischemia from prolonged spermatic cord occlusion. If the entire mass cannot be excised with testis sparing, then perform radical orchiectomy.

g. In adults with a germ cell tumor, obtain multiple biopsies of the normal ipsilateral testis tissue to check for GCNIS (the surrounding ipsilateral testis parenchyma contains GCNIS in over 80% of cases). The presence of GCNIS increases the risk of local recurrence of germ cell cancer. See page 138 for biopsy technique and treatment of NGCIS.

After Excision of a Germ Cell Testis Cancer

1. Obtain post-orchiectomy serum tumor markers

   a. Monitor serum tumor markers until the nadir values are reached. Postoperatively, it usually takes ≥ 5 half lives to eliminate excess circulating markers. Five half lives are 1-2 weeks for B-HCG ($T\frac{1}{2}$ = 1-3 days), 3 weeks for LDH ($T\frac{1}{2}$ = 4.0-4.5 days), and 5 weeks for AFP ($T\frac{1}{2}$ = 5-7 days). *S stage is determined using the nadir value of the post-orchiectomy markers.*

   b. Small post-orchiectomy elevations of tumor markers may not be caused by testis cancer, especially in patients with no visible metastatic disease. Evaluate these patients for an alternate etiology of marker elevation (see page 137) and monitor the marker levels. Patients with microscopic or undiscovered metastatic disease typically have a consistent rise in the tumor marker, whereas patients with a non-malignant source of the marker elevation usually have a relatively stable marker level.

2. Imaging for staging

   a. For cross sectional imaging, CT with IV contrast is preferred, but MRI with Gadolinium may be used if iodinated contrast is contraindicated.

   b. Abdomen and pelvis cross sectional imaging—performed on all patients with testis cancer, preferably by CT with IV contrast.

   c. Chest imaging—for clinical stage IA or IB pure seminoma (i.e. normal tumor markers and normal CT abdomen/pelvis), chest x-ray is preferred over chest CT (if chest x-ray is abnormal, then obtain a chest CT with IV contrast). Chest CT with IV contrast is preferred in all other patients, including patients with nonseminoma, abnormal chest x-ray, metastasis on physical exam or on abdomen/pelvis CT (i.e. stage II or III), or an elevated post-orchiectomy tumor marker (including stage IS).

   d. Brain MRI with and without contrast should be done when any of the following criteria are present.
      i. Neurologic signs or symptoms are present.
      ii. B-HCG > 5000 IU/L
      iii. AFP > 10,000 ng/ml
      iv. Extensive lung metastases
      v. Non-pulmonary visceral metastasis

   e. Bone scan can be performed when clinically indicated.

   f. In patients with normal post-orchiectomy serum tumor markers but imaging is inconclusive for metastasis, then consider repeat imaging in 4 to 8 weeks. This additional imaging may clarify the extent of disease before management is finalized.

3. In patients with pure seminoma in the orchiectomy specimen, there are two findings on post-orchiectomy tumor markers that suggest the patient also has nonseminoma.
   a. B-HCG > 1000 IU/L—B-HCG elevation over 1000 IU/ml is rare with pure seminoma. Review the orchiectomy specimen to see if nonseminoma may have been missed on the initial evaluation.
   b. Elevated AFP—elevated AFP can occur for two main reasons.
      i. AFP source is not from testis cancer—evaluate the patient for other causes of AFP elevation (see page 137).
      ii. AFP source is from nonseminoma testis cancer—in this case, there is nonseminoma present somewhere in the patient. Review the orchiectomy specimen to see if nonseminoma may have been missed on the initial evaluation. Also, conduct a thorough evaluation for metastatic disease.
4. Assign a TNM stage and group. For patients with stage IIC or III cancer, assign a IGCCCG risk category (page 136).
5. The AUA 2019 guidelines recommends that treatment decisions be based on imaging that was performed within the previous 4 weeks and tumor markers performed within the previous 10 days.
6. Evaluation and treatment of adults—see page 155.
7. Evaluation and treatment of children—see page 145.

After Excision of a Non-Germ Cell Testis Cancer
1. Testis lymphoma—treated with systemic therapy (lymphoma is considered a systemic disease even if it is present only in the testis).
2. For treatment of gonadal stromal tumors, see page 137 (e.g. Leydig cell tumors, sertoli cell tumors, granulosa cell tumors).
3. For patients with stage I or stage II non-seminoma germ cell cancer whose orchiectomy specimen contains teratoma with somatic type malignancy, then the preferred treatment is full template bilateral RPLND. These tumors are typically resistant to chemotherapy and radiation.

Scrotal Violation in Testicular Malignancy
1. Scrotal violation occurs with pT4 (tumor invades the scrotum), trans-scrotal orchiectomy, or trans-scrotal biopsy. Scrotal violation can alter the normal lymphatic drainage from the testis, which means lymphatic spread from testis cancer can go to the superficial inguinal nodes. Previous inguinal surgery may also alter the lymphatic drainage from the testicle, allowing cancer to spread to the ipsilateral inguinal and iliac nodes.
2. Trans-scrotal biopsy and trans-scrotal orchiectomy
   a. *If there is a suspicion of testis cancer, trans-scrotal biopsy and trans-scrotal orchiectomy are avoided* because they increase the risk of local recurrence compared to radical orchiectomy and they can alter the lymphatic drainage so that cancer can spread to the inguinal nodes.
   b. *Although trans-scrotal biopsy and trans-scrotal orchiectomy increase the risk of local recurrence, they do not alter systemic relapse or overall survival.* Local recurrence occurs in 2.5% in men with scrotal violation compared to 0% in men without scrotal violation.
   c. Among men who underwent excision of the scrotal scar after scrotal violation, only 9.3% had residual tumor in the resected specimen.
3. Treatment—the optimal treatment is unclear, but consider the following.
   a. If stage T4 is suspected at the time of orchiectomy, then orchiectomy should probably been done with en bloc excision of the involved portion of the scrotum.
   b. After trans-scrotal biopsy, perform a radical inguinal orchiectomy and consider en bloc excision the biopsy tract and the scrotal scar.

      c. After trans-scrotal orchiectomy, the AUA 2019 guideline states that adjunctive therapy "may rarely be considered...for local control..." because only 2.5% of these patients have local recurrence. Adjunctive treatment options include excision of the scrotal scar or radiation of the ipsilateral hemiscrotum (for seminoma only).

      d For patients with seminoma and scrotal violation who will be undergoing radiation, the field can be modified to include the ipsilateral iliac and inguinal lymph nodes, and the ipsilateral hemiscrotum.

  4. Follow up—include inguinal lymph node palpation in the physical examination and include the inguinal and pelvic lymph nodes on imaging.

Testis Tumors in Prepubertal Boys

1. For testis cancer, a child is defined as a prepubertal male.
2. Compared to adults, testis tumors in children are:
   a. More likely to be benign (> 50% in children versus 1% in adults).
   b. Usually pure (germ cell tumors in adults are usually mixed).
   c. Less likely to present with metastases.
   d. Teratoma almost always behaves in a benign fashion (teratoma can have malignant behavior in adults).
   e. Seminoma is exceedingly rare in children (but it is common in adults).
3. *Most testis tumors in children are yolk sac tumors or teratomas.*
   Embryonal carcinoma, choriocarcinoma, and seminoma are rare.
   a. Yolk sac tumors can secrete AFP and/or B-HCG. Note that it is normal for infants less than one year of age to have an elevated AFP.
   b. *Teratoma is almost always benign in prepubertal children.*
   c. Treatment of nonseminoma in children (see Part 4 below)
      i. Not pure teratoma—these tumors have malignant behavior. Stage IA or IB cancers are treated with radical inguinal orchiectomy and surveillance. Stage IS, II, or III are treated with radical inguinal orchiectomy and chemotherapy.
      ii. Pure teratoma—in prepubertal boys, teratoma is almost always benign and usually presents as stage IA (confined within the testis); thus, testis sparing is an option. Teratomas are treated with orchiectomy (radical or testis sparing) and surveillance.
4. Granulosa cell tumor—a rare benign stromal tumor that usually presents in the newborn. 75% of these tumors present within one month of birth. Orchiectomy is curative.
5. If desired, a testicular prosthesis may be placed after puberty.

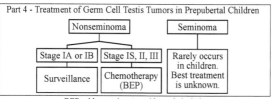

Part 4 - Treatment of Germ Cell Testis Tumors in Prepubertal Children

Nonseminoma		Seminoma
Stage IA or IB	Stage IS, II, III	Rarely occurs in children. Best treatment is unknown.
Surveillance	Chemotherapy (BEP)	

BEP = bleomycin, etoposide, and cisplatin

Seminoma Stage IA or IB—Surveillance, Radiation, or Chemotherapy?

1. *Surveillance is the preferred management for most men with stage IA or IB pure seminoma who will be compliant with follow up.*
   a. Rationale—the retroperitoneal nodes harbor occult cancer in < 20% of men with clinical stage N0 (no adenopathy on CT). If all stage I men receive treatment, over 80% will be treated unnecessarily.
   b. Disadvantages—surveillance has a higher relapse rate than treatment. *Strict compliance and intensive follow up are required.* Patients may have more psychological stress (worry about the higher recurrence rate).
   c. Tumor size > 4 cm and rete testis invasion may increase the risk of relapse, but the data are conflicting. Thus, the NCCN and AUA discourage using these characteristics to guide treatment.
   d. Relapse rate at 5 years is 15-20% for all stage I men undergoing surveillance. Relapse usually occurs in the retroperitoneal lymph nodes. *Most relapses occur within 2 years of orchiectomy, with ≤ 1% of relapses occurring after 5 years.*
   e. Treatment of relapse—restage and treat (XRT or chemotherapy).
2. Abdominal external beam radiation (XRT)—see page 148.
   a. Rationale—occult metastases in the retroperitoneal nodes are treated. XRT requires less intensive follow up than surveillance.
   b. Disadvantages—XRT doubles the risk of death from cardiac disease and doubles the risk of secondary (non-germ cell) cancer.
   c. Relapse rate at 5 years is 3-5%. Relapses usually occur outside the retroperitoneum (i.e. outside the radiation field), primarily in the thorax (lung, mediastinal nodes, supraclavicular nodes). When the iliac nodes are not radiated, the pelvic nodes are also a common site of relapse.
   d. Treatment of relapse—chemotherapy.
3. Chemotherapy—one or two cycles of carboplatin.
   a. Rationale—occult metastases will be treated and it requires less intensive follow up than surveillance. *Chemotherapy results in a lower incidence of contralateral germ cell testis tumors compared to XRT.*
   b. Disadvantages—myelosuppression, worse fertility, and possible small risk of cardiovascular toxicity. Other long-term side effects of chemotherapy are not well defined.
   c. Relapse rate at 5 years is 4-6% for 1 cycle and 2% for 2 cycles of carboplatin. Relapses usually occur in the retroperitoneal lymph nodes. Optimal treatment of relapse is unknown.

Stage I Seminoma	Surveillance	External Beam Radiation	Chemotherapy: Carboplatin x 1 or 2
Morbidity	Low	Low	Low
Cancer specific survival	99%	99%	99%
Relapse rate at 5 years	15-20%	3-5%	4-6% (1 cycle) 2% (2 cycles)
Usual location of relapse	Retroperitoneal Nodes	Outside Retroperitoneum*	Retroperitoneal Nodes
Treatment of relapse	XRT or Chemo	Chemo	XRT or Chemo

XRT = external beam radiation; chemo = systemic chemotherapy

* Relapses occur primarily in the thorax (mediastinal or supraclavicular nodes, lung). When iliac nodes are not radiated, pelvic nodes are also a common site of relapse.

Nonseminoma Stage IA or IB—Surveillance, RPLND, or Chemotherapy?

1. *Surveillance is preferred for compliant men with stage IA. Options for management of stage IB include surveillance, chemotherapy, or RPLND.*
2. Surveillance
   a. Rationale—the retroperitoneal nodes harbor occult cancer in 30% of men with clinical stage N0 (no adenopathy on CT). If all stage I patients receive treatment, 70% will be treated unnecessarily.
   b. Disadvantages–surveillance has a higher relapse rate than treatment. *Strict compliance and intensive follow up are required.* Patients may have more psychological stress (worry about the higher recurrence rate).
   c. Risk factors for relapse include lymphovascular invasion (LVI), stage pT2 or higher, > 50% of the tumor is embryonal cell carcinoma, absence of yolk sac tumor, and proliferation rate > 70% based on MIB-1 staining. *LVI is the most important factor for predicting occult metastasis in the retroperitoneal lymph nodes.* Risk factors other than LVI probably do not contribute independent prognostic information; therefore, they are usually not used for clinical management.
   d. Relapse rate is 25% among all stage I men, 15-20% when LVI is absent, and 50% when LVI is present. Most relapses (60%) occur in the retroperitoneum. *Most relapses occur within 2 years of orchiectomy, with ≤ 1% of relapses occurring after 5 years.*
   e. Treatment of relapse—chemotherapy.
3. Retroperitoneal lymph node dissection (RPLND)—see page 148.
   a. Rationale—occult retroperitoneal metastases are treated and less intensive follow up is required compared to surveillance.
   b. Disadvantages—it is invasive, has a risk of ejaculatory dysfunction, and small long-term risk of bowel obstruction with transperitoneal RPLND.
   c. Relapses occur in 10% of men who are pN0. Relapses usually occur outside the retroperitoneum (*retroperitoneal relapses are rare*).
   d. Treatment of relapse—chemotherapy.
4. Chemotherapy—stage IA receives 1 cycle of bleomycin, etoposide, and cisplatin (BEP). Stage IB receives 1 or 2 cycles of BEP.
   a. Rationale—it is less invasive than RPLND, occult metastases are treated (even those outside the retroperitoneum), relapse is lower than the other options, and less intensive follow up is needed compared to surveillance.
   b. Disadvantages—it does not treat teratoma (see page 150), it may cause infertility, there is small risk of secondary malignancy with etoposide, there is a small long term risk of cardiovascular disease, and many long-term effects of chemotherapy not well defined.
   c. Relapse rate is ≤ 3%. Relapses usually occur in the retroperitoneum.
   d. Treatment of relapse—RPLND and/or chemotherapy. Retroperitoneal relapses usually contain teratoma and should be treated with RPLND.

Stage I Nonseminoma	Surveillance	RPLND	Chemotherapy (BEP x 1 or 2)
Morbidity	Low	Low	Low
Cancer specific survival	≥ 98%	≥ 98%	≥ 98%
Relapse rate	25%†	10%*	≤ 3%
Usual location of relapse	Retroperitoneal Nodes	Outside Retroperitoneum	Retroperitoneal Nodes
Treatment of relapse	Chemo	Chemo	RPLND‡ or chemo

† Relapse rate is 25% among all men, 15-20% when lymphovascular invasion is absent (pT1), and 50% when lymphovascular invasion is present (pT2).

* In men undergoing surveillance after RPLND, the relapse rate is approximately 10% for stage pN0, 25% for stage pN1, 50% for stage pN2, and >90% for stage pN3.

‡ Relapses usually contain teratoma; therefore, they often require surgical excision.

Abdominal External Beam Radiation Therapy (XRT) for Pure Seminoma

1. XRT is utilized for treating stage IA, IB, IIA, or IIB pure seminoma.
2. For stage I, 20 Gy appears to be as effective as 30 Gy and seems to reduce acute toxicity. Thus, the recommended dose for stage I seminoma is 20 Gy.

Stage	XRT Dose	XRT Field
IA or IB	20 Gy	Abdominal retroperitoneal nodes below diaphragm* (including the ipsilateral iliac nodes† is optional)
IIA	30 Gy	Abdominal retroperitoneal nodes below diaphragm* and ipsilateral iliac nodes†
IIB	36 Gy	

* Include para-aortic nodes. Shield contralateral testis if it is not involved.
† Fields that include the ipsilateral iliac nodes are referred to as "dog leg fields."

3. For men with scrotal violation undergoing XRT, see page 144.
4. When the ipsilateral iliac nodes are not radiated, 2% of cases will recur in pelvic nodes; thus, follow up in these men must include pelvic imaging.
5. Toxicity from abdominal XRT
   a. Acute toxicity—the most common side effect is nausea. Uncommon side effects include vomiting, fatigue, and bone marrow suppression.
   b. Late toxicity—rare cases of peptic ulcer, gastritis, and secondary non-germ cell cancers (e.g. leukemia). XRT appears to double the risk of death from cardiac disease and double the risk of secondary cancer.
6. The kidney is radiosensitive and can be damaged when it is radiated.
7. In patients with prior abdominal radiation, inflammatory bowel disease, or a kidney in the expected radiation field (e.g. adenopathy near the kidney, horseshoe kidney, ectopic kidney), consider surveillance for stage IA or IB and chemotherapy (EP x 4) for stage IIA or IIB.

Retroperitoneal Lymph Node Dissection (RPLND)

1. RPLND is surgical removal of the regional retroperitoneal lymph nodes.
2. Surgical technique
   a. *The remnant spermatic cord that is ipsilateral to the testis tumor should always be removed during RLND.*
   b. For nerve sparing (see below), the nerves are *identified prospectively* and preserved.
   c. *"Split and roll"* technique—lymphatic tissue is split on the anterior surface of the great vessel and then rolled off. Ligate the lumbar vessels and remove the lymphatic tissue en bloc.
   d. If necessary, the inferior mesenteric artery can be ligated when the marginal colonic artery is intact.
3. *Postoperative tachycardia is common and is caused by sympathetic discharge.* Complications include ejaculatory dysfunction, chylous ascites (2%), renal vascular injury (3%), and bowel obstruction (1-3%). The mortality rate of RPLND is approximately 0.3%.
4. The morbidity is higher for post-chemotherapy RPLND than for primary RPLND.
5. The morbidity of post-chemotherapy RPLND is higher for seminoma than for nonseminoma because chemotherapy for seminoma induces a desmoplastic reaction that makes dissection difficult.
6. One of the most important side effects from RPLND is impaired ejaculation. Impaired ejaculation after RPLND is caused by injury to post ganglionic sympathetic nerves (T2-L4) and to the hypogastric plexus (sympathetic nerve plexus near the origin of the inferior mesenteric artery [IMA]).

7. Injury to the nerves and the resulting ejaculatory dysfunction can be reduced by two techniques. These two techniques can be used together.
   a. Modified template RPLND—avoids dissection on the contralateral side (especially below the IMA); therefore, it prevents injury to contralateral nerves that are *outside* the template. The modified template without nerve sparing maintains ejaculation in 70-90% of cases.
   b. Nerve sparing—preserves nerves *within* the template.
      i. Nerve sparing is indicated to preserve ejaculatory function.
      ii. Nerve sparing can be performed with any template (even after chemotherapy) if it does not compromise tumor resection.
      iii. Nerve sparing RPLND maintains ejaculatory function in 99% of appropriately selected men (without compromising tumor removal).
8. Modified RPLND Templates
   a. *Modified templates are an option for men with clinical stage I nonseminoma when there is no somatic type malignancy in the orchiectomy specimen and when intraoperative findings reveal no suspicious retroperitoneal lymphadenopathy. If suspicious palpable lymph nodes are found within a modified template, then a full bilateral template should be performed.*
   b. Modified templates decrease the risk of ejaculatory dysfunction by limiting dissection on the contralateral side below the IMA; however, *modified templates have a higher risk of pelvic and retroperitoneal relapse than a full bilateral template.* Thus, some experts recommend performing a nerve sparing bilateral full template in all men.
   c. *Left sided modified RPLND templates are performed for left sided testicular tumors, whereas right sided modified RPLND templates are performed for right sided testicular tumors.*
   d. *Lymphatic metastasis often spread from the right to the left retroperitoneum, but they usually do not spread from left to right.* Therefore, modified templates for right sided testis tumors typically extend further toward the contralateral side than modified templates for left sided tumors.
   e. Various modified templates have been described, but the AUA 2019 guideline recommends that templates remove the following nodes (at a minimum):
      i. Right sided modified template: right common iliac, paracaval, pre-caval, retrocaval, interaortocaval, pre-aortic, and retro-aortic. There was disagreement among the AUA panel as to whether para-aortic nodes above the IMA must be removed.
      ii. Left sided template: left common iliac, para-aortic, pre-aortic, and retro-aortic. There was disagreement among the AUA panel as to whether the interaortocaval nodes above the IMA must be removed.
   f. The example modified templates that are shown in the figure below include removal of the para-aortic nodes for the right sided template and the interaortocaval nodes for the left template. The limits of dissection for these example templates are
      i. Superior limit—renal vessels.
      ii. Inferior limit—where the ipsilateral ureter crosses the common iliac artery.
      iii. Ipsilateral lateral limit—ipsilateral ureter.
      iv. Contralateral lateral limit inferior to the IMA—aorta and ipsilateral common iliac artery.
      v. Contralateral lateral limit superior to the IMA—contralateral ureter for right sided template; vena cava for left sided template
   g. *Surgical margins should not be compromised to maintain a template or to preserve ejaculation.*

RPLND Templates & The Clinical Scenario in Which They Are Used

Modified Templates: indicated for stage I nonseminoma (with no suspicious intraoperative retroperitoneal nodes and no somatic malignancy in the testicle)

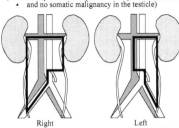

Right   Left

Legend

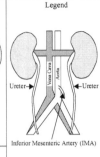

Ureter→   ←Ureter

Inferior Mesenteric Artery (IMA)

Full Bilateral Template: indicated for clinical stage II nonseminoma, suspicious intraoperative retroperitoneal nodes, post-chemotherapy RPLND, or somatic malignancy in the testicle (may also be used for stage I nonseminoma)

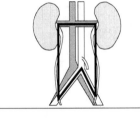

━━ = limits of dissection

For all templates:
1. The ipsilateral spermatic cord and gonadal vein should be resected.
2. The template should be extended to include nodes suspected of harboring cancer. Margins of resection should never be compromised to maintain the template.

Risk of Teratoma in Retroperitoneum with Nonseminoma

1. *Teratoma may be present in the retroperitoneal lymph nodes despite its absence in the orchiectomy specimen. However, the risk of teratoma in the retroperitoneal nodes is higher when teratoma was present in the testicle.*

Nonseminoma Orchiectomy Pathology	Chance of Teratoma in the Retroperitoneal Lymph Nodes in Adults	
	Clinical Stage I	Clinical Stage IIA
Teratoma absent	5% - 7%	8%
Teratoma present	2% - 19%	33%

2. Teratoma requires surgical excision because it is unresponsive to chemotherapy and radiation.
3. For clinical stage II, a predominance of teratoma in the orchiectomy specimen supports using RPLND instead of chemotherapy because teratoma in the testis increases the risk of teratoma in the retroperitoneum.
4. The rational for resecting nodes that have a high likelihood of containing teratoma includes
   a. Teratoma is resistant to chemotherapy and radiation, but can be effectively treated with surgical excision.
   b. If teratoma is not removed, it can grow rapidly and encase or invade nearby structures ("teratoma growth syndrome").
   c. If teratoma is not removed, it can undergo malignant transformation into somatic malignancy, such as sarcoma or adenocarcinoma.
   d. Untreated teratoma can lead to late recurrence of germ cell tumor.

Primary Chemotherapy for Stage II and Stage III Germ Cell Cancers

1. *Platinum (cisplatin) is the most effective agent against germ cell tumors.* However, multi-agent regimens containing cisplatin are more effective than a single agent.

2. Primary chemotherapy refers to the first-line regimen that is administered to treat the cancer. Salvage chemotherapy refers to a regimen that is delivered after failure of primary chemotherapy (second-line, third-line, etc.)

3. The standard primary (first-line) chemotherapy regimen for stage II or III germ cell cancer is either bleomycin, etoposide, and cisplatin (BEP) or etoposide and cisplatin (EP).

   a. *In good risk patients, BEP x 3 cycles is as effective as EP x 4 cycles.* In men with sufficient renal function, carboplatin should not be substituted for cisplatin in good risk patients because it results in a lower complete remission rate.

   b. *Intermediate and poor risk patients should receive BEP x 4 cycles.* VIP x 4 can be utilized for intermediate and poor risk patients who have a contraindication to bleomycin. VIP is VP-16 (etoposide), ifosfamide with Mesna, and cisplatin.

4. Bleomycin

   a. Antitumor antibiotic that binds to and breaks DNA.

   b. Side effects—pneumonitis, pulmonary fibrosis, nail and skin changes.

   c. Bleomycin induced pulmonary toxicity increases the risk of respiratory complications during surgery. These perioperative pulmonary complications can be reduced by aggressive monitoring, avoiding over-hydration, preferential use of colloids, judicious use of crystalloids, and keeping fraction of inspired oxygen less than 25% ($FIO_2 < 0.25$).

   d. Relative contraindications for bleomycin are reduced pulmonary function (e.g. COPD), renal insufficiency, and age > 50 years old.

5. Etoposide (VP-16)

   a. Alkylating agent (covalently binds to DNA).

   b. Dose limiting toxicity = myelosuppression, mucositis. Other side effects include vomiting, alopecia, and *dose related risk of leukemia* (0.8% risk with a mean latency period of 2-4 years).

6. Cisplatin

   a. Cross links DNA.

   b. Dose limiting toxicity = nephrotoxicity. Other side effects include neurotoxicity, hearing loss, *diminished cardiac function*, nausea, and vomiting.

   c. In patients with metastatic germ cell cancer and sufficient renal function, *carboplatin should not be substituted for cisplatin in good risk patients because it results in a lower complete remission rate.* In cases when renal function must be preserved, carboplatin (dose limiting toxicity is myelosuppression) may be substituted for cisplatin (dose limiting toxicity is nephrotoxicity).

7. Carboplatin

   a. One or two cycles of carboplatin is a treatment option for stage IA or IB pure seminoma.

   b. Dose limiting toxicity = myelosuppression. Other side effects of carboplatin include nausea, vomiting, and neuropathy.

Salvage Chemotherapy
1. Salvage chemotherapy is indicated for men who progress during primary chemotherapy or who relapse after primary chemotherapy.
2. Conventional dose salvage chemotherapy
   a. Regimens include
      i. VeIP: Velban (vinblastine), ifosfamide (with Mesna), and cisplatin.
      ii. TIP: Taxol (paclitaxel), ifosfamide (with Mesna), and cisplatin.
   b. 50% achieve a complete response, but only 25% sustain remission.
3. High dose salvage chemotherapy and autologous bone marrow transplant
   a. High dose chemotherapy (HDC) kills bone marrow. Thus, an autologous bone marrow transplant is given after HDC to reconstitute the marrow.
   b. Durable remissions are achieved in 10-20% of patients.
   c. Treatment related mortality is as high as 5-10%.

Post-Chemotherapy Residual Retroperitoneal Mass
1. *Residual retroperitoneal masses rarely contain teratoma after primary chemotherapy for seminoma, but 40% contain teratoma after primary chemotherapy for nonseminoma.*
2. A residual mass is more likely to contain malignancy after salvage chemotherapy than after primary chemotherapy.
3. After primary chemotherapy—when the patient has a good response to chemotherapy and normalization of tumor markers, retroperitoneal surgery may be indicated based on the size of the residual retroperitoneal mass.
   a. Non-seminoma or mixed germ cell tumors—after primary chemotherapy for stage II and III nonseminoma, a residual mass < 1 cm is unlikely to contain teratoma or malignancy (only 9% of these patients recur, with only 4% recurring in the retroperitoneal nodes). A residual mass > 1 cm in size has a significant risk of containing either cancer or teratoma. Therefore, patients with a residual mass > 1 cm in size undergo a full template RPLND with resection of the residual mass.
   b. Pure seminoma—after primary chemotherapy for stage II and III seminoma, a residual mass ≤ 3 cm is unlikely to contain malignancy, whereas a residual mass > 3 cm contains cancer in 30-50% of cases. Patients with a residual mass > 3 cm in size should undergo a PET/CT scan, and if the mass is metabolically active, perform biopsy or excision of the residual mass. RPLND is not done because chemotherapy for seminoma induces a desmoplastic reaction that makes dissection difficult and substantially increases the morbidity of a template RPLND.
4. After salvage chemotherapy—when the patient has a good response to chemotherapy and normalization of tumor markers, residual mass resection (with RPLND for non-seminoma and mixed tumors) is indicated for any residual retroperitoneal mass (regardless of the tumor type or the size of the residual mass) because residual masses in this setting have a significant risk of containing cancer (50%) or teratoma (40%).

Orchiectomy Pathology	Chemotherapy Type	Composition of Post-Chemotherapy Residual Retroperitoneal Mass		
		Germ Cell Malignancy	Pure Teratoma (no viable GCT)	Necrosis or Fibrosis
Pure Seminoma	Primary	10-20%*	Rare	80-90%
Nonseminoma or Mixed GCT	Primary	<10%	40-50%	40-50%
Any GCT	Salvage	50%	40%	10%

GCT = Germ cell tumor
* Overall, malignancy occurs in 10-20% of residual masses. When stratified by size, malignancy occurs in 30-50% of masses > 3 cm, but is rare in masses ≤ 3 cm.

Follow up

1. Follow up depends on the type of testis tumor and the mode of therapy delivered. Follow up protocols for stage I patients undergoing surveillance can be found in the legends on page 156 and page 159.
2. For germ cell tumors, follow up usually consists of regularly performed serum tumor markers, imaging, and physical exam. *The remaining testicle should always be examined routinely because the cumulative risk of malignancy in the remaining testicle is 2-5% by 15 years after orchiectomy.*
3. Follow up physical exams should include examination of the testicle by the physician and by the patient (self exams).
4. After surveillance for stage I germ cell cancer, recurrence after 5 years occurs in ≤ 1% of patients. For this reason, obtaining serum markers and imaging beyond 5 years of follow up are typically done only as clinically indicated.
5. If recurrence occurs, the patient should be re-staged and treated.
6. *Patients with testicular cancer should be monitored for signs and symptoms of hypogonadism.* If hypogonadism is suspected, measure morning serum testosterone level and luteinizing hormone (see page 536).
7. For patients whose treatment included radiation and/or chemotherapy
   a. Advise these patients that they have an increased risk for cardiovascular disease (they are 1.5 to 2.0 times more likely to develop cardiovascular disease compared to those who did not receive chemotherapy or radiation). They should be monitored by a primary care physician so that modifiable risk factors that contribute to cardiovascular disease can be identified and treated.
   b. Advise these patients that they have an increased risk of secondary malignancy (they are 2 times more likely to develop another malignancy compared to those who did not receive chemotherapy or radiation). They should be monitored by a primary care physician and have appropriate cancer screening.

Survival

Stage	IGCCCG Risk Status*	5-Year Overall Survival	
		Seminoma	Nonseminoma
I	—	≥ 98%	≥ 98%
IIA or IIB	—	≥ 95%	≥ 95%
IIC or III	Good	86%	92%
	Intermediate	72%	80%
	Poor	—	48%

Note: Seminoma does not have a poor risk category.
* For definitions of these risk categories, see page 136.

Stage	IGCCCG Risk Status*	5-Year Progression Free Survival	
		Seminoma	Nonseminoma
IIC or III	Good	82%	89%
	Intermediate	67%	75%
	Poor	—	41%

Note: Seminoma does not have a poor risk category.
* For definitions of these risk categories, see page 136.

Evaluation of Suspected Testis Mass

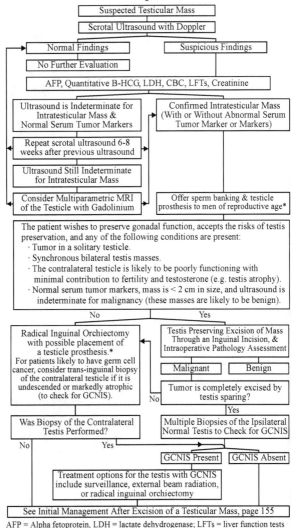

AFP = Alpha fetoprotein, LDH = lactate dehydrogenase; LFTs = liver function tests
CBC = complete blood count; B-HCG = beta human chorionic gonadotropin
GCNIS = germ cell neoplasia in situ; MRI = magnetic resonance imaging
* For children, a testicular prosthesis can be placed after the child completes puberty.

Initial Management After Excision of a Testicular Mass

No Tumor, No GCNIS, & Benign
→ No further treatment

Lymphoma
→ Referral to Medical Oncologist
→ Systemic Therapy

Sertoli or Leydig Cell Tumor
- CT abdomen/pelvis with IV contrast*
- Chest x-ray (if chest x-ray is abnormal then obtain a chest CT with IV contrast*)
- When clinically indicated: bone scan

→ Surveillance if no metastasis

Germ Cell Tumor
- Serum AFP‡, HCG‡, LDH‡;
- CT abdomen and pelvis with IV contrast*
- Chest imaging:
  - For stage IA/IB pure seminoma: chest x-ray (if chest x-ray is abnormal then obtain a chest CT with IV contrast*)
  - For nonseminoma, mixed GCT, or Stage IS/II/III: chest CT† with IV contrast*
- When clinically indicated: brain MRI, bone scan

If serum tumor markers are normal and imaging is inconclusive for metastasis, then repeat imaging in 4 to 8 weeks

Germ Cell Tumor branches to:

Pure Seminoma & Normal AFP
- Adult: See page 156
- Child: See page 145

Nonseminoma, Mixed Germ Cell Tumor, or Elevated AFP

Somatic malignancy Absent
- Adult: See page 158
- Child: See page 145

Somatic malignancy Present°
- See page 144

T½ = half life;
CT = computerized tomography;
MRI = magnetic resonance imaging;
GCNIS = germ cell neoplasia in situ;
IV = intravenous; AFP = alpha-fetoprotein;
B-HCG = beta-human chorionic gonadotropin; LDH = lactate dehydrogenase

* If there is a contraindication to iodinated contrast, then MRI with Gadolinium may be used.

† For clinical stage IA or IB pure seminoma, chest x-ray is preferred over chest CT. Chest CT with IV contrast is preferred in patients with abnormal chest x-ray, nonseminoma, metastasis on physical exam or on CT of the abdomen/pelvis (stage II or III), or an elevated post-orchiectomy tumor marker (including stage IS).

‡ Monitor serum tumor markers until the nadir values are reached. Postoperatively, it usually takes ≥ 5 half lives to eliminate excess circulating markers. Five half lives is 1-2 weeks for B-HCG (T½ = 1-3 days), 3 weeks for LDH (T½ = 4.0-4.5 days), and 5 weeks for AFP (T½ = 5-7 days). *S stage is determined using the nadir value of the post-orchiectomy markers.* When indicated, rule out causes of marker elevation that are not related to germ cell cancer (see page 137).

° Teratoma can de-differentiate into somatic cancer (e.g. sarcoma, adenocarcinoma). These are treated differently than germ cell tumors without somatic cancer.

Initial Treatment of PURE SEMINOMA in Adults

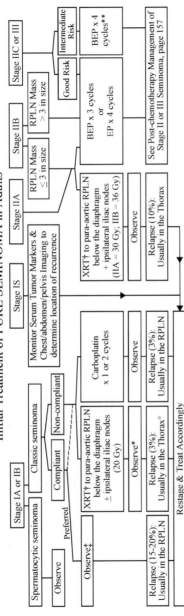

Stage IA or IB

- Spermatocytic seminoma → Observe
- Classic seminoma
  - Compliant (Preferred) → Observe‡
  - Non-compliant → XRT† to para-aortic RPLN below the diaphragm ± ipsilateral iliac nodes (20 Gy)

Observe‡
- Relapse (15-20%): Usually in the RPLN

XRT† to para-aortic RPLN below the diaphragm ± ipsilateral iliac nodes (20 Gy)
- Observe*
- Relapse (3%): Usually in the Thorax°

Carboplatin x 1 or 2 cycles
- Observe
- Relapse (3%): Usually in the Thorax°

Stage IS → Monitor Serum Tumor Markers & Chest/abdomen/pelvis Imaging to determine location of recurrence

Stage IIA → XRT† to para-aortic RPLN below the diaphragm + ipsilateral iliac nodes (IIA = 30 Gy; IIB = 36 Gy)
- Observe
- Relapse (10%): Usually in the Thorax

Stage IIB
- RPLN Mass ≤ 3 in size
- RPLN Mass > 3 in size
→ BEP x 3 cycles or EP x 4 cycles

Stage IIC or III
- Good Risk → BEP x 3 cycles or EP x 4 cycles
- Intermediate Risk → BEP x 4 cycles**

See Post-chemotherapy Management of Stage II or III Seminoma, page 157

Restage & Treat Accordingly

Dashed line = non-preferred option; EP = Etoposide and cisplatin; BEP = Bleomycin and cisplatin; RPLN = Retroperitoneal lymph nodes; XRT = External beam radiation;

† XRT should be avoided in men with inflammatory bowel disease, prior abdominal radiation, or kidney in the radiation field (e.g. horseshoe kidney, ectopic kidney, adenopathy near the kidney). Shield the contralateral testis if it is not involved. For men with scrotal violation, include the ipsilateral iliac and inguinal lymph nodes in the radiation field. If there is gross tumor spillage or positive margins during orchiectomy, include the ipsilateral hemiscrotum in the radiation field.

* When the ipsilateral iliac nodes are not radiated, follow up must include imaging of the pelvic nodes.

** VIP x 4 may be used when there is a contraindication to bleomycin. VIP is etoposide, ifosfamide, and cisplatin.

° When the iliac nodes are not radiated, the iliac nodes are also a common site of relapse.

‡ Example surveillance protocol: history, physical exam, and cross sectional imaging (CT or MRI) of the abdomen ± pelvis (with or without contrast) every 4-6 months for the first 2 years, every 6-12 months for years 3 to 5. Beyond 5 years, cross sectional imaging is performed when clinically indicated. Chest x-ray and serum tumor markers are obtained when clinically indicated.

Post-chemotherapy Management of Stage II or III PURE SEMINOMA in Adults

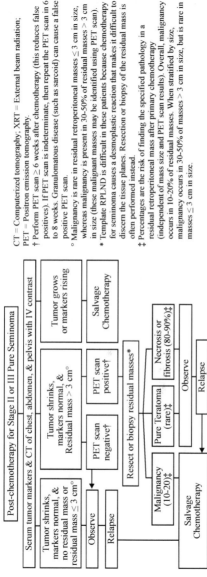

CT = Computerized tomography; XRT = External beam radiation; PET = Positron emission tomography.

† Perform PET scan ≥ 6 weeks after chemotherapy (this reduces false positives). If PET scan is indeterminate, then repeat the PET scan in 6 to 8 weeks. Granulomatous disease (such as sarcoid) can cause a false positive PET scan.

° Malignancy is rare in residual retroperitoneal masses ≤ 3 cm in size, whereas malignancy is present in 30-50% of residual masses > 3 cm in size (these malignant masses may be identified using PET scan).

* Template RPLND is difficult in these patients because chemotherapy for seminoma causes a desmoplastic reaction that makes it difficult to discern the tissue planes. Resection or biopsy of the residual mass is often performed instead.

‡ Percentages are the risk of finding the specified pathology in a residual retroperitoneal mass after primary chemotherapy (independent of mass size and PET scan results). Overall, malignancy occurs in 10-20% of residual masses. When stratified by size, malignancy occurs in 30-50% of masses > 3 cm in size, but is rare in masses ≤ 3 cm in size.

Initial Treatment of NONSEMINOMA/MIXED GERM CELL TUMOR in Adults

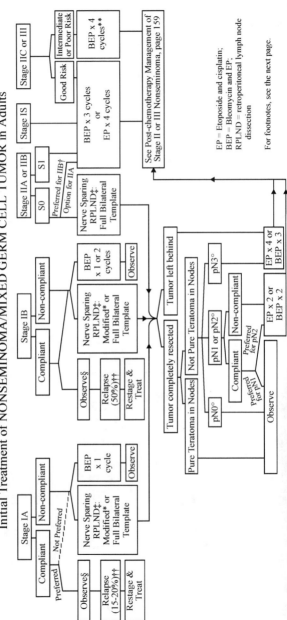

EP = Etoposide and cisplatin;
BEP = Bleomycin and EP;
RPLND = retroperitoneal lymph node dissection

For footnotes, see the next page.

Post-chemotherapy Management of Stage II or III NONSEMINOMA/MIXED GERM CELL TUMOR in Adults

CT = Computerized tomography; RPLND = retroperitoneal lymph node dissection

† RPLND is an option on S0 stage IIB when there are no cancer related symptoms, no potential for aberrant lymphatic drainage (such as scrotal violation or prior inguinal surgery), and retroperitoneal tumor mass is unifocal & small (e.g. < 3 cm).

†† 60% of relapses occur in the retroperitoneum.

§ Example surveillance protocol: history, physical exam, and serum tumor markers every 2-3 months for the first year, every 2-4 months for year 2, every 4-6 months for year 3, every 6-12 months for years 4 and 5, and as clinically indicated beyond 5 years. In patients at low risk for relapse (e.g. stage IA), obtain chest x-ray and cross sectional imaging (CT or MRI) of the abdomen ± pelvis (with or without contrast) every 3-6 months for the first year, every 4-12 months for year 2, once in year 3, once in year 4 or 5, and as clinically indicated beyond 5 years. For patients at high risk for relapse (e.g. Stage IB), obtain imaging more often.

° For surveillance after primary RPLND, relapse occurs in approximately 10% with stage pN0, 25% with stage pN1, 50% with stage pN2, and > 90% with stage pN3. Most relapses occur outside the retroperitoneum, primarily in the lungs

°° After primary chemotherapy, patients who undergo surveillance for a residual mass < 1 cm have a 9% recurrence rate, but only 4% recur in the retroperitoneum. So, if all of patients with a residual mass < 1 cm undergo RPLND, 96% will be subjected to unnecessary surgery. After salvage chemotherapy, the risk of residual malignancy is much higher; therefore, resection of a residual retroperitoneal mass (regardless of size) is recommended after salvage chemotherapy.

* If palpable nodal metastases are discovered during a modified template, a full bilateral template should be performed. Resect all palpable regional nodes.

** VIP x 4 may be used when there is a contraindication to bleomycin.

‡ A predominance of teratoma in the orchiectomy specimen supports using RPLND over chemotherapy because it increases the risk of teratoma in the retroperitoneum.

‡‡ Percentages are the risk of the specified pathology after primary chemotherapy.

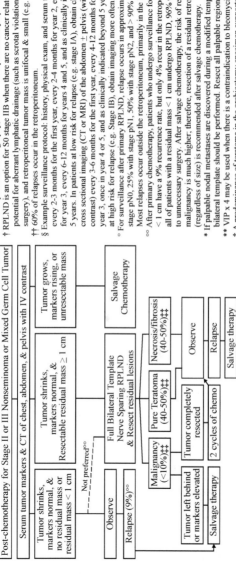

REFERENCES

General

AUA—Stephenson A, et al: **Diagnosis and treatment of early stage testicular cancer guideline: AUA Guideline. AUA Education and Research, Inc., 2019. (www.auanet.org).**

Carver BS, Sheinfeld J: Germ cell tumors of the testis. Ann Surg Oncol, 12(11): 871, 2005.

Donohue JP, Foster RS: Management of retroperitoneal recurrences, seminoma and nonseminoma. Urol Clin North Am, 21(4), 1994.

EAU—Laguna MP, et al: **Guidelines on testicular cancer. European Association of Urology. 2021. (www.uroweb.org/guidelines).**

ICUD—International Consultation on Urologic Diseases: **testicular cancer. Urology, 78(4A), S423-S474, 2011.**

International Germ Cell Cancer Collaborative Group. **International germ cell consensus classification: a prognostic factor-based staging system for metastatic germ cell cancers. J Clin Oncol, 15(2): 594, 1997.**

Krege S, et al: **European consensus conference on diagnosis and treatment of germ cell cancer: a report of the second meeting of the European Germ Cell Cancer Consensus Group: Part I. Eur Urol, 53: 478, 2008.**

Krege S, et al: **European consensus conference on diagnosis and treatment of germ cell cancer: a report of the second meeting of the European Germ Cell Cancer Consensus Group: Part II. Eur Urol, 53: 497, 2008.**

NCCN—National Comprehensive Cancer Network clinical practice guidelines in oncology: **Testicular cancer. V.2.2021, 2021. (www.nccn.org).**

Ross JH, et al: Clinical behavior and a contemporary management algorithm for prepubertal testis tumors: a summary of the prepubertal testis tumor registry. J Urol, 168: 1675, 2002.

Tsili AC, et al: MRI of the scrotum: recommendations of the ESUR scrotal and penile imaging working group. Eur Radiol, 28(1): 31, 2018.

van den Belt-Dusebout AW, et al: Treatment specific risks of second malignancies and cardiovascular disease in 5 year survivors of testicular cancer. J Clin Oncol, 25(28): 4370, 2007.

Walsh TJ, et al: Increased risk of testicular germ cell cancer among infertile men. Arch Intern Med, 169(4): 351, 2009.

Williamson SR, et al: The World Health Organization 2016 classification of testicular germ cell tumors: a review and update from the International Society of Urological Pathology Testis Consultation Panel. Histopathology, 70(3): 335, 2017.

Testicular Microlithiasis

Richenberg J, et al: Testicular microlithiasis imaging and follow up: guidelines of the ESUR scrotal imaging subcommittee. Eur Radiol, 25: 323, 2015.

Scrotal Violation

Capelouto CC, Clark PE, et al: A review of scrotal violation in testicular cancer: is adjuvant local therapy necessary? J Urol, 153: 981, 1995.

Patel HD, et al: Testis sparing surgery and scrotal violation for testicular masses suspicious for malignancy: a systematic review and meta-analysis. Urol Oncol, 38(5): 344, 2020.

Testis Sparing Excision of Mass

Heidenreich A, et al: Organ sparing surgery for malignant germ cell tumor of the testis. J Urol, 166: 2161, 2001.

Patel HD, et al: Testis sparing surgery and scrotal violation for testicular masses suspicious for malignancy: a systematic review and meta-analysis. Urol Oncol, 38(5): 344, 2020.

Germ Cell Neoplasia In Situ

Dieckmann KP, et al: Treatment of testicular intraepithelial neoplasia (intratubular germ cell neoplasia unspecified) with local radiotherapy or with platinum based chemotherapy: a survey of the German Testicular Cancer Study Group. Ann Oncol, 24(5): 1332, 2013.

Dieckmann KP, et al: Diagnosis of contralateral testicular intraepithelial neoplasia (TIN) in patients with testicular germ cell cancer: systematic two site biopsies are more sensitive than a single random biopsy. Eur Urol, 51: 175, 2007.

Gupta M, et al: Diagnosis and management of intratubular germ cell neoplasia in situ: a systematic review. J Urol, 204(1): 33, 2020.

van der Maase H, et al: Carcinoma in situ of the contralateral testis in patients with testicular germ cell cancer. Br Med J, 293: 1398, 1986.

Nonseminoma - Teratoma

Heidenreich A, Moul JW, et al: The role of retroperitoneal lymphadenectomy in mature teratoma of the testis. J Urol, 157(1): 160, 1997.

Herr HW, et al: Management of teratoma. Urol Clin North Am, 20(1): 145, 1993.

Sheinfeld J, Motzer RJ, et al: Incidence and clinical outcome of patients with teratoma in the retroperitoneum following primary retroperitoneal lymph node dissection for clinical stages I and IIA nonseminomatous germ cell tumors. J Urol, 170: 1159, 2003.

Nonseminoma - General

Alpers P, et al: Randomized phase III trial comparing retroperitoneal lymph node dissection with one course of bleomycin and etoposide plus cisplatin chemotherapy in the adjuvant treatment of clinical stage I nonseminomatous testicular germ cell tumors. J Clin Oncol, 26(18): 2966, 2008.

Colls BM, et al: Late results of surveillance of clinical stage I nonseminoma germ cell testicular tumors: 17 years experience in a national study in New Zealand. BJU Int, 83: 76, 1999.

Large MC, et al: Retroperitoneal lymph node dissection: reassessment of modified templates. BJU Int, 104: 1369, 2009.

Pizzocaro G, et al: Adjuvant chemotherapy in resected stage II nonseminomatous germ cell tumors of the testis. Eur Urol 10: 151, 1984.

Pohar KS, et al: Results of retroperitoneal lymph node dissection for clinical stage I & II pure embryonal carcinoma of the testis. J Urol, 170: 1155, 2003.

Richie JP: Complications of retroperitoneal lymph node dissection. AUA Update Series, Vol. 12, Lesson 16, 1993.

Saxman SB, Nichols CR, Foster RS, et al: The management of patients with clinical stage I nonseminomatous testicular tumors and persistently elevated serologic markers. J Urol, 155: 587, 1996.

van Dijk MR, et al: Survival of non-seminomatous germ cell cancer patients according to the IGCC classification: an update based meta-analysis. Eur J Cancer, 42(7): 820, 2006.

Williams SD, et al: Immediate adjuvant chemotherapy versus observation with treatment at relapse in pathological stage II testicular cancer. N Engl J Med, 317(23): 1433, 1987.

Seminoma

Aparicio J, et al: Multicenter study evaluating a dual policy of post-orchiectomy surveillance and selective adjuvant single agent carboplatin for patients with clinical stage I seminoma. Ann Oncol, 14: 867, 2003.

Dieckmann KP, et al: Adjuvant treatment of clinical stage I seminoma: is a single course of carboplatin sufficient? J Urol, 55(1): 102, 2000.

Fossa SD, et al: Optimal planning target volume for stage I testicular seminoma. A Medical Research Council Randomized Trial. J Clin Oncol, 17: 1146, 1999.

Jones WG, et al: Randomized trial of 30 versus 20 Gy in the adjuvant treatment of stage I testicular seminoma. J Clin Oncol, 23(6): 1200, 2005.

Martin JM, et al: Evidence based guidelines for following stage 1 seminoma. Cancer, 109: 2248, 2007.

Mead GM, et al: Randomized trials in 2466 patients with stage I seminoma: patterns of relapse and follow up. J Natl Cancer Inst, 103: 241, 2011.

Oliver RT, et al: Randomized trial of carboplatin versus radiotherapy for stage I seminoma. J Clin Oncol, 29(8): 957, 2011 [update of Lancet, 366(9482): 293, 2005].

Zagars GK, et al: Mortality after cure of testicular seminoma. J Clin Oncol, 22(4): 6540, 2004.

Postchemotherapy Residual Mass

Ehrlich Y, et al: Long term follow up of cisplatin combination chemotherapy in patients with disseminated nonseminomatous germ cell tumors: is a postchemotherapy retroperitoneal lymph node dissection needed after complete remission? J Clin Oncol, 28(4): 531, 2009.

Sheinfeld J, Bajorin D: Management of the postchemotherapy residual mass. Urol Clin North Am, 20(1): 133, 1993

Sheinfeld J, et al: Management of postchemotherapy residual masses in advanced germ cell tumors. AUA Update Series, Vol. 17, Lesson 3, 1997.

PROSTATE CANCER

General Information
1. Prostate cancer is the most common internal malignancy in U.S. males. Approximately 12% of U.S. men will be diagnosed with prostate cancer in their lifetime.
2. Prostate cancer is the second leading cause of cancer-related death in U.S. men. However, *the approximate lifetime risk of dying from prostate cancer is only 3% (when including men of all races). In men of African ancestry, the lifetime risk of dying from prostate cancer is approximately 2 times higher. Nonetheless, most prostate cancers do not cause death.*
3. The most common type of prostate cancer is adenocarcinoma.

Presentation
1. Age—usually presents at age $\geq$ 65, but it can occur at any age.
2. Most patients are asymptomatic. Advanced cancer may present with bone pain, voiding symptoms, hematuria, urine retention, or hydronephrosis.

Metastasis from the Prostate Cancer
Common metastatic locations (listed from most common to least common): pelvic lymph nodes, bone, lung, liver.

Incidental Prostate Cancer
1. 28-61% of patients undergoing radical cystectomy are found to have incidental prostate adenocarcinoma.
2. Up to 10% of patients undergoing transurethral resection of the prostate (TURP) are found to have incidental prostate cancer.
3. During autopsy, older subjects have a higher chance of having incidental prostate cancer. Most of the incidental prostate cancers that are discovered during autopsy are microscopic and low grade.

Age (years)	Chance of Incidental Prostate Cancer	
	Deceased Subjects, Diagnosed at Autopsy† (PSA & DRE unknown)	Live Subjects, Diagnosed by Prostate Biopsy‡ (PSA ≤ 4 & normal DRE)
20-29	0-8%	—
30-39	6-31%	—
40-49	13-43%	—
50-59	22-55%	—
60-69	32-70%	14%
70-79	33-83%	17%*
≥ 80	48-87%	

DRE = digital rectal exam of the prostate; PSA = prostate specific antigen

† Data from J Urol 150: 379, 1993; Eur Urol 30: 138, 1994; In vivo 8: 439, 1994; Urol Oncol 5: 274, 2000; Prostate 54: 238, 2003; Eur Urol 48: 739, 2005; J Urol 179:892, 2008.

‡ Based on 6 or more cores obtained during transrectal prostate biopsy in live subjects. Data from N Engl J Med, 350: 2239, 2004.

* This data is based on men age 71-91 years.

Risk Factors for Prostate Cancer

Risk Factors for Developing Prostate Cancer
1. Family history of prostate cancer
2. African ancestry
3. Age > 40-50
4. Genetic mutations or syndromes that increase the risk of prostate cancer (e.g. BRCA 2 mutations, CHEK2 mutations, Lynch syndrome).

Family History of Prostate Cancer
1. *Family history of prostate cancer can increase the chance of developing prostate cancer and increase the chance of dying from prostate cancer.*
2. Each of the following family characteristics increases the risk of *developing* prostate cancer.
   a. The family member with cancer is closer in relation—first degree relatives (brother, father, or son) with prostate cancer impart a higher risk of cancer than second degree relatives (grandfather, uncle, nephew, or grandson) and third degree relatives (cousin or great grandfather).
   b. The family member was diagnosed at a younger age (particularly age < 65 years).
   c. A greater number of family members have prostate cancer.
3. *Having a first degree relative with prostate cancer increases the risk of dying from prostate cancer.* Each of the following characteristics contributes to increasing the risk of *dying* from prostate cancer.
   a. First degree relative was diagnosed at age < 60 years.
   b. A greater number of first degree relatives have prostate cancer.

# of 1st-Degree Relatives with Prostate Cancer	Relative Increase in Risk of Dying from Prostate Cancer*
1	2-3 x greater
2	3-6 x greater
3	8-10 x greater

* Compared to men whose 1st degree relatives did not have prostate cancer.
Data from Eur Urol 58(2): 275, 2010.

African Ancestry
1. Men of African ancestry have been referred to in some studies as Black men or, for studies conducted in the Unites States, as African American men.
2. Men of African ancestry are more likely to develop prostate cancer and are more likely to be diagnosed at an earlier age.
3. Men of African ancestry are more likely to have an advanced stage of cancer at diagnosis, to have a more aggressive cancer, and to die from their cancer.

Age at Diagnosis
1. Prostate cancer is rare in men < 40 years of age.
2. The risk of prostate cancer increases after age 40-50.
3. More than 90% of prostate cancers are diagnosed in men > 50 years of age.
4. Median age of diagnosis in the United States is 66 years.

Genetic Mutations & Prostate Cancer

General Information on Genetic Mutations

1. Mutations can be classified based on whether they are inherited from the parent's gametes at the time of conception (germline mutation) or whether they arise in non-gamete cells after conception (somatic mutation).

2. Germline mutations—these genetic mutations are *inherited* from a parent at the time of conception and are copied into *all cells in the body* (although it may not be present in all gametes). *The mutation can be passed from generation to generation.*

   a. Tissue required for germline testing—theoretically, testing can be performed using any nucleated diploid (non-gamete) cell because they contain a full compliment of inherited DNA; however, testing is typically done using lymphocytes (from a blood sample) and/or buccal mucosa cells (from a saliva sample or a buccal swab).

   b. Population in which germline testing is utilized—patients with or without cancer.

   c. Reasons to test for germline mutations—in a person without cancer, testing can determine the risk of subsequently developing cancer and the risk they may pass a mutation to their children. In a person with cancer, testing may guide treatment (some therapies may be more effective when a certain mutation is present), may help refine the prognosis of existing cancer, may help establish a patient's personal risk for other cancers (some genetic syndromes are associated with multiple cancers), may determine the risk of passing a mutation to their children, and may ascertain if family members may be at risk for having the same mutation.

3. Somatic mutation—these genetic mutations are acquired after conception; therefore, they are *not inherited* and *cannot be passed to the next generation*. Somatic mutations arise only in *some cells in the body* (such as within a cancer cell). In a cancer with somatic mutations, the genes involved and percent of cells affected may change over time because of genetic instability within the cancer and selective pressure from cancer treatment. *Most mutations in prostate cancer are somatic rather than germline.*

   a. Tissue required for somatic testing—*a sample of the malignant tissue is required.*

   b. Population in which somatic testing is utilized—patients with cancer.

   c. Reasons to test for somatic mutations—to guide treatment (some therapies may be more effective when a certain mutation is present) or to help better define the prognosis.

4. If a cancer has a certain mutation, the mutation may have arisen from either genetic aberrations in the cancer (somatic mutation) or from the patient's inherited genes (germline mutation).

5. If a patient has a certain germline mutation, the same mutation will be present in that patient's cancer (unless genetic instability in the cancer has removed the mutation).

Comparison of Mutations Associated with Cancer

	Germline Mutation	**Somatic Mutation**
Origin of the Mutation	Inherited from a parent	Spontaneous mutation within the cancer
Can be Transmitted to Offspring	Yes	No
Cells in Which the Mutation is Present	All nucleated diploid cells in the body	Some or all cancer cells
Population in Which Testing is Utilized	With or without cancer	With cancer
Tissue Sources Typically Used for Testing	Lymphocytes, buccal cells	Cancer cells
Predicts Risk of Developing Cancer in the Future	Yes	No
May Help Guide Treatment of Existing Cancer	Yes	Yes
May Help Define Prognosis of an Existing Cancer	Yes	Yes

Genetic Mutations that Increase the Risk of Prostate Cancer

1. Certain genetic mutations can increase the risk of developing prostate cancer. The genes in which these mutations occur can be categorized according to their function (in some cases, the gene may be involved in more than one function). When in their normal (unmutated) form, many of these genes repair errors in DNA, such as genes involved in homologous recombination repair (HRR) or mismatch repair. When one of these DNA repair genes undergoes mutation, it loses its normal function; therefore, DNA errors are perpetuated rather than corrected. These unrepaired errors in DNA can cause cancer.

Examples of Genes That Increase the Risk Prostate Cancer, Categorized by Function

DNA Homologous Recombination Repair (HHR)				DNA Mismatch Repair	Regulation of Other Genes
ATM	BRIP1	MRE11A	PALB2	MLH1	HOXB13
ATR	CHEK2	MSH2	PMS2	MSH2	
BRCA1	FAM175A	MSH6	RAD51C	MSH6	
BRCA2	GEN1	NBN	RAD51D	PMS2	

2. *More aggressive prostate cancers are associated with a higher likelihood of having a germline mutation. Also, men with intraductal, ductal, or cribriform prostate cancer are more likely to have germline or somatic mutations.*

Cancer Stage	**Chance of a Germline Mutation Related to Prostate Cancer**
Localized, Low/Intermediate Risk	2%
Localized, High Risk	6%
Metastatic	12-16%

Data from N Engl J Med 375: 443, 2016 & J Clin Oncol 37: 490, 2019.

3. BRCA1 and BRCA2 mutations
    a. Both BRCA1 and BRCA2 mutations increase the risk of multiple cancers including prostate cancer, male breast cancer, female breast cancer, ovarian cancer, and pancreatic cancer.
    b. BRCA mutations are inherited in an autosomal dominant fashion.
    c. BRCA1 mutation—there is conflicting evidence as to whether a germline BRCA1 mutation increases the risk of developing prostate cancer. Also, evidence is insufficient to determine if BRCA1 mutations influence the aggressiveness or lethality of prostate cancer.
    d. BRCA2 mutation—compared to men with normal BRCA2 genes, men with a germline BRCA2 mutation are 2 to 6 times more likely to develop prostate cancer. They are also more likely to be diagnosed with prostate cancer at an earlier age, to have a more advanced stage at diagnosis, to have a more aggressive cancer, and to die from their cancer. *BRCA2 mutations are the most common germline mutations in men with metastatic prostate cancer.*
    e. Compared to the general population, *Jews of Eastern European ancestry (Ashkenazi Jews) are 10 times more likely to have a BRCA mutation* (BRCA1 or BRCA2 mutations occur in 2% Ashkenazi Jews and in 0.2% of the general population).
    f. Men with a BRCA mutation and metastatic castration resistant prostate cancer may be candidates for treatment with a PARP inhibitor (see page 248).
4. DNA mismatch repair genes (MLH1, MSH2, MSH6, PMS2)—a mutation in any of these genes can increase the risk of developing prostate cancer.
    a. A mutation in these genes causes a loss of their normal function, resulting in deficient mismatch repair (dMMR) of DNA. The presence of dMMR leads to microsatellite instability (MSI), which is a predisposition to developing further mutations.
    b. Testing for mutations in these genes can be performed using assays for either dMMR or for MSI (mutations are present when dMMR or MSI are present). The degree of MSI can be classified as MSI high (MSI-H), MSI low (MSH-L), MSI-indeterminate (MSI-I), or MSI absent (MSI absent is also called microsatellite stable, MSS). A higher risk for prostate cancer is mainly associated with MSI-H.
    c. Lynch syndrome (hereditary nonpolyposis colorectal cancer)—an autosomal dominant syndrome that increases the risk of developing multiple malignancies, including cancer of the prostate, upper urinary tract, colon, rectum, small bowel, stomach, biliary tract, pancreas, endometrium, ovary, and brain. It arises from a germline mutation in any of several genes, including DNA mismatch repair genes such as MLH1, MSH2, MSH6, and PMS2. *Lynch syndrome increases the risk of developing prostate cancer by 2 to 6 fold;* however, it does not appear to alter the age of onset or the aggressiveness of the cancer. *Men with dMMR or MSI are at risk for Lynch syndrome.*
    d. *When MSI or dMMR is present, the patient is a candidate for treatment with pembrolizumab (see page 251).*
5. CHEK2 mutation (particularly I157T)—this mutation increases the risk of developing cancers of the prostate, kidney (specifically clear cell cancer), breast (male or female), colon, and thyroid.
6. *If a patient has known or suspected genetic susceptibility to prostate cancer, he should be referred for genetic counseling.*

Testing for Genetic Abnormalities in Men with Prostate Cancer

1. *Germline* genetic testing should include testing for BRCA1, BRCA2, ATM, PALB2, CHEK2, MLH1, MSH2, MSH6, and PMS2. Germline testing *is recommended* in men with prostate cancer and any of the following characteristics:
   a. High risk localized prostate cancer.
   b. Regional or distant metastasis from prostate cancer (stage N1 or M1).
   c. Ductal, intraductal, or cribriform pattern prostate cancer.
   d. Family history that meets any of the following criteria:
      i. Brother, father, or multiple family members diagnosed at age < 60 years with Grade Group ≥ 2 prostate cancer.
      ii. Brother, father, or multiple family members who died of prostate cancer.
      iii. Ashkenazi Jewish ancestry
      iv. Family history of germline mutations that increase the risk of prostate cancer (e.g. BRCA2, Lynch syndrome, CHEK2).
      v. Family history of three or more of the following cancers on the same side of the family (especially when diagnosed at age ≤ 50 years): prostate with Grade group ≥ 2, urothelial, kidney, gastric, bile duct, pancreatic, small bowel, colorectal, breast, ovarian, endometrial, or melanoma.

2. *Somatic* testing of malignant tissue
   a. Men with regional node metastasis (N1M0)—consider tests of homologous recombination repair genes (BRCA1, BRCA2, ATM, etc.) and tests for deficient DNA mismatch repair (using an assay for either MSI-H or dMMR).
   b. Castration naive men with distant metastasis (M1)
      i. Recommended—tests for homologous recombination DNA repair genes (BRCA1, BRCA2, ATM, etc.).
      ii. Consider—tests for deficient DNA mismatch repair (using an assay for either MSI-H or dMMR).
   c. Castration resistant men with distant metastasis (M1)—recommended tests include assays for homologous recombination repair genes (BRCA1, BRCA2, ATM, etc.) and tests for deficient DNA mismatch repair (using an assay for either MSI-H or dMMR).
   d. Untreated men who have very low risk, low risk, or favorable intermediate risk prostate cancer and life expectancy > 10 years—somatic testing in these men may help determine if they have a higher risk of progression on surveillance. There are several assays available, including Decipher Prostate Biopsy, Oncotype DX Prostate, Prolaris, and Promark. See page 202 for more information on these tests.
   e. Men who underwent radical prostatectomy that have a positive surgical margin, stage pT3 (seminal vesicle invasion, extraprostatic extension, or bladder neck invasion), or rising PSA—the Decipher Prostate RP test can help predict which of these men may be best managed by surveillance (with salvage XRT as needed). See page 222 for more information.

3. *Somatic* testing of benign tissue—in men with a previous benign biopsy who are still suspected of having prostate cancer, ConfirmMDx or Mitomic Prostate Core Test can be performed to help predict the risk of prostate cancer. See page 189, for more information on these tests.

Pathology

Prostatic Intraepithelial Neoplasia (PIN)

1. PIN is a dysplasia of the prostate epithelial cells. These dysplastic cells are inside glands that *have a basal cell layer.*
2. PIN is categorized as low grade or high grade.
3. PIN often coexists with prostate cancer.
4. The presence of PIN does not seem to raise the serum PSA.
5. Focal high grade PIN is typically defined as 1 or 2 sites of involvement. Multifocal high grade PIN is typically defined as ≥ 3 sites of involvement.
6. *Low grade PIN and focal high grade PIN do not increase the risk of developing prostate cancer.*
7. Multifocal high grade PIN increases the risk of developing prostate cancer. *After a 10-12 core systematic prostate biopsy, approximately 30% of men with multifocal high grade PIN will develop prostate cancer.* A greater number of foci with high grade PIN correlates with a higher risk of developing cancer.
8. It is important to distinguish high grade PIN from ductal and intraductal prostate cancer because they can have a similar appearance on histology. When the pathology report reveals extensive high grade PIN but no prostate cancer, consider having the biopsy reviewed by a pathologist with expertise in prostate cancer to rule out ductal and intraductal carcinoma.
9. Management of PIN (see Management of Biopsy Results, page 197)
   a. Low grade PIN or focal high grade PIN—monitor digital rectal exam (DRE) and PSA. Biopsy again if indicated based on the PSA and DRE.
   b. Multifocal high grade PIN (≥ 3 sites)—monitor PSA and DRE, and re-biopsy the prostate in 1-3 years with increased sampling from the high grade PIN region and from adjacent regions. When extensive high grade PIN is present, confirm the absence of ductal and intraductal cancer, and then re-biopsy in 1 year. (see Management of Biopsy Results, page 197).

Atypical Tissue

1. The terms atypia, atypical glands, and atypical hyperplasia are not specific and should be avoided.
2. Atypical adenomatous hyperplasia (adenosis)—although weak circumstantial data links this entity to prostate cancer, follow up of a limited number of cases suggests a benign outcome. Therefore, *isolated atypical adenomatous hyperplasia is generally considered benign. Re-biopsy is usually unnecessary, but clinical follow up is warranted.*
3. Atypical small acinar proliferation (ASAP)—also called "atypia suspicious for carcinoma" or "atypical glands suspicious for carcinoma".
   a. ASAP is a gland or glands suspicious for cancer, but there is insufficient architectural and/or cytologic atypia for a diagnosis of cancer.
   b. ASAP has a well documented association with prostate cancer. *40-60% of men with ASAP have prostate cancer on subsequent biopsy* (the cancer is usually found in the same region where the ASAP was found, and 80-90% of the cancers are Gleason score ≤ 6).
   c. The chance of developing cancer is more likely with ASAP than with multifocal high grade PIN.
   d. The presence of ASAP does not seem to alter PSA.
   e. Management of ASAP—re-biopsy within 3-6 months with increased sampling from the atypical region and from adjacent regions (see Management of Biopsy Results, page 197).

Diagnostic Criteria for Prostate Adenocarcinoma
1. Prostate adenocarcinoma originates from prostate *epithelial cells* and stains positive for prostatic acid phosphatase (PAP) and for PSA.
2. Normal prostate glands always have a basal cell layer. *Prostate adenocarcinoma never has a basal cell layer* (not even an incomplete layer). Basal cells stain positive for high molecular weight keratin (HMWK) but negative for PSA and PAP. Therefore, when it is difficult to determine if the cells are malignant, stain the slide with HMWK. If glandular structures lack basal cells (negative HMWK), cancer is present.
3. For grading of prostate adenocarcinoma, see page 198.

Types of Prostate Cancer
1. Adenocarcinoma—arises from the prostate gland epithelial cells.
   a. Acinar adenocarcinoma (>95%)—this is the common variant, and the term "prostate cancer" generally refers to this entity.
   b. Prostatic ductal adenocarcinoma—a rare aggressive prostate cancer that arises from within the prostate ducts. It is assigned a Gleason score of 4+4. It usually arises from the peripheral zone, but it tends to grow into the urethral lumen; therefore, *patients commonly have a normal prostate digital examination and tend to present with obstructive voiding symptoms or gross hematuria.* PSA is often normal. It has a propensity to metastasize to the lung, liver, testicle, and penis. Ductal type is treated the same as acinar adenocarcinoma. Acinar and ductal variants often occur together. Genetic mutations appear to be more common in ductal cancers. Occasionally, ductal adenocarcinoma may be misdiagnosed as high grade PIN because they can have a similar appearance on histology.
   c. Intraductal carcinoma of the prostate (IDCP)—IDCP arises from the spread of acinar adenocarcinoma into the prostate ducts. Therefore, its presence on a biopsy typically indicates that aggressive acinar adenocarcinoma is present somewhere else in the prostate. Genetic mutations appear to be more common in IDCP. IDCPs may be misdiagnosed as high grade PIN because they can have a similar appearance on histology.
2. Non-adenocarcinomas (< 5%)—transitional cell carcinoma is the most common non-adenocarcinoma. Others cancer types include small cell carcinoma and sarcoma.

Location of Prostate Cancer
1. *The most common location of prostate cancer is the peripheral zone.*
2. Prostate cancer tends to be multifocal.
3. More than 65% of cancers are within 5 mm and 35-45% are within 1 mm of the urethra. Thus, ablative therapy that spares the periurethral tissue may leave cancer behind.

Location of Prostate Cancer	
Peripheral Zone	70%
Transition Zone	20%
Central Zone	5-10%
Anterior Fibromuscular	Rare

Local Cancer Spread
1. *Capsular penetration is most common in the posterior-lateral prostate, near the neurovascular bundle.*
2. Capsular penetration is twice as common in peripheral zone cancers as in transition zone cancers.
3. Capsular penetration is more common in patients with higher clinical stage, higher grade group (Gleason score), and higher preoperative PSA.

Prevention of Prostate Cancer

Smoking Cessation

1. Smoking within 10 years of being diagnosed with prostate cancer appears to increase the risk of high stage, high grade, metastasis, biochemical recurrence, castration resistance, and prostate cancer specific mortality. Men who quit smoking > 10 years before the diagnosis of prostate cancer have a similar prostate cancer specific mortality as non-smokers.
2. It is unclear if smoking cessation reduces the risk of developing prostate cancer; however, if a man quits smoking, he may reduce the risk of having aggressive features if a prostate cancer does develop.

Dietary Supplements for Prostate Cancer Prevention

1. *Vitamin C, vitamin D, Vitamin E, multivitamins, selenium, lycopene, soy, and omega-3 fatty acids appear to be ineffective for prevention of prostate cancer. In men with high grade PIN, oral green tea catechins may decrease the risk of developing prostate cancer. A Mediterranean diet may reduce the risk of developing aggressive prostate cancer.*
2. Vitamin E—multiple randomized trials (including SELECT, HOPE, and PHS II) showed that oral supplementation with vitamin E does not reduce the risk of prostate cancer after 7 to 10 years of follow up.
    a. SELECT trial—randomized 35,533 men age ≥ 50 with a PSA < 4 and normal prostate exam into 4 groups: placebo, vitamin E (α-tocopherol 400 IU po q day), selenium (L-selenomethionine 200 mcg po q day), or both vitamin E and selenium. After a median follow up of over 8 years, none of the interventions reduced the incidence of prostate cancer, but *vitamin E significantly increased the risk of prostate cancer.*
    b. HOPE trial—randomized 9641 men age > 55 to placebo or vitamin E (α-tocopherol 400 IU po q day). After a median follow up of 7 years, vitamin E did not reduce the incidence of prostate cancer.
    c. Physicians Health Study II (PHS II)—randomized 14,641 men age ≥ 50 to placebo, vitamin E (α-tocopherol 400 IU po qod), vitamin C (500 mg po q day), or both vitamin E and C. After a median follow up of 8 years, none of the interventions reduced the incidence of prostate cancer.
3. Vitamin C—several studies (including PROtEus and PHS II) showed that oral supplementation with vitamin C does not reduce the risk of prostate cancer after long term follow up.
4. Vitamin D—the VITAL study showed that oral supplementation with vitamin D does not reduce the risk of prostate cancer after 5 years of follow up. A higher serum vitamin D level does not reduce the risk of developing prostate cancer nor the risk of dying from prostate cancer.
5. Multivitamin—a component of PHSII randomized 14,641 men age ≥ 50 to placebo or an oral daily multivitamin. After a median follow up of 11.2 years, the multivitamin did not reduce the incidence of prostate cancer.
6. Selenium—multiple randomized trials (including SELECT, and NBT) showed that oral supplementation with selenium does not reduce the risk of prostate cancer after 2 to 10 years of follow up.
7. Soy protein—a few small randomized studies suggest that oral soy protein does not reduce the risk of prostate cancer after 2 to 3 years of follow up.
8. Omega-3 fatty acids—the VITAL study showed that oral omega-3 fatty acid does not reduce the risk of prostate cancer after 5 years of follow up.
9. Lycopene—randomized and non-randomized trials suggest that lycopene may decrease PSA, but it does not prevent prostate cancer.
10. Green tea catechins—limited data suggests that oral intake of green tea catechins in men with high grade PIN may decrease the development of prostate cancer within 1-2 years of follow up.

11. Mediterranean diet—limited retrospective data suggests that men are less likely to develop an aggressive prostate cancer when they are have a diet rich in fruits, vegetables, fish, legumes, and olive oil.

Medications for Prostate Cancer Prevention

1. Metformin—only non-randomized studies have been done. The quality of data is poor and the data are conflicting as to whether metformin can prevent prostate cancer.
2. Statins—retrospective data indicate that statins do not reduce the risk of developing prostate cancer.
3. 5α-reductase inhibitors—see below.

5α-Reductase Inhibitors (5ARI)

1. PCPT (Prostate Cancer Prevention Trial)—over 18,000 men age ≥ 55 with a normal prostate exam and PSA ≤ 3.0 were randomized to a 7 year course of placebo or finasteride 5 mg po daily.
2. REDUCE trial (Reduction by Dutasteride of Prostate Cancer Events)—over 8,000 men age > 50 with a negative prostate biopsy, prostate volume < 80 cc, and PSA = 2.5 to 10 were randomized to a 4 year course of placebo or dutasteride 0.5 mg po daily.
3. In these studies, 5ARIs reduce the relative risk of developing prostate cancer by nearly 25%. However, subgroup analyses shows that 5ARIs reduce the risk of developing cancer with Gleason score ≤ 6, but slightly increase the risk of developing cancer with Gleason score = 8-10. Despite the slight increased risk of Gleason 8-10 cancer, long term follow up (13 to 15 years) shows equivalent overall and prostate cancer specific survival in men with prostate cancer whether they took a 5ARI or placebo.
   a. Approximately 75% of the prevented cancers are very low risk (see page 201) and perhaps clinically insignificant.
   b. The absolute risk of developing a Gleason score = 8-10 cancer is increased by less than 1% in men taking a 5ARI.
   c. Putting the data into perspective—*out of 200 men receiving a 5ARI, one man will be more likely to develop a Gleason 8-10 cancer, 3 men will be less likely to develop a potentially clinically meaningful Gleason ≤ 6 cancer, and approximately 8 men will be less likely to develop a very low risk (and potentially clinically insignificant) Gleason ≤ 6 cancer. The greater risk of developing high grade cancer while taking a 5ARI did not increase mortality. Conversely, the greater chance of preventing a low grade cancer while taking a 5ARI did not reduce mortality.*
4. Taking a 5ARI increases the risk of erectile dysfunction and low libido.
5. *The FDA did not approve 5ARIs for the prevention of prostate cancer.*

Screening for Prostate Cancer

General Information

1. Over 90% of prostate cancers detected by screening are organ-confined.
2. Screening means that testing is done in *asymptomatic* patients to detect cancer at an earlier point in time.
3. PSA detects more organ confined cancers than digital rectal exam (DRE). When used together, PSA and DRE detect more cancers than DRE alone.
4. Cancers detected by PSA are more likely to be organ confined and less likely to be metastatic; therefore, screening with PSA detects prostate cancer at an earlier stage.
5. *PSA elevation typically occurs 6 to 13 years before prostate cancer causes symptoms.*

Is Prostate Cancer Screening Beneficial?

1. Screening for prostate cancer is controversial because of disagreement regarding the balance between its benefits and its harms.
    a. Harms
        i. Overdiagnosis—some prostate cancers do not cause morbidity or mortality, even when they are untreated (i.e. they are "clinically insignificant"). In other words, an insignificant cancer is unlikely to cause harm in a patient's lifetime, even if the cancer remains undiagnosed. Overdiagnosis means that a man is diagnosed with an insignificant cancer. Current estimates suggest that *overdiagnosis typically occurs in 23% to 50% of all prostate cancer cases.* Older age increases the risk of overdiagnosis.
        ii. Overtreatment—when overdiagnosis occurs, the patient may be subjected to unnecessary tests (e.g. prostate biopsy), unnecessary treatments, and added morbidity (e.g. treatment related side effects).
        iii. Increased psychologic stress—from cancer, tests, treatments, etc.
        iv. Increased medical costs.
    b. Benefits—*screening results in diagnosing cancer at a lower stage and grade, reduces the risk of developing metastatic cancer, and reduces the risk of dying from prostate cancer. The 2013 Prostate Cancer World Congress consensus concluded that "For men aged 50-69, level 1 evidence demonstrates that PSA testing reduces prostate cancer specific mortality and the incidence of metastatic prostate cancer."*
2. *Randomized studies indicate that screening for prostate cancer can reduce the relative risk of dying from prostate by approximately 30%. Screening does not reduce all-cause mortality.*
3. The main screening trials and their findings are discussed below. *Note that these studies do not provide adequate information for groups that were under-represented, such men with non-white ethnicity, age < 50-55, or family history of prostate cancer.*
4. PLCO (Prostate, Lung, Colorectal, Ovarian cancer screening trial)—76,683 men age 55 to 74 in the Unites States were randomized to routine screening (annual PSA and digital rectal exam) or to "usual care" (control group in which patients could elect to undergo screening). After 15 years, the risk of death from prostate cancer was similar between the groups. Problems with this study include
    a. PSA testing was very common in the "usual care" control group (86% underwent at least one PSA and 46% underwent annual PSA testing). This contamination of the control group likely diluted any advantage from screening. *When the data were adjusted to account for contamination of the control group, screening reduced the relative risk of death from prostate cancer by 27-32%.*
    b. Approximately 44% of men in the trial underwent PSA testing before enrolling in the study. This pre-study screening may have purged cancers from the study population and altered the results of the trial.
    c. Only 30-40% of men with an abnormal PSA underwent prostate biopsy.
    d. This trial compared organized screening to opportunistic screening (it did not compare screening to not screening).
    e. All of the problems listed above severely limit the relevance of the PLCO for determining if screening saves lives. The ERSPC and Goteborg trials are more methodologically sound and have fewer shortcomings; therefore, they are more germane for determining if screening saves lives.

5. CAP (Cluster Randomized Trial of PSA Testing for Prostate Cancer)—408,825 men age 50 to 69 in the United Kingdom were randomized to a group in which all men were offered a single PSA test or to a group in which PSA testing was only offered if the patient asked about PSA. After a median follow up of 10 years, the risk of death from prostate cancer was similar between the groups. Screening did not reduce all-cause mortality. Problems with this study include

   a. This trial compared routinely offering a single PSA test to offering a PSA test at the request of the patient (it did not compare screening to not screening).

   b. CAP offered only one PSA test per patient. ERSCP, PLCO, & Goteborg utilized periodic PSA testing. Periodic screening with PSA is more sensitive for detecting prostate cancer than a single PSA test.

   c. A valid PSA test was obtained in only 34% of men in the "screened" group, which was not that much different than the ~15% PSA testing rate in the control group. This limits the relevance of the CAP trial in determining if PSA screening saves lives.

6. ERSPC (European Randomized Study for screening Prostate Cancer)—182,000 men age 50 to 74 in 7 European countries were randomized to PSA screening or no PSA screening. A predefined core group of 162,388 men age 55-69 was the main focus of the study. Screening interval varied among the countries, and ranged from 2 to 7 years. After 16 years of follow up, *screening significantly reduced the relative risk of death from prostate cancer by 20%; however, this reduction in mortality was only seen in men age 55-69 and not in men age $\leq$ 70. Screening did not reduce all-cause mortality.* 570 men had to be screened and 18 men had to be diagnosed with cancer to prevent one death from prostate cancer. Also, *PSA screening decreased the risk of developing metastatic prostate cancer.* Problems with this study include

   a. Based on data from the Netherlands, approximately 19% of the control group underwent PSA testing (but this is far less than 86% in PLCO). However, *when the data were adjusted to account for contamination of the control group, screening reduced the relative risk of death from prostate cancer by 25-31%.*

   b. The screening interval (2, 4, or 7 years) and biopsy trigger (PSA range $\geq$ 3.0-4.0) varied between countries.

   c. When data were analyzed by country, the relative risk of death from prostate cancer ranged from 0% to 51%.

7. Goteborg Trial—20,000 men age 50 to 64 in Sweden were randomized to routine PSA screening (PSA every 2 years) or no screening (control group). After 18 years of follow up, *PSA screening significantly reduced the relative risk of death from prostate cancer by 35% in men who started screening at age 50-64 (all men in the study), and by approximately 53% in the subgroup of men who started screening at age 50-59.* 231 men had to be screened and 10 men had to be diagnosed with cancer to prevent one death from prostate cancer. *PSA screening decreased the risk of developing metastatic prostate cancer.* A subset of the men in the Goteborg trial were enrolled in the ERSPC. Key advantages of this study include

   a. Presumably, few men in the control group underwent PSA testing.

   b. Few men underwent PSA testing before enrolling in this study.

   c. Most men with an abnormal PSA underwent prostate biopsy.

Comparison of Screening Trial Design & Study Population

Trial	Study Population				Screening Protocol		
	# of Men	Age Range	Age Mean	% White° Race	Screening Test(s)	Testing Interval (years)	Biopsy Trigger
PLCO	76,683	55-74	?	85%	Periodic PSA & DRE	1	PSA > 4.0 or abnormal DRE
CAP	408,825	50-69	59	?**	Single PSA	–	PSA ≥ 3.0
ERSPC	182,000	50-74	61	?**	Periodic PSA	2-7	PSA ≥ 3.0-4.0
Goteborg	20,000	50-64	?	?**	Periodic PSA	2	PSA ≥ 2.5-3.4

DRE = digital rectal exam; PSA = prostate specific antigen in ng/ml; ? = unknown
° Specifically, non-hispanic white men.
**The percentage of non-hispanic white men is likely very high because the proportion of non-white men in Europe was low during the study period.

Comparison Of Screening Trial Results, Contamination, and Compliance

Trial	Relative Reduction in PC Mortality with Screening°		Median Follow Up (years)	Had PSA* before Trial‡	Contamination in the Control Group (had PSA* during Trial)	Compliance in the Screened Group	
	Unadjusted	Adjusted				With PSA*	With Biopsy§
PLCO	0%	27-32%	17	44%	86%	99%	30-40%
CAP	0%	–	10	?	10-15%	34%	85%
ERSPC	20%	25-31%	16	13%†	19%†	83%	86%
Goteborg	35%	–	18	3%	? (Likely Low)	77%	94%

* Men that had a least one PSA test.   PC = prostate cancer; ? = unknown
‡ Percentage of entire study population.   PSA = prostate specific antigen
§ Percent of men with an abnormal PSA who underwent prostate biopsy.
† Data from Netherlands cohort (J Urol 164: 1216, 2000, Eur Urol 65: 329, 2014).
° Unadjusted rates did not account for contamination in the control group and were calculated at the median follow up. Adjusted rates correct for contamination in the control group and were calculated at 11 years of follow up. Contamination in the control group (when not accounted for) can dilute the benefit of screening.

What Should Patients Know Before Deciding to be Screened?

1. In United States, prostate cancer is the most common internal malignancy diagnosed in men. Approximately 12% of U.S. men will be diagnosed with prostate cancer in their lifetime.
2. In the United states, prostate cancer is the second most common cause of cancer-related death in men. However, *the approximate chance of dying from prostate cancer is only 3%* (when all races are included, the risk is 2.4% in the U.S. and 4.3% in the United Kingdom). Thus, *most prostate cancers do not cause death.*
3. Screening can reduce the *relative risk* of dying from prostate cancer by 30%, which means it decreases the *actual lifetime risk* by about 1%.
4. Information specific to men of African ancestry
   a. Men of African ancestry are more likely to develop prostate cancer.
   b. Men of African ancestry are more likely to develop the cancer at an earlier age, to have more advanced cancers, to have more aggressive cancers, and to die from prostate cancer.
   c. In men of African ancestry, *the lifetime risk of dying from prostate cancer is approximately 2 times higher than other races* (for men of African ancestry, the risk of dying from prostate cancer is 3.9% in the U.S. and 8.7% in the United Kingdom).

5. Before screening is offered, physicians should discuss the benefits, risks, and limitations of prostate cancer screening with the patient. *The decision to screen should be a shared decision between the patient and physician.*
    a. Harms include overdiagnosis and overtreatment. Some prostate cancers do not cause morbidity or mortality, even when they are untreated (i.e. they are "clinically insignificant"). In general, a man with insignificant cancer will have no harmful effects if his cancer remains undiagnosed. When an insignificant cancer is discovered, the patient may be subjected to unnecessary tests (e.g. prostate biopsy), unnecessary treatments ("overtreatment"), and additional morbidity (e.g. psychologic stress, treatment related side effects). Screening can increase medical costs.
    b. Benefits include diagnosing cancer at a lower stage and grade, reduced risk of developing metastatic cancer, and reduced risk of dying from prostate cancer.
6. Screening typically consists of PSA testing with or without a digital rectal exam (DRE).
7. Screening with PSA and/or DRE is not 100% accurate. False positive results are common with PSA and DRE (i.e. benign processes often elevate the PSA or make the DRE feel abnormal). In fact, PSA generates a false positive result approximately 60% of the time (depending on the PSA level that is used to trigger a biopsy). Also, screening can miss some cancers (false negative results).
8. If screening is abnormal, additional tests (such as risk calculators, imaging, or other biomarkers) may help better define the risk of prostate cancer and the risk of an aggressive cancer.
9. The diagnosis of prostate cancer requires a prostate biopsy. Prostate biopsy is an invasive procedure associated with a low risk of serious side effects (see Side Effects of Prostate Biopsy, page 197).
10. If cancer is diagnosed, management options include surveillance or treatment, both of which entail potentially harmful risks.
    a. Some prostate cancers are less likely to cause harm (even when they are untreated). Although there are tests that can estimate the chance that a cancer will be harmful, these tests are not 100% accurate. Cancers that are less likely to cause harm may be managed with surveillance. Surveillance may include subsequent blood tests, prostate exams, imaging, and repeat prostate biopsies.
    b. Treatment of the cancer can cause side effects, such as erectile dysfunction, urinary incontinence, and bowel problems.

Which Tests Are Used For Prostate Cancer Screening?

1. *Prostate cancer screening consists of periodic PSA measurements with or without a digital rectal exam (DRE) of the prostate.* A combination of PSA and DRE appears to detect more cancers than either test alone, although the benefit of adding DRE is marginal because most cancers are detected by PSA. *If the PSA is abnormal, then a DRE should be performed* if it was not done recently. For more details on using these tests for screening, see page 181 for PSA and page 182 for DRE.
2. *Prostate imaging is not recommended for prostate cancer screening* because it does not improve cancer detection. However, prostate imaging is useful for guiding prostate biopsies.
3. Currently, there is insufficient information regarding the use of other tests (such as PCA3, PHI, etc.) as an initial screening modality.

Who Should Be Screened And Starting At What Age?

1. *Screening should be offered to men of appropriate age who have a life expectancy of more than 10 years.*
2. Men with average risk for prostate cancer—many guidelines recommend screening starting at age 50-55 in these men.
3. Men at higher risk for prostate cancer—many guidelines recommend screening starting at age 40-45 in men with a higher risk of lethal prostate cancer and/or a high risk for developing prostate cancer at an early age (such as such as men with a family history of prostate cancer, African ancestry, or the presence of germline mutations associated with prostate cancer). Many guidelines recommend starting at age 40 in men at very high risk.
4. The 2013 Prostate Cancer World Congress consensus states *"Baseline PSA testing for men in their 40's is useful for predicting the future risk of prostate cancer."* For men age 40-49, the median PSA is 0.7 ng/ml. Men with PSA above this median (especially PSA $\geq$ 1.0, which is above the 75th percentile for this age) have a higher risk for prostate cancer and for aggressive prostate cancer. Men age 45-49 with a PSA $\geq$ 1.6 have 9 fold higher risk of dying from prostate cancer within 25 years compared to men with PSA $\leq$ 1.0.

At What Interval Should The Screening Tests Be Performed?

1. Periodic screening with PSA is more sensitive for detecting prostate cancer than a single PSA test. Therefore, serial PSA measurements are recommended for screening.
2. Screening is often performed annually; however, the custom of annual screening is not evidence-based.
3. Many guidelines suggest determining the screening interval based on PSA values. Men whose PSA suggests a low risk of developing metastasis and lethal prostate cancer can be screened less often.
   a. The 2021 ACS guideline recommends screening every 2 years in men with PSA < 2.5 and every year in men with PSA $\geq$ 2.5.
   b. The EAU 2021 guideline recommends a screening interval of 2 years for men with PSA > 1 at age 40 or PSA > 2 at age 60 (because these men have a higher risk of metastatic and lethal prostate cancer) and an interval of 8 years for all other men.
   c. The CUA 2017 guideline recommends a screening interval of 4 years in men with PSA < 1, 2 years in men with PSA = 1-3, and consider more frequent PSA testing or adjunctive tests to decide if biopsy is warranted in men with PSA > 3.
   d. The NCCN 2021 guideline recommends screening every 2-4 years if PSA < 1, every 1-2 years if PSA = 1-3, and consider adjunctive tests to decide if biopsy is warranted in men with PSA > 3.
4. The 2018 AUA guideline states *"...a routine screening interval of two years or more may be preferred over annual screening...it is expected that screening intervals of two years preserve the majority of the benefits and reduce overdiagnosis and false positives."*
5. A screening interval of 1 year may be more appropriate for men with a higher risk of developing lethal prostate cancer, whereas a longer interval may be appropriate for men with a lower risk. *Risks for developing lethal prostate cancer include: baseline PSA above the median for the patient's age group, family history of prostate cancer, African ancestry, and the presence of germline mutations associated with prostate cancer.*

At What Age Should Screening Be Stopped?

1. There is no universally accepted age after which prostate cancer screening should be stopped. *Many guidelines recommend that screening should cease when the patient's life expectancy is less than 10-15 years, regardless of the patient's current age.* However, it can be difficult to accurately predict life expectancy. Thus, some guidelines specify an age when screening should be discontinued.

2. Several guidelines suggest that *routine* screening should be halted at age 70, but *screening may be reasonable in men over age 70 when they have excellent health and minimal comorbidities (especially if they have a family history of longevity, a rising PSA, or have never had PSA testing).*

   a. The 2013 Prostate Cancer World Congress consensus states "Older men in good health with over 10 year life expectancy should not be denied PSA testing on the basis of their age."

   b. The 2021 ACS guideline states that "men without symptoms of prostate cancer who do not have a 10 year life expectancy should not be offered testing since they are not likely to benefit."

   c. The AUA 2018 guideline recommends against *routine* screening in men age > 70, but states "Some men over age 70 years who are in excellent health may benefit from prostate cancer screening."

   d. The NCCN 2021 guideline states that screening "...after 75 years of age should be done only in very healthy men with little or no comorbidity (especially if they have never undergone PSA testing or have a rising PSA)..."

   e. The USPSTF discourages the screening of men ≥ 70 years old.

3. Clinicians can utilize PSA level at age 70-75 to help determine which healthy men may benefit from further screening. *Men age 70-75 with PSA ≥ 3 are more likely to benefit from further PSA testing.*

   a. PSA < 3 at age 70-75—these men have a very low risk of dying from prostate cancer (≤ 3%); therefore, further screening in these men is unlikely to be beneficial.

   b. PSA ≥ 3 at age 70-75—these men have a 7% risk of dying from prostate cancer, but the risk increases as they get older. So, the older these men get, the higher their risk of dying from prostate cancer.

Screening PSA and Subsequent Risk of Dying from Prostate Cancer

1. Men age 40-50—for men without risk factors for prostate cancer (e.g. no family history, not of African ancestry, no genetic predisposition), some physicians think that using PSA to predict future risk is of marginal value because it does not confer a clinical advantage over testing starting at age 50. Nonetheless, PSA can predict future risk in this age group.

   a. PSA ≤ 1.0 at age 45-49—these men have the lowest risk of dying from prostate cancer.

   b. PSA ≥ 1.6 at age 45-49—these man have 9 fold higher risk of dying from prostate cancer within 25 years compared to men with PSA ≤ 1.0.

2. Men age 60—men with PSA ≤ 1 at age 60 have a very low risk of developing metastasis (0.5%) or dying from prostate cancer (0.2%) by the age of 85.

3. Men age 70-75

   a. PSA < 3 at age 70-75—these men have a very low risk of dying from prostate cancer (≤ 3%).

   b. PSA ≥ 3 at age 70-75—these men have a 7% risk of dying from prostate cancer, but the risk increases as they get older.

4. *PSA elevation typically occurs 6 to 13 years before prostate cancer causes symptoms.*

AUA 2018 Guidelines For Prostate Cancer Screening

1. If screening is offered, physicians should discuss the benefits, risks, and limitations of prostate cancer screening with the patient and then offer testing. The decision to screen should be a shared decision between the patient and the physician.
2. Screening consists of PSA with or without digital rectal exam (DRE).
3. Who should be screened?
   a. Men with life expectancy < 10-15 years—routine screening is not recommended.
   b. Men with life expectancy > 10-15 years
      i. Age < 40—the AUA recommends against screening in these men because they have a very low risk of prostate cancer.
      ii. Age 40-54—routine screening is not recommended for men with average risk of prostate cancer. Consider screening in men at higher risk, such as men with African ancestry or a family history of lethal adenocarcinoma (such as prostate, ovary, pancreas, male or female breast cancer).
      iii Age 55-69—offer screening through shared decision making.
      iv. Age ≥ 70—routine screening is not recommended, but may be reasonable in men who are in excellent health (minimal comorbidities) and who have a life expectancy > 10 years, especially if they have family history of longevity.
4. Screening interval
   a. A screening interval of 2 or more years may be preferred over screening every year.
   b. Screening interval can be individualized according to baseline PSA. For example, *men age 60 with PSA < 1, the risk of subsequently dying from prostate cancer was only 0.2%*; therefore, these men may benefit from less frequent screening.

U.S. Preventative Service Task Force (USPSTF) 2018 Guideline

1. In 2018, the USPSTF suggested that clinicians can offer or provide PSA testing for selected patients depending on individual circumstances and that there is at least moderate certainty that the benefit is small (grade C recommendation).
2. The USPSTF discouraged the use of PSA in man age > 70 (grade D recommendation).

Example Screening Protocol

1. Guidelines on prostate cancer screening are highly variable (see table on the next page). The reader is encouraged to read guidelines that are relevant to the country in which you practice.
2. In order to account for the variation in guideline recommendations, an example screening protocol (shown on page 183) was synthesized from multiple guidelines.

Comparison of Screening Recommendations for Prostate Cancer

| Guideline | Age to Start Screening Men with Life Expectancy > 10 Years Based on Prostate Cancer Risk | | | Age to Stop Screening | Suggested Screening Tests |
	Average Risk	High Risk	Very High Risk		
AUA 2018	55	40-54§		70, but Individualize°	PSA with or without DRE
NCCN 2021	45	40‡‡		Individualize°	PSA with or without DRE*
ACS 2021	50	45**	40**	Individualize°	PSA with or without DRE
CUA 2017	50‡	45‡		60 if PSA<1, all others at 70	PSA
EAU 2021	≥ 50	≥ 45†	≥ 40†	<15 years of life expectancy	PSA and DRE
PCFA 2016	50	45††	40††	Not specified	PSA
USPSTF 2018	55			70	PSA

AUA = American Urologic Association; EAU = European Association of Urology
NCCN = National Comprehensive Cancer Network; ACS = American Cancer Society
CUA = Canadian Urological Association; PSA = prostate specific antigen
PCFA = Prostate Cancer Foundation of Australia and Cancer Council Australia
USPSTF = United States Preventative Service Task Force; DRE = digital rectal exam
§ For men age 40 to 54 years at higher risk (e.g. family history of prostate cancer or African ancestry), decisions regarding prostate cancer screening and when to start screening should be individualized.
* NCCN guideline states "Strongly consider a baseline digital rectal examination."
** Start at 40 in men at very high risk (e.g. more than one first-degree relative who had prostate cancer before the age of 65). Start at age 45 in men at high risk (e.g. African ancestry or men with a father or brother diagnosed with prostate cancer before the age of 65). Start at age 50 in men with average risk of prostate cancer.
‡ Start at 45 in men with higher risk (e.g. African ancestry or family history of prostate cancer), and at age 50 in men with average risk. These starting ages do not apply to men with germline mutations that increase the risk of prostate cancer, who may need to be tested at a younger age.
‡‡ Consider screening starting at age 40 in men with African ancestry, family history of prostate cancer, and/or germline mutations that increase the risk of prostate cancer. Start at age 45 in men with average risk of prostate cancer.
† Start at age ≥ 40 in men with BRCA2 mutations. Start at age ≥ 45 in men with African ancestry or a family history of prostate cancer. Start at age ≥ 50 in men with average risk.
†† Start at age 40 in men with a 9-10 times higher risk of death from prostate cancer (e.g. three 1st degree relatives diagnosed with prostate cancer). Start at age 45 in men with at least 2.5-3.0 times the risk of death from prostate cancer (e.g. one or two 1st degree relatives diagnosed with prostate cancer). The guidelines did not specify a risk category for men of African decent, but these men have 2 times the risk of death from prostate cancer compared to Caucasian men. Therefore, it seems reasonable to include men of African ancestry in the high risk category and to start screening them at age 45. Start at age 50 in men with average risk. These guidelines are endorsed by the Urological Society of Australia and New Zealand (USANZ).
° Screening may be reasonable in men age > 70 with excellent health (minimal comorbidities) and life expectancy > 10 years, especially if they have family history of longevity, a rising PSA, or have never had a PSA test. Few men over the age of 75 benefit from prostate cancer screening.

PSA for Prostate Cancer Screening

1. PSA is not capable of diagnosing prostate cancer. PSA only estimates the risk of prostate cancer (the higher the PSA, the higher the risk of prostate cancer). Cancer can be present even when the PSA is very low. Therefore, the term "normal" should probably not be utilized for PSA (the terms "low risk" or "lower risk" may be more appropriate). For more details on PSA, see page 300.

2. Cancers detected by PSA are more likely to be organ confined and less likely to be metastatic; therefore, screening with PSA detects prostate cancer at an earlier stage. *PSA elevation typically occurs 6 to 13 years before prostate cancer causes symptoms.*

3. *The decision to perform a biopsy is often based on many criteria, not just the total PSA value (see page 183).*

4. A single abnormal PSA should not prompt prostate biopsy. The abnormal PSA level should be verified after a few weeks (using the same assay at the same lab). Minimize confounding causes of elevated PSA, such as genitourinary infection, ejaculation, and prostate trauma (e.g. urethral instrumentation, prostate massage, cycling, motorcycle riding, long plane, long car rides, etc.). Also, *approximately 10% to 30% of elevated PSA tests will decline to a normal value within the following year (however, PSA returning to normal does not eliminate the possibility of prostate cancer, so these men should be monitored closely).*

5. *In asymptomatic men, attempting to reduce PSA with a course of antibiotics is not recommended (using antibiotics in this setting does not appear to alter the PSA).*

6. Hemodialysis and peritoneal dialysis do not alter total PSA significantly.

7. Abnormal total PSA value—there is no universally accepted threshold value above which the total PSA is considered abnormal. Higher PSA thresholds reduce unnecessary biopsies, but increase the risk of missing cancer. Lower PSA thresholds reduce the risk of missing cancer, but increase the detection of "clinically insignificant" cancer.

   a. Age and ethnicity specific reference ranges—these may help account for variation in the risk for prostate cancer between different populations.

Age (years)	"Normal" Serum PSA Range (ng/ml)		
	Caucasian	African-American	Asian-American
40-49	0-2.5	0-2.0	0-2.0
50-59	0-3.5	0-4.0	0-3.0
60-69	0-4.5	0-4.5	0-4.0
70-79	0-6.5	0-5.5	0-5.0

   b. It is important to realize that *PSA reference numbers used in most screening and diagnostic algorithms are based on men not taking a 5α-reductase inhibitor.*

   c. *5α-reductase inhibitors (finasteride, dutasteride) typically reduce total PSA by approximately 50% within 12 months. After 12 months of treatment, clinicians can double the PSA (to estimate what the PSA would be in the absence of a 5α-reductase inhibitor) in order to compare it to reference PSA values.*

8. Abnormal change in total PSA
   a. In men taking a 5α-reductase inhibitor—these mediations reduce total PSA by approximately 50% after 6-12 months of treatment, although the maximum PSA reduction and the time to reach it are highly variable. *Men whose total PSA does not decline by 50% within 12 months of starting a 5α-reductase inhibitor or whose PSA rises while on a 5α-reductase inhibitor have a higher risk for prostate cancer; therefore, prostate biopsy is often recommended in these men.* Using a 5α-reductase inhibitor appears to improve the ability of PSA to predict the presence of prostate cancer, particularly high grade cancers. 5α-reductase inhibitors usually do not alter the percent free PSA.
   b. In men not taking a 5α-reductase inhibitor—in these men, PSA velocity (PSAV) may help determine the risk of prostate cancer (although the evidence is conflicting as to whether PSA velocity is useful for predicting the presence of prostate cancer).
      i. For total PSA < 4 ng/ml, PSA velocity > 0.35 ng/ml/year suggests the presence of a clinically significant prostate cancer. Men with PSA velocity > 0.35 and PSA < 4 have a higher risk of dying from prostate cancer 5-15 years later.
      ii. For total PSA = 4-10 ng/ml, PSA velocity > 0.75 ng/ml/year suggests the presence of prostate cancer.
      iii. For total PSA > 10, PSA velocity is not useful.
   c. PSAV requires at least 3 PSA levels taken at least 6 months apart.

$$PSAV = 0.5 \times \left(\frac{PSA_2 - PSA_1}{Time_1} + \frac{PSA_3 - PSA_2}{Time_2} \right)$$

PSA_1 = 1st PSA (ng/ml)
PSA_2 = 2nd PSA (ng/ml)
PSA_3 = 3rd PSA (ng/ml)
$Time_1$ = years from PSA_1 to PSA_2
$Time_2$ = years from PSA_2 to PSA_3

Digital Rectal Exam (DRE) for Prostate Cancer Screening

1. Screening for prostate cancer should not be performed using only DRE. DRE is used as an adjunct to PSA testing. If the PSA is abnormal, then a DRE should be performed if it was not done recently.
2. There is no universal agreement on what constitutes an abnormal DRE. A nodule or firm (indurated) area is usually considered suspicious.
3. If the clinician concludes that the DRE is *suspicious* for cancer, then a prostate biopsy is indicated.
4. Abnormal DRE increases the likelihood of prostate cancer compared to a normal DRE.
5. When the DRE is abnormal, the risk of prostate cancer is only 4% with PSA < 1, but is at least 40% when PSA is between 4 and 10.

PSA (ng/ml)	Chance of Finding Prostate Cancer in Men with an Abnormal Prostate Exam
< 1.0	4%
≤ 4.0	15%
4.1 - 9.9	40%
≥ 10	75%

The rates were calculated by combining data from 5 studies
(J Urol 152: 1506, 1994; J Urol 151: 1283, 1994; J Urol 151: 1571, 1994;
J Natl Cancer Inst 90: 1817, 1998; BJU Int 102: 1524, 2008).

Example Prostate Cancer Screening Protocol Derived from Multiple Guidelines

For men age 40-45 & life expectancy > 10 years,
Discuss risks and benefits of screening for prostate cancer

Factors that suggest the need for biopsy:

1. Suspicious prostate exam
2. Abnormal total PSA—there is no universally accepted cutoff that defines an abnormal total PSA. Clinicians may use age & ethnicity adjusted cutoffs (see below).
3. Abnormal change in total PSA
   a. For men *not* taking a 5-alpha-reductase inhibitor, consider biopsy when
      - PSA velocity ≥ 0.35 ng/ml/year for total PSA < 4 ng/ml.
      - PSA velocity ≥ 0.75 ng/ml/year for total PSA = 4-10 ng/ml [PSA velocity is not helpful for PSA >10 ng/ml].
   b. For men taking a 5-alpha-reductase inhibitor (5ARI), consider biopsy when
      - PSA consistently rises (by any amount)
      - Total PSA does not decline ≥ 50% by 12 months after starting the 5ARI

Other tests that may be considered:

- Prediction from a risk calculator
- Other markers (e.g. free PSA, Prostate Health Index, PCA3, 4K score, etc.).
- Prostate MRI
- PSA density (PSAD)—PSAD ≥ 0.15 suggests the presence of prostate cancer. PSAD has not been adequately studied in men taking a 5ARI. See page 185.

Other factors that may be considered:

- Pathology results from previous biopsies
- Family history of prostate cancer
- Ethnicity—men of African ancestry have a higher risk of prostate cancer.
- Life expectancy—typically predicted by age and comorbidities.

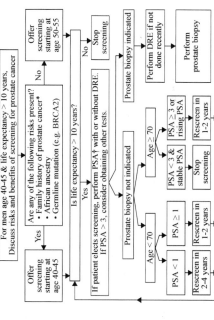

PSA = prostate specific antigen in ng/ml; DRE = digital rectal exam of prostate
NOTE: PSA levels shown above are for men not taking a 5α-reductase inhibitor.
* The risk for developing prostate cancer increases when the family members with cancer are closer in relation, diagnosed at a younger age, or greater in number.
† For ≥ 2 days before testing, avoid activities that can increase PSA (e.g. ejaculation, long plane/car/motorcycle/bicycle/horse rides, urethral manipulation, etc.)

Age & Ethnicity Adjusted Total PSA Values

Age (years)	"Normal" Total PSA Range (ng/ml)			
	Caucasian	African Ancestry	Asian Ancestry	
40-49	0-2.5	0-2.0	0-2.0	
50-59	0-3.5	0-4.0	0-3.0	
60-69	0-4.5	0-4.5	0-4.0	
70-79	0-6.5	0-5.5	0-5.0	

Risk When Total PSA = 4-10

% Free PSA	Probability of Cancer
< 10%	56%
10-15%	28%
15-20%	20%
20-25%	16%
> 25%	8%

Risk of Prostate Cancer Based on PSA and DRE

A combination of PSA and DRE appears to detect more cancers than either test alone, although the benefit of adding DRE is marginal because most cancers are detected by PSA.

Prostate Exam	Total PSA (ng/ml)	% of Men with Prostate Cancer	
		Any Gleason Score	Gleason Score ≥ 7
Normal	≤ 0.5	6.6%	<1%
Normal	0.6-1.0	10%	1%
Normal	1.1-2.0	17%	2%
Normal	2.1-3.0	24%	4.6%
Normal	3.1-4.0	27%	6.7%
Normal	4.1-10.0	20-25%	?
Abnormal	4.1-10.0	40%	?
Normal or Abnormal	> 10	> 50%	?

Data from N Engl J Med 350(22): 2239, 2004; J Urol 151: 1283, 1994;
J Natl Cancer Inst 90: 1817, 1998.

Other Tests to Determine the Need for Prostate Biopsy

General Information

1. PSA with or without DRE is the only regimen that is recommended for prostate cancer screening (there are not enough data to determine if other tests are useful for routine screening).
2. PSA and DRE are also the initial tests that are used to determine whether a prostate biopsy may be warranted. If PSA and/or DRE are abnormal, then other tests may used to help decide on the need for biopsy. Examples of these other tests include risk calculators, prostate MRI, and other biomarkers (free PSA, PCA3, PHI, 4K score, etc.).
3. These other tests can better define the risk of prostate cancer. They cannot diagnose prostate cancer (a prostate biopsy is required for diagnosis).

Risk Calculators

These calculators help determine the need for biopsy by incorporating many criteria to predict the risk of prostate cancer. Examples include the ERSPC risk calculator and the PCPT risk calculator.

Percent Free PSA (% Free PSA)

1. This blood test measures the amount of free PSA (PSA that is not bound to other proteins) and the amount of total PSA (all circulating PSA, bound or unbound). From these measurements, percent free PSA is calculated using the following equation: % free PSA = (free PSA ÷ total PSA) x 100.
2. The higher the percent free PSA, the lower the risk for prostate cancer.
3. Percent free PSA does not seem to be altered by 5α-reductase inhibitors.
4. Percent free PSA is FDA approved only for men with total PSA = 4-10 and a normal prostate exam.
5. Hemodialysis and peritoneal dialysis do not alter total PSA, but they do alter free PSA. Thus, *% free PSA should not be used in dialysis patients.*

% Free PSA	Probability of Prostate Cancer in Men with *Normal* Prostate Exam and Total PSA = 4-10 ng/ml
< 10%	56%
10-15%	28%
15-20%	20%
20-25%	16%
> 25%	8%

Complexed PSA

1. This blood test measures the amount of PSA that is bound (or complexed) to other proteins. The higher the complexed PSA, the higher the risk of prostate cancer.
2. PSA is complexed mostly with α1-antichymotrypsin. A smaller amount is complexed with α2-macroglobulin.
3. Complexed PSA has not gained widespread acceptance.

Prostate Health Index (PHI)

1. PHI is a blood test. *A higher PHI score indicates a higher PHI score indicates a higher risk of prostate cancer.*
2. PHI uses a combination of total PSA, free PSA, and [-2]proPSA to calculate the PHI score. [-2]proPSA is an isoform of free PSA.
3. PHI is FDA approved for men with PSA from 4 to 10, age $\geq$ 50 years, and normal prostate exam.

PHI Score	Risk of Cancer
<27	9.8%
27.0-35.9	16.8%
36.0-54.9	33.3%
$\geq$ 55	50.1%

PSA Density (PSAD)

1. PSAD $\geq$ 0.15 suggests the presence of prostate cancer.
2. PSAD requires measurement of total PSA and prostate volume. Prostate volume is typically calculated from a transrectal ultrasound of the prostate.
3. PSAD has not been adequately studied in men taking a 5α-reductase inhibitor. Also, there is conflicting evidence as to whether PSA density is useful for predicting the presence of prostate cancer.

$$PSAD = \frac{PSA \ (ng/ml)}{Prostate \ Volume \ (cc)}$$

4Kscore

1. The 4Kscore is a blood test. It incorporates four kallikreins (free PSA, total PSA, intact PSA, and human kallikrein 2) and clinical characteristics (patient age, DRE findings, and prior biopsy results) to predict the risk of group grade $\geq$ 2 (Gleason score $\geq$ 7) prostate cancer. The higher the 4K score, the higher the risk of prostate cancer.
2. 4Kscore also predicts the risk of developing metastatic prostate cancer. In men age 60 with PSA $\geq$ 3, the risk of developing metastatic prostate cancer at 15 years after the 4Kscore test is almost 10 fold higher in men with 4Kscore $\geq$ 7.5% compared to men with 4Kscore < 7.5%.
3. 4Kscore also predicts the risk of dying from prostate cancer. In men age 60-73 with PSA $\geq$ 2, the risk of dying from prostate cancer at 15 years after the 4Kscore test is 1.7% in men with 4Kscore < 7.5%, and 13% in men with 4Kscore $\geq$ 7.5%.
4. No optimal cut point has been established above which biopsy is indicated; however, prostate biopsy for 4Kscore $\geq$ 7.5 has been suggested because this score indicates a higher risk of current Gleason $\geq$ 7 cancer, a higher risk of subsequently developing metastasis, and a higher risk of dying from prostate cancer. Also, performing prostate biopsy in men with 4Kscore $\geq$ 7.5 detects essentially all Gleason score $\geq$ 8 cancers.
5. 4K score is indicated in men with elevated PSA and/or abnormal DRE (including men who are biopsy naive or who have had a prior benign biopsy). The test should be avoided in the following circumstances:
   a. Digital rectal examination within the previous 96 hours.
   b. Use of medications that influence PSA within the previous 6 months.
   c. Prostate procedure within the previous 6 months.
   d. Recent use of biotin supplements > 5mg/day—biotin can interference with the test and may cause erroneous results.

ExoDx Prostate Intelliscore (EPI)

1. EPI is a urine test that evaluates 3 genes (PCA3, ERG, and SPDEF) using the RNA in urinary exosomes. Higher levels of urinary RNA from PCA3 and ERG are associated with an increased risk of prostate cancer. SPDEF is used as an internal reference. Exosomes are membrane bound vesicles that are created within a cell and then released into the extracellular environment. The exosome contains markers (such as PCA3 and ERG) from the cell in which it originated.
2. DRE is not necessary before the test. In fact, the patient should not undergo DRE within the 24 hours before the test.
3. A higher EPI score indicates a higher risk of Gleason ≥ 7 cancer.
4. A cut point of EPI > 15.6 can be used to select men for prostate biopsy; however, 9% of men with EPI ≤ 15.6 have a Gleason ≥ 7.
5. EPI is indicated for men age ≥ 50 with PSA = 2 to 10 (with or without an abnormal DRE). There is no evidence to suggest that sexual activity before EPI will impact the results. The test has not been validated in men using medications that influence PSA within the previous 3-6 months or in men that had a prostate procedure within the previous 6 months. The test should be avoided in the following circumstances:
   a. Digital rectal examination within the previous 24 hours.
   b. Urinated within the past 60 minutes.
   c. Prostatitis within the past 3 to 6 months.

SelectMDx

1. This test is performed on a post-DRE urine sample.
2. SelectMDx evaluates 3 genes (DLX1, HOXC6, and KLK3) by measuring their RNA in the urine. Higher levels of urinary RNA from DLX1 and HOXC6 are associated with an increased risk of prostate cancer. KLK3 RNA is used as an internal reference.
3. SelectMDx results are generated from the 3 gene assay and clinical data (patient age, PSA, prostate volume, DRE findings, and family history).
4. SelectMDx predicts the likelihood of finding any prostate cancer and of finding Gleason ≥ 7 prostate cancer. If the results indicate "very low risk", then the risk of Gleason ≥ 7 is 5% and the risk of Gleason ≥ 8 is less than 1%.
5. This test is indicated in men with a PSA = 4-10 (with or without and abnormal DRE). The test has not been validated in men using medications that influence PSA within the previous 6 months or in men that had a prostate procedure within the previous 6 months.

Multiparametric MRI (mpMRI) of the Prostate

1. Prostate mpMRI may be used to help determine the need for prostate biopsy in men with abnormal PSA or DRE.
2. The PIRADS system uses prostate mpMRI to determine the risk of having clinically significant prostate cancer (for details on prostate MRI and the PIRADS system, see page 459). PIRADS category ranges from 1 to 5, with a higher PIRADS category indicating a higher risk of prostate cancer and a higher risk of aggressive prostate cancer. *PIRADS 1 indicates a completely normal prostate mpMRI.*
   a. PIRADS 1 or 2—the risk of grade group ≥ 3 cancer (Gleason score $\geq 4+3$) is very low (approximately 2%); therefore, these lesions are rarely biopsied (although a clinician may consider biopsy if other factors indicate a high suspicion of cancer). Not performing a biopsy of PIRADS ≤ 2 lesions will miss a grade group 2 (Gleason score = 3+4) approximately 9% of the time.

b. PIRADS 3—the risk of Gleason score $\geq$ 4+3 cancer is approximately 4%. Some clinicians believe that the risk is high enough to warrant a biopsy of all PIRADS 3 lesions, while others believe that the decision to biopsy these lesions should be based on additional testing (such as PSA density, PSA velocity, 4Kscore, Prostate Health Index, etc.).

c. PIRADS 4 or 5—the risk of Gleason score $\geq$ 4+3 cancer is relatively high (at least 13-37%); therefore, most clinicians recommend biopsy of these lesions.

PIRADS Version 2 Category	Risk of Finding Clinically Significant† Prostate Cancer in the Prostate Lesion when using Targeted Biopsy*	
	Gleason Score $\geq$ 3+4 (Grade Group $\geq$ 2)	Gleason Score $\geq$ 4+3 (Grade Group $\geq$ 3)
1 or 2	9%	< 2%
3	14%	4%
4	33%	13%
5	66%	37%

† There is debate regarding the exact criteria that define a clinically significant cancer. See page 201 for the definition of "clinically significant."

* Data includes men who had no previous biopsy, men with a previous benign systematic biopsy, and men with a previous malignant systematic biopsy. Calculations for PIRADS 3-5 were restricted biopsies that targeted the lesion seen on MRI (and excluded systematic biopsy results), whereas calculations for PIRADS 1-2 included systematic biopsies and (if done) targeted biopsies. The rates were calculated by combining data from 14 studies: Transl Androl Urol 7(1): 132, 2018; J Urol 200: 767, 2018; NEJM 378(19): 1767, 2018; J Urol 196(3): 690, 2016; Cancer 122: 884, 2016; Int Braz J Urol 45: 713, 2019; Radiology 283(1): 130, 2017; Eur Urol 73(3): 353, 2018; J Urol 198: 583, 217; Eur Uol 75: 570, 2019; Can Urol Assoc J 12(12): 401, 2018; J Urol 201: 510, 2019; BJU Int 120: 631, 2017; Cancer Res Treat 52(3): 714, 2020.

3. Inflammation, basal cell hyperplasia, and high percentage of stroma are all more common in MRI lesions than in normal appearing prostate. In fact, these benign pathologic conditions may present as a suspicious lesion on prostate MRI (producing a false positive MRI).

4. Biopsy naive men (i.e no prior biopsy)—prospective studies (e.g. PECISION, MRI-FIRST, and 4M) show that *mpMRI guided prostate biopsies reduce the detection of clinically insignificant cancer compared to systematic biopsies (thus, reducing overdiagnosis). Also, mpMRI guided biopsies increase the detection of Gleason score $\geq$ 7 cancer compared to systematic biopsies*, but the difference was not significant in all studies.

5. Guidelines for use of mpMRI in biopsy naive men

a. American Urological Association (AUA) 2018 guideline—mpMRI "…imaging…can be considered in men with a suspicious PSA level to inform prostate biopsy decisions."

b. European Association of Urology (EAU) 2021 guideline—when screening suggests a risk of cancer, the clinician should "Perform mpMRI before prostate biopsy." Also, "When mpMRI is negative (i.e. PIRADS $\leq$ 2) and clinical suspicion of prostate cancer is low, omit biopsy based on shared decision making with the patient…When mpMRI is positive (i.e. PIRADS $\geq$ 3), combine targeted and systematic biopsy."

c. Canadian Urological Association (CUA) 2017 guideline—states "…mpMRI should not be routinely used in the biopsy naive setting", and that "In patients…who are biopsy naive, mpMRI followed by targeted biopsy…should not be considered the standard of care."

     d. National Comprehensive Care Network (NCCN) 2021 guideline— "It is recommended that MRI should proceed biopsy, and image guided biopsy techniques be employed routinely." The guideline also states that "most [experts] advocate for a combined approach [both targeted and systematic sampling] as some high grade cancers are uniquely detected using the systematic approach."

6. Guidelines for use of mpMRI in men with prior benign biopsy

    a. AUA/SAR 2016 guideline—mpMRI "should strongly be considered in any patient with a prior negative biopsy who has persistent clinical suspicion for prostate cancer...a case specific decision must be made whether to also perform concurrent systematic sampling."

    b. EAU 2021 guideline—in men whose testing suggests a risk of cancer, the clinician should "Perform mpMRI before prostate biopsy." Also, "When mpMRI is negative (i.e. PIRADS $\leq$ 2) and clinical suspicion of prostate cancer is high, perform systematic biopsy based on shared decision making with the patient...When mpMRI is positive (i.e. PIRADS $\geq$ 3), perform targeted biopsy only."

    c. CUA 2017 guideline—"In men who had a prior negative TRUS guided systematic biopsy who demonstrate increasing risk of having clinically significant prostate cancer since prior biopsy...mpMRI followed by targeted biopsy may be considered..."

    d. NCCN 2021 guideline—multiparametric MRI with targeted biopsies "...are recommended after at least 1 negative prostate biopsy and high suspicion for cancer based on PSA and/or biomarkers."

7. For mpMRI guided biopsy technique, see page 194.
8. For using mpMRI during prostate cancer surveillance, see page 216.
9. For more details on prostate MRI and MRI in general, see page 459.

Tests Specifically Indicated for Men with a Prior Benign Prostate Biopsy

1. When there is suspicion of prostate cancer despite a prior benign biopsy, several tests are approved for use in this specific setting to help better stratify the risk of cancer. These include a urine test (PCA3), tissue based tests (ConfirmMDx and Mitomic Prostate Test), and imaging (mpMRI).
2. Some of these tests are described below.

PCA3 (Prostate Cancer Gene 3)

1. PCA3 is performed an a post-DRE urine sample. Prostate exam pushes prostate cells into the urethra, which are then expelled in the voided urine. Prostate cells in the voided urine are analyzed for overexpression of the PCA3 gene.

2. *A higher PCA3 score indicates a higher risk of prostate cancer.*

PCA3 Score	Risk of Cancer*
< 5	12%
5-19	17%
20-34	23%
35-49	32%
50-100	45%
>100	50%

* In men with at least one previous benign prostate biopsy

3. The PCA3 assay is not influenced by prostatitis, 5α-reductase inhibitors, α-blockers, saw palmetto, quinolones, doxycycline, or sildenafil.

4. PCA3 is FDA approved for men age $\geq$ 50 with one or more previous benign prostate biopsies (but should not be used in men with atypical small acinar proliferation on their most recent biopsy). Although PCA3 is not FDA approved for men that are biopsy naive, some clinicians still use the test in these men.

ConfirmMDx

1. ConfirmMDx is performed on benign prostate tissue from a prior biopsy.
2. Cancer can induce molecular changes in the surrounding benign tissue (a field effect or "halo"). When a benign core contains a field effect, there is a higher risk of cancer near the site from which the core was taken.
3. ConfirmMDx measures DNA methylation of 3 genes (GSTP1, APC, and RASSF1). Methylation in any of these genes suggests an increased risk of prostate cancer near the site from which the core was taken.
4. If DNA methylation is absent, then the risk is 4% for Gleason score ≥ 7 prostate cancer and 10% for any grade cancer. If methylation is present, then the risk of any grade prostate cancer is approximately 30-50%.
5. ConfirmMDx is indicated for men with a previous benign biopsy who are being considered for repeat prostate biopsy. The test can be used in men with high grade PIN or atypical small acinar proliferation (atypia suspicious for cancer). If rebiopsy is indicated, then consider performing a systematic biopsy (see page 196) with increased sampling of the methylated regions and perhaps the adjacent regions.

Mitomic Prostate Core Test (MPCT)

1. MPCT is performed on benign prostate tissue from a prior biopsy.
2. MPCT measures a specific deletion in mitochondrial DNA to determine the risk that prostate cancer may have been missed on a previous biopsy. It is similar to ConfirmMDX in that it tests for a field effect and provides information regarding the risk for prostate cancer.

Diagnosis and Work Up

Indications for Prostate Biopsy

1. See page 183 for details regarding the indications for prostate biopsy.
2. *The 2013 Prostate Cancer World Congress Consensus states that "PSA testing should not be considered on its own, but rather as part of a multivariable approach to early prostate cancer detection..." and that "...digital rectal examination, prostate volume, family history, ethnicity, risk prediction models...can help to better risk stratify men."* Prior biopsy results, life expectancy, age, and comorbidities may also be considered when deciding on the need for prostate biopsy.

Prostate Biopsy—General Concepts

1. Cores are usually obtained transrectally under local anesthesia using transrectal ultrasound guidance. Transperineal biopsies have a lower risk of infection than transrectal biopsies, however, transperineal biopsies are often more painful and require more local anesthesia.
2. *In men with an elevated PSA, a 10-12 core systematic prostate biopsy has a false negative rate of approximately 20% to 30%.*
3. For men without an anus (e.g. after abdominoperineal resection), prostate biopsies can be obtained by the following routes.
   a. Transperineal biopsies using ultrasound, CT, or MRI guidance. Ultrasonic imaging can be performed transabdominal or transperineal.
   b. Transgluteal biopsies using CT or MRI guidance.

Transrectal Prostate Biopsy

1. Preparation for transrectal prostate biopsy
   a. Bowel preparation—The EAU recommends using a povidone-iodine rectal preparation (in addition to systemic antibiotic prophylaxis) because it decreases the risk of infectious complications. Administering an enema prior to the procedure does not reduce the risk of infection. However, it may minimize the chance that gross stool in the rectum hinders placement of the transrectal probe.

    b. Culture based antibiotic prophylaxis—this optional strategy involves obtaining a rectal culture so that bacterial sensitivity profiles are available before the biopsy. Prophylaxis is then adjusted as needed to cover organisms that are resistant to the recommended prophylaxis regimen. The data are conflicting as to whether this reduces the rate of sepsis over empiric antibiotics.

    c. Empiric antibiotic prophylaxis (based on the AUA guidelines)

       i. Preferred antibiotic regimen—fluoroquinolone alone or a combination of an aminoglycoside and a cephalosporin (1st, 2nd, or 3rd generation).

       ii. Alternative antibiotic: Aztreonam or consider infectious disease consultation.

      iii. For oral administration, the antibiotic should usually be taken 2 to 4 hours before the procedure. For intramuscular or intravenous administration, the antibiotic should be given within 1 hour of the procedure.

      iv. If the patient has a high risk of having a resistant organism (see below), then consider adding an appropriate additional antibiotic to the prophylaxis regimen or consider performing culture based antibiotic prophylaxis.

       v. Risk factors for being colonized with and developing an infection from a multidrug resistant organism—antibiotic use within the last 6 months, hospitalization within the last 6 months, infection after a previous prostate biopsy, history of prostatitis, history of urinary tract infections, recent international travel, and known colonization with an organism resistant to the recommended prophylaxis regimen.

      vi. Taking a greater number of cores and injecting local anesthesia does not appear to increase infection rate.

2. Transrectal ultrasound (TRUS) for prostate biopsy

    a. Most prostate cancers are isoechoic. *When prostate cancer is visualized on TRUS, it is usually hypoechoic.* Rarely, prostate cancers are hyperechoic.

    b. Color Doppler and power Doppler ultrasound can improve biopsy targeting by helping localize areas than may contain cancer.

    c. *TRUS cannot reliably identify prostate cancer.* When a biopsy is indicated based on other factors, the biopsy should be performed even if the TRUS is normal. Obtaining only TRUS targeted biopsies (from areas that appear suspicious) is ineffective. However, TRUS targeted biopsies may be useful when combined with systematic biopsies.

3. Local anesthetic for prostate biopsy (prostate block)

    a. Prostate innervation—the prostate nerves arise from sympathetic and parasympathetic branches of the inferior hypogastric plexus. They course along the posterior-lateral prostate from the base toward the apex.

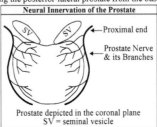

Neural Innervation of the Prostate

SV

SV

◄—— Proximal end

Prostate Nerve & its Branches

Prostate depicted in the coronal plane
SV = seminal vesicle

    b. Some urologists apply lidocaine jelly topically to the anus before the biopsy to help decrease discomfort from inserting the probe.

    c. Prostate block anesthetizes the prostatic nerves (which are sympathetic and parasympathetic branches from the inferior hypogastric plexus).

    d. Prostate block technique—on each side (near the lateral edge of the prostate), inject 2-5 cc of 1% plain lidocaine between the prostate base and the seminal vesicle. Alternatively, place the needle into the lateral prostate (at the base, mid, and apex) and inject 1% plain lidocaine as the needle is withdrawn. These two techniques can be combined.

Injecting Local Anesthetic for Prostate Biopsy

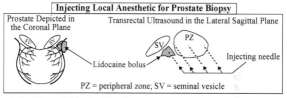

Prostate Depicted in the Coronal Plane

Transrectal Ultrasound in the Lateral Sagittal Plane

PZ

Injecting needle

Lidocaine bolus

PZ = peripheral zone; SV = seminal vesicle

---

4. Avoiding painful apical biopsies

    a. The dentate line (also called the pectinate line or anorectal junction) is the anatomic division between the anus and the rectum (figure 1). Cephalad to the dentate line, tissue is innervated by branches of the inferior hypogastric plexus (prostate branches are anesthetized by prostate block). Below the dentate line, tissue is innervated by branches of the inferior rectal nerve (*not* anesthetized by prostate block). When obtaining a biopsy near the apex, the needle may pass below the dentate line, causing severe pain (figure 2).

    b. To avoid painful apical biopsies, place the tip of the ultrasound posterior to the mid prostate and position the tip of the biopsy needle just inside the end of the probe (figure 3). Then, angle the probe so that its tip sweeps anterior and toward the prostate apex (figure 4). This maneuver retracts the dentate line away from the prostate apex and allows the biopsy needle to pass above the dentate line. Then, fire the biopsy gun.

    c. The dentate line is not well visualized on transrectal ultrasound.

Avoiding Anal Pain During Prostate Biopsy

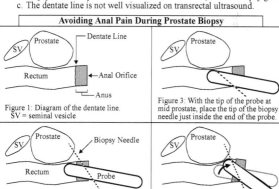

Figure 1: Diagram of the dentate line. SV = seminal vesicle

Figure 2: Painful apical biopsy that passes below the dentate line.

Figure 3: With the tip of the probe at mid prostate, place the tip of the biopsy needle just inside the end of the probe.

Figure 4: Angle and sweep the probe anterior toward the apex to retract the dentate line away from the needle path.

Initial Systematic Prostate Biopsy

1. Prostate cancer can arise anywhere in the prostate, but it usually arises in the peripheral zone (PZ); therefore, biopsies are concentrated in the PZ.
2. Summary of the AUA and NCCN recommendations.
   a. Systematic cores—obtain at least 12 systematic cores that sample the lateral PZ and para-sagittal PZ. Taking > 12 cores may slightly increase cancer detection, slightly increase negative predictive value (NPV), and slightly reduce undergrading, but it increases detection of "insignificant cancer." Taking 18-21 cores increases cancer detection by < 4%.
   b. Lesion directed cores—obtain cores from suspicious regions detected on prostate imaging or digital rectal examination (DRE). Prostate cancer is found in 30% of hypoechoic lesions and in 30% of palpable nodules.
   c. Transition zone sampling is not recommended during the initial systematic biopsy because of its low yield in this setting.
3. Lateral PZ—sampling the lateral PZ improves NPV and cancer detection (thus, most guidelines recommend sampling the lateral PZ).
4. Anterior-apical PZ—*sampling of the anterior-apical PZ is prudent. In fact, the AUA guideline states that "clinicians should use templates that incorporate adequate sampling of the apex or anterior apex."*
   a. When the anterior-apical PZ is not sampled, 5% of men will have benign pathology despite the presence of cancer in the anterior-apical PZ (i.e. the patient will receive a false benign diagnosis in 5% of cases).
   b. 25-50% of cancers are present in both the anterior-apical PZ and other areas of the prostate. Thus, *biopsy patterns that do not sample the anterior-apical PZ will underestimate the amount of cancer in 25-50% of cases.* Sampling the anterior-apical PZ is especially important in men on surveillance because it more accurately assesses the extent of cancer.
5. *Lateral and anterior-apical cores must be obtained to effectively sample the anterior horn of the PZ (see diagram below).*
6. The author's initial systematic prostate biopsy pattern (see diagram below)
   a. 14 systematic cores—4 para-sagittal cores (anterior-apical, apex, mid, base) and 3 lateral cores (apex, mid, base) on each side. This protocol detects more cancers than protocols that do not sample the anterior-apical PZ and protocols that take fewer cores (Moussa, 2010).
   b. Additional systematic cores are obtained in large prostates (e.g. > 50 cc).
   c. Cores are obtained from suspicious areas detected on imaging or DRE.

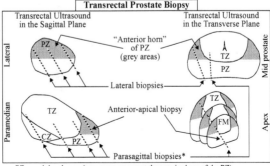

Transrectal Prostate Biopsy

PZ = peripheral zone (grey areas represent the anterior horn of the PZ)
TZ = transition zone; FM = fibromuscular stroma; CZ = central zone; ⅄ = urethra
* Biopsies in the sagittal paramedian plane are also called "parasagittal biopsies."

Anterior-Apical Biopsy

1. In the sagittal plane (e.g. midway between the urethra and the lateral edge of the prostate), insert the biopsy needle so that its tip is 1.5 cm from the anterior capsule and then fire the biopsy gun (this core samples all the way to the anterior capsule).
2. A large transition zone (TZ) may compress the anterior apical peripheral zone; thus, prostates with a large TZ may require a steeper biopsy angle.

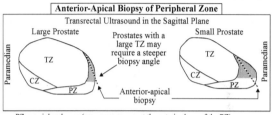

PZ = peripheral zone (grey areas represent the anterior horn of the PZ)
TZ = transition zone; CZ = central zone

Transition Zone (TZ) Biopsy

1. Transition zone sampling is not recommended during the initial systematic biopsy because of its low yield in this setting. Transition zone biopsy may be more useful during repeat biopsies.
2. *Prostate cancer can occur anywhere in the TZ, but it is usually located in the distal two-thirds of the TZ near the anterior midline* (see diagram); therefore, transition zone biopsies should be concentrated in this region.
3. Insert the biopsy needle through the PZ and into the TZ. When the needle tip is in the TZ, fire the biopsy gun. With a large TZ, insert the needle far enough to adequately sample the anterior TZ.

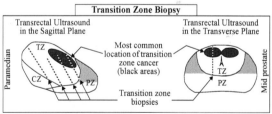

PZ = peripheral zone (grey areas represent the anterior horn of the PZ)
TZ = transition zone (black areas represent the most common location of transition zone cancers); CZ = central zone; ʎ = urethra

Seminal Vesicle (SV) Biopsy

1. *Men who are considering salvage cryotherapy after radiation should undergo SV biopsy (in addition to prostate biopsy) because cancer in the SV occurs in up to 42% of men who recur after radiation.*
2. The indication for SV biopsy in other circumstances is not well defined. Consider performing SV biopsy in the following situations.
   a. A large cancer in the base of the prostate—SV invasion is more likely when there is a large cancer in the base of the prostate.
   b. PSA > 15—seminal vesicle involvement is 20-25% with PSA > 15.

c. A nomogram predicts a high risk of SV invasion (e.g. Koh H, et al: J Urol, 170: 1203, 2003).

d. Imaging suggests the presence of cancer in the SV—SV invasion is more likely in men whose ultrasound shows a hypoechoic lesion in the base of the prostate, a hyperechoic lesion in the SV, loss of the normal echogenic fat between the prostate base and SV, the posterior (rectal) surface of the SV is convex toward the rectum, or the SV is displaced anteriorly > 1 cm from the rectal wall.

3. Biopsies should be concentrated in the proximal third of the SV (the part closest to the prostate). Sample as close as possible to the junction of the SV and the prostate without sampling the prostate.

   a. When prostate cancer invades into the SV, the initial site of invasion is almost always the proximal SV.

   b. Distal SV invasion in the absence of proximal SV invasion is rare.

   c. Spread of prostate cancer into the distal 1 cm of the SV is rare.

4. In the paramedian plane, the biopsy needle tip is advanced through the rectal wall and positioned a few millimeters posterior to the proximal seminal vesicle. Then, the biopsy gun is fired. Attempt to sample the entire anterior-posterior distance of the SV. The needle should not penetrate into the prostate, the bladder lumen, or the peritoneum.

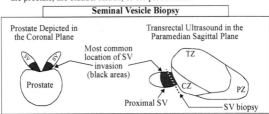

Seminal Vesicle Biopsy

Prostate Depicted in the Coronal Plane

Most common location of SV invasion (black areas)

Prostate

Transrectal Ultrasound in the Paramedian Sagittal Plane

TZ

CZ

PZ

Proximal SV

SV biopsy

SV = seminal vesicle; PZ = peripheral zone; TZ = transition zone; CZ = central zone

Multiparametric MRI (mpMRI) Guided Prostate Biopsy

1. A normal prostate mpMRI does not exclude prostate cancer. *If the prostate mpMRI is normal, but there is a suspicion of prostate cancer, then a systematic biopsy should be performed.*

2. There are 3 techniques for performing mpMRI guided biopsies (i.e. biopsies that target suspicious areas on mpMRI).

   a. In-bore mpMRI guided biopsies—biopsies are done with the patient in the MRI gantry. MRI images confirm that the biopsy needle is placed into the target. The procedure is time consuming and requires the patient to be in the prone position for a prolonged period.

   b. TRUS/mpMRI fusion guided biopsies—using the mpMRI, an outline of the prostate and the suspicious lesions are constructed within a computer. Prior to the biopsy procedure, this data is loaded into a fusion system. At the time of the biopsy procedure, the urologist uses the fusion system to align the prostate on the TRUS images and the mpMRI images so that they track together in real time. The lesion outline from the mpMRI is then overlaid onto the real time TRUS images, which allows the clinician to target the lesion that was seen on mpMRI.

   c. Cognitive fusion guided biopsies—the clinician looks at the mpMRI images and creates a mental map of the lesion's location within the prostate. Then, the clinician performs TRUS guided biopsy and targets suspicious area based on the mental map.

3. The detection of clinically significant cancer is similar regardless of which mpMRI guidance technique is used. Although, TRUS/mpMRI fusion and in-bore guided biopsies appears to be more reliable for targeting small lesions or lesions that are in a difficult to reach location.

4. Minimum number of cores per lesion—the AUA/SAR 2016 guideline suggests taking a minimum of 2 cores per lesion because the majority of cancer can be detected with 2 cores. However, at least 9% of clinically significant cancers are missed using only 2 cores. The EAU 2021 guideline recommends taking at least 3 cores per lesion. *To improve the diagnostic yield of mpMRI guided biopsies, taking 3-5 cores per lesion may be best, especially for small lesions or lesions that are PIRADS ≤ 3.*

5. Detection of significant cancer—mpMRI guided biopsies detect fewer Gleason ≤ 6 cancers and more Gleason ≥ 7 cancers compared to systematic biopsies (although in biopsy naive men, the trend toward higher detection of Gleason ≥ 7 cancer was not significant in all studies). In other words, *mpMRI guided biopsies detect fewer clinically insignificant cancers (reducing over-detection) and detect more clinically significant cancers (reducing the chance of missing a threatening cancer) compared to systematic biopsies.* Nonetheless, MRI guided biopsies can still miss some clinically significant cancers. In fact, mpMRI guided biopsy alone will miss approximately 5% of Gleason ≥ 7 cancers compared to a combination of systematic and mpMRI guided biopsy. To maximize detection of clinically significant cancer, systematic and mpMRI guided biopsies can be combined.

6. *Many studies have shown that performing systematic and targeted biopsies together increase the detection of clinically significant cancer compared to either type of biopsy alone (but it will also increases the number of clinically insignificant cancers that are detected).*

7. For men who are biopsy naive—the AUA/SAR 2019, EAU 2021, and NCCN 2021 guidelines recommend combining systematic and mpMRI guided prostate biopsies.
   a. AUA/SAR 2019—"use of systematic biopsy in conjunction with mpMRI targeted sampling is advisable until the time that individual experience demonstrates a low risk of missed clinically significant cancers."
   b. EAU 2021—"When mpMRI is positive (i.e PIRADS ≥3), combine targeting and systematic biopsy."
   c. NCCN 2021—"...most [experts] advocate for a combined approach [both targeted and systematic sampling] as some high grade cancers are uniquely detected using the systematic approach."

8. For men with a prior negative biopsy—the EAU 2021 guideline recommends performing only a targeted biopsy, whereas the AUA/SAR 2019 guideline states that combined systematic and mpMRI guided biopsies should be performed until "quality assurance efforts have validated the performance of prostate mpMRI interpretations with results consistent with the published literature" (and if this is the case, then only targeted biopsies can be performed).

9. For more details about prostate mpMRI and its use in prostate biopsy, see page 186.

Re-biopsy After Previous Negative Biopsy
1. Re-biopsy is performed in men suspected of having prostate cancer despite a previous benign biopsy. Reasons for suspecting prostate cancer in this setting may include a rising total PSA, a change in DRE, previous biopsy findings (e.g. multifocal high grade PIN, atypical small acinar proliferation), or other test results (e.g. ConfirmMDx, PCA3, etc.).
2. *A typical systematic 12 core biopsy will miss a clinically significant cancer approximately 20-30% of the time* (a 20-30% false negative rate).
3. *When cancer is missed on the initial systematic biopsy, the cancer is usually "hiding" in one of the following locations: anterior-apical peripheral zone, midline peripheral zone, or anterior transition zone.* The minimum sampling on systematic re-biopsy should include the same scheme recommended for an initial biopsy (see page 192), but also consider obtaining cores from the transition zone, midline peripheral zone, and anterior-apical prostate.
4. Transurethral biopsy—transurethral resection of the prostate is usually not utilized to biopsy for prostate cancer because it has a low diagnostic yield (it detects prostate cancer in ≤ 8% cases). The transition zone can usually be sampled adequately by transrectal or transperineal biopsy.
5. Systematic saturation biopsy—an abundance of cores (e.g. > 20) are taken throughout the prostate. Saturation biopsy may be performed transperineal (using a brachytherapy template) or transrectal. Saturation biopsy is an alternative to repeating a standard 10-12 core systematic biopsy.
6. Methods to help determine the need for repeat biopsy after a prior benign systematic biopsy
   a. Multiparametric MRI (mpMRI) of the prostate—in men with a rising PSA or a high risk for prostate cancer despite a previous benign prostate biopsy, prostate mpMRI may help identify cancer that has been missed. mpMRI can also be used to guide biopsies into the suspicious region. Several studies show that the cancer detection rates are higher with targeted biopsies than with systematic biopsies. Although cancer detection rates are highest when systematic and targeted biopsies are performed together. *If the biopsy of a PIRADS 5 lesion is benign, consider repeating the mpMRI and the mpMRI guided biopsy (take at least 3 to 5 cores from the lesion) because there is still high likelihood of cancer (even when the repeat mpMRI shows that the lesion has improved to a PIRADS 2 or 3, the risk of finding cancer on repeat biopsy is nearly 25%; if the repeat mpMRI shows that the lesion is still PIRADS 4 or 5, then the risk of finding cancer on repeat biopsy is 62%).*
   b. Molecular tests—for details on these tests, see page 188.
      i. PCA3—a test that analyzes urine for overexpression of the PCA3 gene. PCA3 is FDA approved to determine the risk of cancer in men age ≥ 50 with a previous benign prostate biopsies.
      ii. Tests for tumor field effects—cancer can induce changes in the surrounding benign tissue. These changes are called a field effect or "halo". When a benign core contains a field effect, there is a higher risk of cancer elsewhere in the prostate. If there is suspicion of prostate cancer despite a previous benign biopsy, then testing for a field effect can help determine the risk that cancer may be present. Examples of tests that check for a field effect include ConfirmMDx and Prostate Core Mitomic Test.

Confirmatory and Surveillance Biopsies for Men with Prostate Cancer
1. Confirmatory Prostate Biopsy—see page 213.
2. Surveillance Prostate Biopsy—see page 216.

Side Effects Of Prostate Biopsy

1. Most side effects are minor. Major side effects are rare.
2. Severe rectal bleeding—this is initially managed by applying pressure to the prostate using one of the following methods: hold pressure with a finger or with the ultrasound probe, rectal packing (place a lubricated pack in the rectum), or place a Foley catheter in the rectum and inflate the balloon (often done after rectal packing). If bleeding persists

Prostate Biopsy Side Effect	Risk
Minor gross hematuria	Common
Minor rectal bleeding	Common
Hematospermia	Common
Bleeding requiring intervention	0.7%
Transient fever	$\leq 6.2\%$
Epididymitis	0.7%
Prostatitis	1.0%
Sepsis	$\sim 1\%$
Vasovagal episode	5.3%
Voiding symptoms (transient)	$\leq 25\%$
Urinary retention	$\leq 2.6\%$
Erectile dysfunction (transient)	<1%

despite holding pressure, consider applying hemostatic agents, anoscopy with suture ligation, or colonoscopy with injection of epinephrine. If bleeding still persists, embolization or surgical interventional may be required.

3. Severe gross hematuria—severe hematuria, especially with clot retention, is initially managed by placement of a urethral catheter and irrigation of the catheter to remove clots. Placing the catheter on light traction for a short period of time may help stop the bleeding. If significant bleeding still persists, then start continuous bladder irrigation using a 3-way catheter. If bleeding still persists or warrants more immediate intervention, then perform cystoscopy with coagulation of the bleeding site.

4. Tumor seeding along the needle tract is extremely rare (only 40 cases were reported from 1953 to 2012). The majority of cases presented with high grade, poorly differentiated cancers.

Management of Biopsy Results

Prostate Biopsy Performed (for indications, see page 183)			
Normal or AAH or Low Grade PIN or Focal High Grade PIN	Multifocal High Grade PIN‡ (≥ 3 sites)§	ASAP‡ or Suspicious for Cancer	Prostate Cancer
Monitor PSA & DRE	Monitor PSA & DRE, Extended† Re-biopsy* in 1-3 Years	Extended† Re-biopsy* in 3-6 Months	Stage & Manage

ASAP = atypical small acinar proliferation; DRE = digital rectal examination
AAH = atypical adenomatous hyperplasia; PIN = prostatic intraepithelial neoplasia

* Re-biopsy consists of at least 12 systematic cores including cores from the lateral peripheral zone and apical anterior prostate. Transition zone biopsies are optional. Also, consider performing multiparametric MRI guided prostate biopsies to target any suspicious lesions.
† Extended means that additional cores should be taken from the abnormal region and its adjacent regions.
‡ Consider obtaining a test that predicts the chance that cancer may have been missed on the previous biopsy (such as ConfirmMDx, which is validated in men with high grade PIN or ASAP. See page 189).
§ Focal is defined as present in 1 or 2 sites, whereas multifocal is defined as present in 3 or more sites. A greater number of foci with high grade PIN correlates with a higher risk of developing cancer. When extensive high grade PIN is present, confirm the absence of ductal and intraductal cancer (consider having the pathology reviewed by a prostate specialist), and then re-biopsy in 1 year.

Stage and Grade

Gleason Score

The Gleason score is determined by the *architectural pattern of the prostate glands* (cellular characteristics, such as mitoses, are not considered). The two most abundant patterns are assigned a number from 1 to 5. These two pattern numbers are added to obtain the Gleason score. The Gleason score is reported as the most abundant pattern plus the second most abundant pattern, followed by the sum (e.g. 4+3=7). The higher the Gleason pattern and the higher the Gleason score, the worse the prognosis. A tertiary pattern may be reported when there is a small amount of Gleason pattern 4 or 5 because their presence (even if it is scant) portends a worse prognosis.

Gleason Pattern	Tumor Confined to Well-circumscribed Nodules	Stroma Present Between Each Gland	Variability in Gland Size and Morphology
1	Yes	Yes	None (large uniform glands)
2	Yes	Yes	Minimal
3	No	Yes	Moderate
4	No	No (Fused glands)	Fused ("back to back") glands or cribriform* glands
5	No	Tumor cells don't form glands (solitary tumor cells or cells packed together in sheets or nests)	

* Cribriform pattern means that the tumor appears to have small open spaces or holes when viewed under a microscope.

Group Grade

1. The International Society of Urological Pathology (ISUP) developed a new reporting system for prostate cancer grading, which was subsequently adopted by the World Health Organization. It utilizes the Gleason system to determine a grade group.
2. The higher the grade group, the worse the prognosis.

ISUP/WHO Grade Group	Gleason Score	Gleason Pattern Requirement
1	≤ 6	No pattern 4 or 5
2	7	3+4
3	7	4+3
4	8	Any pattern
5	9-10	Any pattern

PSA to Stage Prostate Cancer

1. Higher pre-treatment PSA increases the risk for capsular penetration, seminal vesicle invasion, lymph node metastasis, and distant metastasis.
2. PSA is part of the criteria used to determine risk category (see page 201).

Imaging to Stage Prostate Cancer

1. The two most common sites of metastasis are the bones and the pelvic lymph nodes; therefore, imaging for metastases are focused on these sites.
   a Distant metastasis—bone scan is the initial imaging exam to check for distant metastasis.
   b. Regional lymph node metastasis—regional lymph nodes are located in the true pelvis below the bifurcation of the common iliac arteries (pelvic, hypogastric, obturator, iliac, and sacral nodes). The risk of cancer in the regional nodes can be assessed using nomograms (such as the Partin tables: BJU Int, 111: 22, 2012). However, N stage is determined by pelvic imaging (CT or MRI) or by pelvic node sampling.

2. Men with symptoms suggestive of metastatic disease—all men with symptoms suggestive of metastatic disease should undergo imaging for metastasis.
3. Men without symptoms of metastatic disease
   a. Imaging the local extent of the cancer—in men who are candidates for curative therapy, prostate mpMRI may be useful to help identify extraprostatic extension (e.g. to assess for involvement of the neurovascular bundles when nerve sparing RP is being considered). TRUS is not accurate for local staging.
   b. Imaging for metastasis—the recommended initial imaging is based on risk level (see the table below).

Recommendations for Initial Imaging to Assess for Metastasis in Men Without Cancer-Related Symptoms (Adapted from NCCN, AUA, and EAU Guidelines)		
Risk Group§	**Technetium-99m Bone Scan**	**Abdominal-pelvic Cross Sectional Imaging (CT or MRI)†**
Very Low Risk	No	No
Low Risk	No	No
Favorable Intermediate risk	Optional*	Recommended if nomogram indicates > 10% risk of regional node metastasis‡
Unfavorable Intermediate risk	Yes	Yes
High Risk	Yes	Yes

* In these men, bone scan was deemed optional by the AUA, but not recommended by the NCCN or EAU.
‡ In these men, cross sectional imaging was deemed optional by the AUA and not recommended the EAU. The NCCN recommends CT or MRI if a nomogram indicates > 10% risk of regional node metastasis.
† Multiparametric MRI may be able to detect nodal metastasis better than CT scan. The NCCN prefers mpMRI over CT for assessment of the pelvic lymph nodes, whereas the AUA and EAU had no preference of one over the other. MRI and CT may be performed with and/or without intravenous contrast.
§ For details of the risk groups, see page 201.

c. Consider obtaining a bone scan in men with elevated alkaline phosphatase.
d. A higher PSA and a higher Gleason score increase the probability of having a positive bone scan.
e. If the bone scan is inconclusive, then additional imaging of the suspect areas can be obtained using plain x-ray, CT scan, MRI, PET/CT, or PET/MRI (PET scan should be done with one of the following agents: NaF-18, PSMA, or fluciclovine). If this additional imaging is still inconclusive, then a bone biopsy may be necessary. For more detailed information on bone scan, CT, MRI, and PET, see page 456.

Total PSA* (ng/ml)	Probability of Positive Bone Scan
< 10	2.3%
10-20	5.3%
20-50	16%
> 50	> 35%

Biopsy Gleason Score*	Probability of Positive Bone Scan
≤ 7	5.5%
≥ 8	28%

* At initial diagnosis. Data from J Urol 171: 2122, 2004.

f. Using PET for the initial metastatic evaluation is not recommended. PET may be useful when the initial metastatic evaluation is inconclusive or negative despite a high risk for metastasis. Although PET scans can detect more small volume metastases, it is unclear if there is a benefit to detecting these metastases at an earlier time (there is minimal data on whether basing a treatment decision on PET improves a patient's outcome). Also, these tests have a significant false positive rate; thus, the NCCN recommends biopsy of PET-positive lesions when feasible.

TNM Stage (AJCC 2017)

The side on which the lymph nodes are involved does not affect the N stage. This classification applies only to adenocarcinoma. Surgical margin status should be specified with pathologic stage.

Primary Tumor (T) - Clinical Stage

Tx	Primary tumor cannot be assessed
T0	No evidence of primary tumor
T1	Clinically inapparent tumor that is not palpable
T1a	Tumor incidental histologic finding in 5% or less of tissue resected
T1b	Tumor incidental histologic finding in more than 5% of tissue resected
T1c	Tumor identified by needle biopsy found in one or both sides, but not palpable
T2	Tumor is palpable and confined within prostate
T2a	Tumor involves one-half of one side or less
T2b	Tumor involves more than one-half of one side but not both sides
T2c	Tumor involves both sides
T3	Extraprostatic tumor that is not fixed or does not invade adjacent structures
T3a	Extracapsular extension (unilateral or bilateral)
T3b	Tumor invades seminal vesicle(s)
T4	Tumor is fixed or invades adjacent structures other than seminal vesicles such as external sphincter, rectum, bladder, levator muscles, and/or pelvic wall

Primary Tumor (T) - Pathologic Stage†

pT2	Organ confined
pT3	Extraprostatic extension
pT3a	Extraprostatic extension (unilateral or bilateral) or microscopic invasion of bladder neck
pT3b	Tumor invades seminal vesicle(s)
pT4	Tumor is fixed or invades adjacent structures other than seminal vesicles such as external sphincter, rectum, bladder, levator muscles, and/or pelvic wall

Regional Lymph Nodes (N)

Nx	Regional lymph nodes cannot be assessed
N0	No positive regional nodes
N1	Metastases in regional node(s)

M Stage*

M0	No distant metastasis
M1	Distant metastasis
M1a	Nonregional lymph node(s)
M1b	Bone(s)
M1c	Other site(s) with or without bone disease

* When more than on site of metastasis is present, the most advanced category is used.

† There is no pathologic T1 classification. Positive surgical margin should be indicated by an R1 descriptor, indicating residual microscopic disease.

Risk Categories

1. *A pretreatment PSA velocity > 2.0 ng/ml per year, high PSA at diagnosis, biopsy Gleason score 8-10, and a palpable nodule all increase the risk of death from prostate cancer.*
2. PSA, biopsy grade, and clinical T stage can be used to stratify the risk for recurrence after treatment and for cancer specific mortality. The following risk levels were adapted from the AUA, EAU, and NCCN guidelines.

Risk Level		Criteria
Very Low		PSA < 10 & PSAD < 0.15 & Clinical stage T1c & Grade group 1* & ≤ 50% cancer per core & ≤ 2 positive cores†
Low		PSA < 10 & Grade group 1 & Clinical stage T1-T2a & does not meet the criteria for very low risk
Intermediate		No high risk characteristics and one or more of the following criteria: PSA = 10-20 or Grade group 2-3 or Clinical stage T2b-T2c
Intermediate	Favorable	Any of the following scenarios‡: · Grade group 1 & PSA < 10 & clinical stage T2b-T2c, or · Grade group 1 & PSA = 10-20 & clinical stage T1-T2a, or · Grade group 2 & PSA < 10 & clinical stage T1-T2a
Intermediate	Unfavorable	Any of the following scenarios: · Grade group 1 & PSA = 10-20 & clinical stage T2b-T2c, or · Grade group 2 & PSA = 10-20 & clinical stage T1-T2a, or · Grade group 2 & PSA ≤ 20 & clinical stage T2b-T2c, or · Grade group 3 & PSA ≤ 20 & clinical stage ≤ T2c
High		PSA > 20 or Grade Group ≥ 4 or Clinical stage ≥ T3

PSA = prostate specific antigen; PSAD = PSA density (see page 185).

* Gleason score ≤ 6 with no pattern 4 or 5.

† When a lesion is biopsied using MRI guided, TRUS guided, or DRE guided targeting, the positive cores from that lesion (regardless of the number of cores involved or the percentage per core involved) count as a single positive core. For systematic biopsies, this criteria assumes that ≥ 10 cores were taken.

‡ The NCCN guideline also includes cancer present in < 50% of the biopsy cores (see † above) as a mandatory criteria for favorable intermediate disease. In other words, the following formula must be true: (# of cores with cancer†) ÷ (# of systematic cores taken + # of lesions biopsied) is < 50%.

Definition of Clinically Significant & Clinically Insignificant Cancer

1. Cancers that are more likely to cause harm are considered clinically significant. However, some prostate cancers are unlikely to cause harm in a patient's lifetime, even when they are undiagnosed and untreated (i.e. they are "clinically insignificant").

   a. Many studies classify any cancer with Gleason score ≤ 6 as clinically insignificant.

   b. The Epstein criteria (JAMA, 271: 368, 1994) for clinically insignificant cancer are clinical stage T1c, Gleason score ≤ 6 (grade group 1), cancer in ≤ 2 biopsy cores from a systematic biopsy, ≤ 50% cancer involvement in any core, and PSA density < 0.15. The criteria using number or percent of cores involved is based on systematic biopsy (for this classification, when a lesion is targeted, the positive cores from that lesion count as a single positive core). *Also, approximately 8% of cancers classified as insignificant by these criteria were not organ confined at the time of RP.* The Epstein criteria were adopted as the definition of very low risk prostate cancer.

2. Clinically significant is typically defined as cancers that do not meet the criteria for insignificant cancer; however, many studies define clinically significant as any cancer with Gleason score ≥ 7 (grade group ≥ 2).
3. In general, no specific set of criteria can be 100% accurate in predicting which cancers will be insignificant (i.e. harmless). When criteria suggest that there is a low risk of harm, surveillance is recommended. Any cancers that ultimately turn out to be potentially harmful, will hopefully be detected during surveillance.

Molecular Testing of Prostate Cancer Before Treatment

General Information
1. These assays measure the state of multiple genes (or their proteins) in cancer tissue to predict various prognostic outcomes.
2. None of these tests have been studied in randomized trials. Also, there is a paucity of data on whether basing a treatment decision on these tests improves a patient's outcome. Nonetheless, the prognostic data supplied by these tests has been utilized to manage patients.
3. Currently, these tests are mainly used to help decide on curative treatment versus surveillance.
4. The AUA 2017, EAU 2021, and NCCN 2021 guidelines recommend against the routine use of these tests, but their use in select patients may be beneficial. Men with very low risk disease are unlikely to benefit from molecular testing, and the NCCN recommends against testing in these men. Also, these tests should be used only in men with life expectancy ≥ 10 years who are candidates for curative treatment.

Prolaris
1. This test examines 31 cell cycle progression genes and 15 control (housekeeping) genes in prostate cancer tissue.
2. The Prolaris report provides data on the following risks:
   a. 10-year prostate cancer specific mortality *with conservative management* (i.e. watchful waiting).
   b. 10-year risk of metastasis after *RP or XRT.*
3. Prolaris is utilized to help decide on curative treatment versus surveillance in untreated men with low risk or favorable intermediate risk prostate cancer and with > 10 year life expectancy. It may also be used to decide on intensity of treatment in men with unfavorable intermediate or high risk disease and with > 10 year life expectancy.

Decipher Prostate Biopsy
1. Decipher Prostate biopsy measures the expression of 22 genes to generate a genomic risk.
2. The Decipher Prostate Biopsy report provides data on the following risks:
   a. 10-year prostate cancer specific mortality *after RP.*
   b. 5-year risk of metastasis *after RP.*
   c. Gleason pattern ≥ 4 at RP
3. Decipher Prostate Biopsy is utilized to help decide on curative treatment versus surveillance in untreated men with low risk or favorable intermediate risk prostate cancer and with > 10 year life expectancy. It may also be used to decide on intensity of treatment in men with unfavorable intermediate or high risk disease and with > 10 year life expectancy.
4. A different Decipher test, Decipher Prostate RP, is used after RP to predict clinical outcome after post-RP radiation. See page 222 for details.

Oncotype DX Prostate
1. This test examines 12 genes related to prostate cancer and 5 control (housekeeping) genes in prostate cancer tissue.
2. The Oncotype DX report provides data on the following risks:
   a. 10-year prostate cancer specific mortality *after RP.*
   b. 10-year risk of metastasis *after RP.*
   c. Local extension outside the prostate (pT3) at RP.
   d. Gleason score $\geq 4+3$ at RP.
3. Oncotype DX is utilized to help decide on curative treatment versus surveillance in untreated men with low risk or favorable intermediate risk prostate cancer and with > 10 year life expectancy.

ProMark
1. This test measures 8 proteins relevant to prostate cancer.
2. The ProMark report provides data on the following risks:
   a. Non-organ confined disease (pT3 or N1 or M1) at RP.
   b. Gleason score $\geq 4+3$ at RP.
3. ProMark is utilized in untreated men with low risk or favorable intermediate risk prostate cancer who have > 10 year life expectancy to help decide on curative treatment versus surveillance.

Treatment of Potentially Curable Prostate Cancer

General Information
1. Localized prostate cancer is defined as cancer present only in the immediate region of the prostate (i.e. N0M0 and stage $\leq$ T3). Localized cancers have a high potential for cure.
2. Regional metastasis is defined as cancer that has spread to regional lymph nodes (stage N1). For N1M0 prostate cancer, cure is possible, but the cure rates are lower than for localized prostate cancer. See page 230.
3. Metastatic prostate cancer is defined as cancer that has spread to areas other than regional nodes (stage M1). Stage M1 is not curable.

Lifestyle Changes as Adjunct to Standard Management
1. Smoking—smoking at the time of prostate cancer diagnosis is associated with higher stage, higher grade, biochemical recurrence, metastasis, earlier onset of castration resistance, and death from prostate cancer. It is unclear if smoking cessation after diagnosis improves outcome.
2. Diet Modification
   a. The randomized MEAL (Men's EAting and Living) study showed that increasing vegetable intake did not alter cancer progression in men with low risk prostate cancer.
   b. Certain dietary elements may slow the growth of prostate cancer; however, it is unknown if diet modification reduces progression or improves survival. Some diet modifications can prolong PSA doubling time, but they may be altering PSA without altering the cancer.
   c. The risk, optimal dose, and efficacy of these substances are unknown.

Dietary Elements that May Slow the Growth of Prostate Cancer			
Low fat	Green tea†	Vitamin E**	Selenium**
High fiber	Lycopene‡	Vitamin D	Soy protein*

* The beneficial effects of soy protein are thought to arise from *isoflavones.*
† The beneficial effects of green tea are thought to arise from *polyphenols.*
‡ Lycopene is present in tomatoes and tomato paste.
** Data indicate that Vitamin E, selenium, soy protein, and lycopene do not prevent prostate cancer. For details, See Prostate Cancer Prevention, page 171.

Which Treatment is Best for Localized Prostate Cancer?
1. There is no universal agreement regarding which treatment is best for localized prostate cancer.
2. Comparison of cure rates
   a. For low risk prostate cancer in men age ≥ 50, RP, XRT, permanent brachytherapy, and cryotherapy appear to have similar cure rates.
   b. For high risk prostate cancer in men age ≥ 50, brachytherapy alone and cryotherapy alone have lower cure rates than RP alone, XRT alone, and XRT with brachytherapy. Therefore, *brachytherapy alone or cryotherapy alone are usually not used to treat high risk prostate cancer.*
3. Comparison of side effects
   a. RP has a higher risk of erectile dysfunction and urinary incontinence than XRT, whereas XRT has a higher risk of bowel dysfunction than RP.
   b. Cryotherapy has a significantly higher risk of erectile dysfunction than XRT, whereas urinary and bowel side effects are similar.
4. Standard treatment options for localized prostate cancer include radical prostatectomy (RP), external beam radiation (XRT), brachytherapy (BT), combined external beam radiation and brachytherapy (XRT+BT), and surveillance. Androgen deprivation therapy (ADT) alone is not recommended for treatment of localized prostate cancer.
   a. RP may be done with or without a pelvic lymph node dissection (RP±PLND).
   b. Radiation may be given with or without a temporary course of androgen deprivation therapy (XRT±ADT, XRT+BT±ADT)
5. Men with distant metastasis or symptoms that are caused by prostate cancer should be treated.
6. For men with no cancer-related symptoms, no distant metastasis, and a short life expectancy (< 5-10 years), watchful waiting is usually the preferred management.
7. For men with no cancer-related symptoms, no distant metastasis, and life expectancy ≥ 10 years, the preferred management is based on risk.
   a. *For very low risk or low risk prostate cancer, active surveillance is preferred for most men.*
   b. *For intermediate risk prostate cancer, curative treatment (with RP, XRT±ADT, BT±XRT±ADT) is preferred for most men.*
   c. *For high risk prostate cancer, curative treatment (with RP, XRT + ADT, or XRT+BT + ADT) is preferred for most men.*
8. Cryotherapy is considered a non-standard option for men with very low, low, or intermediate risk prostate cancer.
9. Other therapies, such as high intensity focused ultrasound (HIFU), are still considered investigational. If HIFU is utilized, it should only be used in men with very low, low, or intermediate risk cancer.
10. Currently, therapies that treat the entire prostate gland are the standard of care. Partial or focal treatments (aimed at the cancer within the gland rather than the entire gland) are considered investigational.
11. *Androgen deprivation alone should not be used to treat men with asymptomatic localized (N0M0) prostate cancer* (unless there is a contraindication to standard management).
    a. Retrospective data shows that using castration as the only treatment for localized prostate cancer does not improve overall survival or prostate cancer-specific survival compared to no treatment. In addition, castration does not delay the need for other palliative therapies.
    b. A randomized trial in men undergoing surveillance for localized prostate cancer showed that treatment with high dose bicalutamide increased the risk of death compared to placebo after median follow up of 10 years.

Non-Randomized Trials Comparing Curative Treatments

1. Non-randomized trials are inherently biased and are utilized to generate a hypothesis, not to prove a hypothesis. The information in this section should be interpreted with this limitation in mind. Clinical practice should be based on prospective randomized trials whenever possible.

2. *With more than 10 years of follow up, many non-randomized studies suggest that RP has a higher long term cure rate, disease specific survival, and overall survival compared to XRT± ADT, primary androgen deprivation, or surveillance. However, XRT+brachytherapy achieves a similar overall and disease specific survival as RP. XRT at a dose of 79-81 Gy appears to have equivalent survival compared to XRT+ brachytherapy.* A few selected examples of these studies are listed below (additional studies are listed in the References section on page 278).

   a. A meta-analysis by Wallis et al (2016) pooled 118,830 patients from 19 studies and found that XRT alone or brachytherapy alone had a higher overall mortality and prostate cancer specific mortality than RP. Caveats: Some studies included in this meta-analysis used a radiation regimen that is considered suboptimal by current standards (e.g. dose < 75 Gy, no ADT for intermediate or high risk cancers).

   b. Robinson et al (2018) compared over 41,000 men in a Swedish database who underwent RP or radiation. In men with low or intermediate risk disease, radiation was associated with a higher rate of death from prostate cancer than RP, although the absolute difference was small.

   c. Pokala and Menon (2009) compared 6906 men age < 50 years and showed that RP resulted in a significantly higher 15 year cancer specific and overall survival than either XRT or no curative therapy, especially in men with moderately or poorly differentiated tumors. This data suggests that RP is the treatment of choice for men age < 50.

   d. Abdel-Rahman (2019) compared 3953 men who were diagnosed with localized prostate cancer during participation in the PLCO screening trial and subsequently received either XRT (with or without androgen deprivation) or RP. Men who underwent RP had a significantly higher overall survival and prostate cancer specific survival.

   e. Huang et al (2019) compared 2228 men with age < 60 years and with localized Gleason score ≥ 8 prostate cancer who underwent either RP (with or without adjuvant XRT), XRT (with or without ADT), or combined XRT+BT (with or without ADT). Prostate cancer specific mortality and overall mortality were higher for XRT than for RP; but similar for RP and XRT+BT.

   f. Westover et al (2012) compared 657 men with localized Gleason score ≥ 8 prostate cancer who underwent either RP or combined XRT+BT+ADT. There was no difference in prostate cancer specific mortality between RP and combined XRT+BT+ADT.

   g. Muralidhar et al (2019) compared 6643 men with Gleason 9 or 10 localized prostate cancer who underwent RP with adjuvant XRT or XRT+BT. There was no difference in overall survival or prostate cancer mortality between the groups.

   h. Shen et al (2012) analyzed 12,745 men with high risk prostate cancer who underwent brachytherapy, XRT, or both. Men who underwent brachytherapy with XRT had a lower prostate cancer specific mortality than men who underwent XRT alone (this study did not account for radiation dose). However, Amini et al (2016) showed no difference in overall survival with XRT at 79 to 81 Gy compared to a combination of XRT an brachytherapy.

Summary of Randomized Trials Comparing Curative Treatments

1. *Treatment with RP or XRT can reduce risk of death from prostate cancer and death from any cause compared to surveillance or watchful waiting (and these benefits are most pronounced in men age < 65 years).* Treatment also reduces local progression, distant metastases, and use of androgen deprivation, but it also increases the risk of side effects.

2. XRT and RP appear to achieve similar cure rates. RP has a higher risk of erectile dysfunction and urinary incontinence than XRT, whereas XRT has a higher risk of bowel dysfunction than RP.

3. Cryotherapy has poor efficacy in high risk localized prostate cancer. Cryotherapy has a significantly higher risk of erectile dysfunction than XRT, whereas urinary and bowel side effects are similar to XRT.

4. It is unclear if combining XRT and brachytherapy is better than XRT alone in men with intermediate or high risk localized prostate cancer.

Surveillance/Watchful Waiting versus RP (Randomized Trials)

1. For definitions of watchful waiting and active surveillance, see page 212.

2. Iversen study & VACURG study—compared watchful waiting to radical prostatectomy. There was no difference in overall survival after 15 to 23 years of follow up. Caveat: Patients were enrolled before 1980; thus, the data are not applicable to current practice because contemporary diagnosis and staging are different than those studied. These studies were conducted before PSA was available. Also, the study populations were rather small.

3. SPCG4 (Scandinavian Prostate Cancer Group 4) compared RP to watchful waiting in 695 men with age < 75, PSA < 50, & clinical stage T1-2 N0M0.
   a. 100% of men in the RP group underwent a PLND.
   b. For the watchful waiting group, only palliative (non-curative) treatment was planned (although 15% eventually underwent curative therapy).
   c. Androgen deprivation was administered at the time of metastasis in both groups. For men undergoing RP, ADT was also initiated for palpable local recurrence during most of the study period.
   d. At a median follow up of 23.6 years, *men undergoing RP had a significantly lower rate of distant metastasis (27% vs. 48%), death from prostate cancer (death rate 21% vs. 35%), and death from any cause (79% vs. 94%).* When patients were stratified by age, RP had a significantly lower rate of distant metastasis and death from prostate cancer regardless of age at randomization, although *the benefit was more pronounced in men < 65.* Death from any cause was lower in men undergoing RP regardless of age at randomization, but the difference was significant only in men age < 65. *RP resulted in a mean of 2.9 years of life gained compared to surveillance.*
   e. Watchful waiting had a significantly higher risk of local progression, distant metastasis, and use of androgen deprivation, but a lower risk of erectile dysfunction and urinary incontinence compared to RP.
   f. Caveats—this study may not be applicable to current practice because its cohort (76% clinical stage T2, 47% PSA > 10, and 5% detected by PSA) is not typical of contemporary patients.

4. PIVOT (Prostate cancer Intervention Versus Observation Trial)—compared watchful waiting to RP in 731 men with age ≤ 75, PSA ≤ 50, and clinical stage T1-T2 NxM0.
   a. 82% of men in the RP group underwent a PLND.
   b. For the watchful waiting group, only palliative (non-curative) treatment was planned (although 20% eventually underwent curative therapy).
   c. For both groups, androgen deprivation was started for symptomatic or metastatic progression, or at the discretion of the treating physician.

    d. At a median follow up of 18.6 years, *men who underwent RP had a significantly lower rate of death from any cause, although the absolute benefit was small (67.6% vs. 73.3%). For RP, the survival benefit was greater in men with any of the following characteristics: age < 65 years, fewer comorbidities, ≥ 34% of cores positive, or intermediate risk disease.* In the most recent update, death from prostate cancer could not be assessed, but an older report showed that RP resulted in a non-significant reduction in death from prostate cancer at a median follow up of 12.7 years (7.4% vs. 11.4%). *RP resulted in a mean of 1 year of life gained compared to watchful waiting.*

    e. Watchful waiting had a higher risk of local progression, bone metastasis, and use of androgen deprivation, but a lower risk of erectile dysfunction and urinary incontinence compared to RP.

    f. Caveats—PIVOT is applicable to current practice because contemporary patients are similar to those studied (the majority were clinical stage T1c, PSA < 10, and detected by PSA). PIVOT may not be applicable to men age < 60 (only 10% of patients were age < 60).

5. PROTECT trial (Prostate Testing for Cancer & Treatment) randomized men with age 50-69, clinically localized prostate cancer, and PSA=3-20 to XRT, RP, or active surveillance. Median follow up was 10 years.

    a. In the RP group, PLND was performed in men who had a higher risk of regional node metastasis (the proportion of these men was not reported).

    b. In the active surveillance group, curative treatment was offered at the discretion of the treating physician. The decision to proceed with curative therapy was usually driven by a rise in PSA, and was not necessarily driven by cancer progression.

    c. *At a median follow up of 10 years, there was no difference in death from prostate cancer or death from any cause between XRT, RP, and surveillance.*

    d. Surveillance resulted in a significantly higher rate of clinical progression and distant metastasis compared to XRT or RP. Surveillance resulted in a lower risk of erectile dysfunction than XRT or RP, a lower rate of urinary incontinence than RP, and a lower risk of bowel dysfunction than XRT.

    e. Caveats

       i. The conclusions of this study cannot be extrapolated to men with intermediate or high risk disease because these groups were under-represented (only 20% had Gleason score = 7 and 2% had Gleason score ≥ 8). The majority of the study population were low risk; thus, there were few deaths from prostate cancer during the 10 years of follow up. The small number of deaths made it difficult to determine any differences in mortality between the study arms.

       ii. In SPCG-4 and PIVOT, the watchful waiting arms received palliative (non-curative) treatment for progression, whereas the active surveillance arm in PROTECT received curative therapy at the discretion of the treating physician. In fact, among men assigned to the active surveillance group, treatment with curative intent was administered to 25% within 3 years and to approximately 55% by 10 years after randomization. So, PROTECT did not compare curative treatment to no curative treatment. Also, 22% of men that were randomized did not undergo their assigned management. *If the data are analyzed based on the treatment actually received (rather than by intention to treat), then treatment with either XRT or RP resulted in a significantly lower risk of death from prostate cancer compared to active surveillance.*

iii. *The main message of this study appears to be that men with low or intermediate risk prostate cancer have small risk of dying within 10 years whether they undergo up front curative treatment or up front active surveillance.* Longer follow up will be required to determine if treatment is better than surveillance or if there is a difference in survival between XRT and RP. A study enrolling a substantial portion of intermediate and high risk men will be required to determine if treatment is better than surveillance in these groups.

6. *Taken together, this data suggests that RP reduces local progression, distant metastases, use of androgen deprivation, death from prostate cancer, and death from any cause compared to watchful waiting, and these benefits are most pronounced in men < 65 years old. RP also increases the risk of erectile dysfunction and urinary incontinence starting early in the course of treatment. For low risk prostate cancer, RP, XRT, and active surveillance (with possible delayed curative treatment) have similar survival at 10 years of follow up.*

Comparison of PIVOT, SPCG-4, and PROTECT

			PIVOT	SPCG-4	PROTECT
Baseline Characteristics of the Study Population	Cancer Detected by PSA		76%	5%	100%
	Clinical Stage	T1a/b	4%	12%	0%
		T1c	50%	12%	76%
		T2	45%	76%	24%
	PSA (ng/ml)	< 10	65%	52%	90%
		10-19.9	24%	28%	10%
		20-50	10%	19%	0%
		Mean	10.1	12.9	4.8*
	Biopsy Gleason Score	≤ 6	70%	61%	77%
		7	18%	23%	21%
		8-10	7%	5%	2%
	Mean Age		67	65	62
Management of Arm Not Initially Treated			WW	WW	AS
% of men in the WW or AS arm who eventually underwent curative treatment			20%	15%	55%
Median follow up			18.6	23.6	10.0
All-cause mortality was lower for RP compared to surveillance			Yes	Yes	No
Cancer specific mortality was lower for RP compared to surveillance			No	Yes	No†
Mean years of life gained from RP compared to surveillance			1	2.9	N/A

PSA = prostate specific antigen; RP = radical prostatectomy

WW = watchful waiting (see page 212); AS = active surveillance (see page 212)

* Mean PSA was estimated from median PSA.

† When data are analyzed based on the treatment received (rather than by intention to treat), then RP resulted in a significantly lower cancer specific mortality.

Note: Key differences in the population & study design are highlighted in grey.

Surveillance versus External Beam Radiation (Randomized Trials)

1. Widmark study—compared watchful waiting to external bean radiation (XRT) at a dose of 64-68 Gy in 214 men with clinical stage T1b-T2 N0M0 prostate cancer. With a minimum follow up of 16 years, there was no difference in disease specific or overall survival. However, XRT reduced biochemical, local, and metastatic progression. Caveat: The radiation dose used in the XRT group (64-68 Gy) is suboptimal by current standards (recurrence is more common with XRT dose ≤ 70 Gy).

2. PROTECT trial (Prostate Testing for Cancer and Treatment)—men age 50-69 years with clinically localized prostate cancer and PSA 3-20 were randomized to XRT (74 Gy), RP, or active surveillance.
   a. *At a median follow up of 10 years, there was no difference in death from prostate cancer or death from any cause between XRT, RP, and active surveillance. If the data are analyzed based on the treatment received (rather than by intention to treat), then treatment with either XRT or RP resulted in a significantly lower risk of death from prostate cancer.*
   b. Active surveillance resulted in a significantly higher rate of clinical progression and distant metastasis compared to men who had XRT or RP. Surveillance resulted in a lower risk of erectile dysfunction than XRT or RP, a lower rate of urinary incontinence than RP, and a lower risk of bowel dysfunction than XRT.
   c. Caveats—the radiation dose used in this study was similar to current regimens. Also, see caveats that were discussed previously on page 207.

RP versus XRT (Randomized Trials)
1. PROTECT trial (Prostate Testing for Cancer and Treatment)—men age 50-69 with clinically localized prostate cancer and PSA 3-20 were randomized to XRT (74 Gy), RP, or active surveillance.
   a. *With a median follow up of 10 years, there was no difference between XRT and RP in terms of clinical progression, metastasis, need for androgen deprivation, death from prostate cancer, and death from any cause.*
   b. RP was associated with a higher rate of erectile dysfunction and urinary incontinence than XRT, whereas XRT was associated with a higher risk of bowel dysfunction than RP.
   c. Caveats—the radiation dose used in this study was similar to current regimens. Also, see caveats that were discussed previously on page 207.
2. Paulson study—randomized 97 men with clinical stage T1-T2 N0M0 prostate cancer to RP or XRT. Subjects were accrued in the late 1970's. Five-year failure free survival was better for RP than for XRT. Caveat: this data is not applicable to current practice because contemporary diagnosis and staging are different than those studied. This study was conducted before PSA was available. The radiation dose used in the XRT group (<70 Gy) is suboptimal by current standards (recurrence is more common with XRT dose ≤ 70 Gy). Also, the study population was rather small.
3. Akakura study—men with clinical stage T2b-T3, N0M0 prostate cancer were randomized to RP or XRT (60-70 Gy). Androgen deprivation (oral estrogen, orchiectomy $\pm$ antiandrogen, or LHRH agonist $\pm$ antiandrogen) was started 2 months before RP or XRT and continued until biochemical or clinical progression.
   a. After 10 years of follow up, the overall survival and disease specific survival were slightly higher for RP, but these differences were not statistically significant.
   b. Caveats—this study is not applicable to current practice because treatment in this study (androgen deprivation continued indefinitely after curative therapy, XRT dose <70 Gy) is considerably different than contemporary treatment.
4. Lennernas study—89 men with PSA ≤ 50 and clinical stage T1b-T3a, N0M0 prostate cancer were randomized to RP or XRT+BT. The study was closed early because of poor accrual. With few participants, the study was underpowered and differences in survival could not be determined.
5. SPCG-15—this study is randomizing men with locally advanced prostate cancer to XRT+ADT or to RP $\pm$ adjuvant XRT. Results are pending.

XRT + ADT Versus ADT Alone (Randomized Trials)

1. *For locally advanced N0M0 disease, XRT with ADT achieves better overall and disease specific survival than ADT alone.*
2. SPCG7 studied 875 men with clinical stage T1-T3, N0M0 prostate cancer and PSA < 70 who were randomized to life long flutamide with XRT (70 Gy) or life long flutamide without XRT. Men receiving XRT and flutamide had a significantly lower 15-year risk of death from prostate cancer. Caveat: Few oncologists utilize life long antiandrogen monotherapy as a standard treatment option for advanced prostate cancer.
3. Warde et al (2011) studied 1205 men with locally advanced N0M0 prostate cancer (clinical stage T3-T4, or T2 with PSA > 40, or T2 with PSA > 20 and Gleason score > 8). Men were randomized to lifelong castration with XRT (65-69 Gy) or to lifelong castration without XRT. After 7 years, adding XRT to castration improved overall survival and disease specific survival. In the short term, quality of life was worse in the XRT group (presumably from radiation related acute side effects), but, in the long term, there was no significant difference in quality of life between groups.

XRT Versus Cryotherapy (Randomized Trials)

1. Both of the studies below did not meet their accrual goal, so definitive conclusions cannot be drawn. However, cryotherapy appears to be less effective than XRT for locally advanced (stage T2c-T3b) prostate cancer.
2. Calgary trial—closed prematurely due to slow accrual. 244 men with stage T1-3, N0M0 prostate cancer and PSA ≤ 20 were enrolled. Men with Gleason score ≥ 8 were enrolled only if pelvic lymph node dissection was pN0. Participants were treated with 3-6 months of neoadjuvant ADT with an LHRH agonist and randomized to cryotherapy or XRT (68-73 Gy to the prostate and seminal vesicles; lymph nodes were not radiated). XRT and cryotherapy had similar overall and disease specific survival at 5 years. Cryotherapy resulted in significantly worse sexual function, whereas other quality of life domains were similar between groups.
3. Ontario trial—this study did not meet its accrual goal. 64 men with clinical stage T2c-T3b N0M0 prostate cancer were randomized to XRT (66 Gy) or cryotherapy. Men with PSA ≥ 25 were enrolled only if pelvic lymph node dissection or biopsy was pN0. Androgen deprivation with an LHRH agonist was started 3 months before XRT or cryotherapy and was continued for 6 months. At 8 years follow up, disease specific and overall survival were similar, but PSA recurrence was significantly more likely with cryotherapy (59% versus 17%).

XRT Alone Versus XRT with Brachytherapy (Randomized Trials)

1. *Randomized studies indicate that XRT+BT may decrease local recurrence and biochemical failure compared to XRT, but there appears to be no difference in overall survival or prostate cancer specific survival.*
2. Hoskin et al (2012)—220 men with PSA < 50 and clinical stage T1-T3 N0M0 prostate cancer were randomized to XRT alone (55 Gy) or XRT+HDR. 76% of patients received androgen deprivation (6 months for intermediate risk and ≤ 3 years for high risk patients). After a mean follow up of 7 years, XRT+HDR reduced biochemical recurrence compared to XRT alone. Overall survival and side effects were similar between groups. Caveat: the radiation dose used in the XRT alone group is suboptimal by current standards (recurrence is more common with XRT dose ≤ 70 Gy).
3. Dayes et al (2017)—men with non-metastatic clinical stage T2-T3 and pathologic stage N0 prostate cancer were randomized to XRT alone (66 Gy) or XRT with temporary brachytherapy (XRT+HDR). Neither

group received androgen deprivation. After a median follow up of 14 years, XRT+HDR significantly lowered biochemical recurrence compared to XRT alone in both intermediate risk and high risk cancers. Local recurrence was also lower after XRT+HDR (based on prostate biopsy 24 months after treatment). There was no difference in overall survival, prostate cancer specific survival, or side effects between the groups. Caveat: radiation dose used in the XRT alone group is suboptimal by current standards (recurrence is more common with XRT dose ≤ 70 Gy).

4. Morris et al (2017)—398 men with intermediate or high risk localized prostate cancer were treated with 12 months of ADT and 46 Gy of pelvic XRT, and then randomized to either XRT boost (total 78 Gy) or brachytherapy boost. Essentially, this study compared XRT+ADT to XRT+BT+ADT. At a median follow up of 6.5 years, men who underwent XRT+ADT had a higher rate of biochemical failure compared to men who underwent XRT+BT+ADT; however, there was no difference in overall survival. Urinary side effects where significantly more common in men treated with XRT+BT+ADT, This study used an XRT dose and brachytherapy dose that is similar to current practice.

RP Versus Brachytherapy (Randomized Trials)

1. Giberti study 1 (open retropubic RP vs. brachytherapy)—men with very low risk or low risk prostate cancer were randomized to bilateral nerve sparing open retropubic RP with bilateral pelvic lymph node dissection or to I-125 brachytherapy (at least 140 Gy). At 5 years of follow up, there was no difference in biochemical disease specific survival ($\sim 91\%$). Within 1 year of treatment, men undergoing RP were more likely to have sexual dysfunction, while men undergoing brachytherapy were more likely to have irritative voiding symptoms. However, at 5 years of follow up, there was no difference in bowel, urinary, or sexual function. Caveat: Although this patient population and the treatments studied are typical of contemporary practice, the follow up is only 5 years. Also, surveillance is now recommended for most men with very low risk or low risk prostate cancer.

2. Giberti study 2 (robotic RP vs. brachytherapy)—men with very low risk or low risk prostate cancer were randomized to bilateral nerve sparing robotic RP or to I-125 brachytherapy (dose not specified). At 2 years of follow up, there was no difference in biochemical disease specific survival ($\sim 97\%$). Men undergoing robotic RP were more likely to have urinary incontinence within 6 months of treatment, while men undergoing brachytherapy were more likely to have irritative voiding symptoms during the entire 2 year follow up period. Caveat: Although this patient population and the treatments studied are typical of contemporary practice, the follow up is only 2 years. Also, surveillance is now recommended for most men with very low risk or low risk prostate cancer.

3. SPIRIT trial (open retropubic RP vs. brachytherapy)—cancelled because of poor accrual, but some quality of life data was published for the men enrolled. At a median follow up of 5.2 years, men treated with brachytherapy reported better urinary and sexual function.

Watchful Waiting (Observation) for Untreated Cancer

Active Surveillance versus Watchful Waiting

1. Active surveillance for untreated prostate cancer involves routine follow up and testing, with the intent of providing *curative* treatment if the cancer increases in risk. This option is typically used in men with low risk or very low risk prostate cancer whose life expectancy is > 10 years.
2. Watchful waiting (also known as observation) for untreated prostate cancer does not necessary involve routine follow up and testing (this is determined on an individual basis). The intent is to administer *palliative* therapy if the patient's cancer progresses to a point where cancer-related symptoms are imminent or already present. Watchful waiting is typically used in men with non-metastatic prostate cancer (M0) whose life expectancy is less than 5 to 10 years.

Which Men are Eligible for Watchful Waiting?

1. For men with very low, low, or intermediate risk N0M0 prostate cancer, observation is the preferred management in men with no cancer-related symptoms and with life expectancy ≤ 5 years (AUA 2017 and ASCO 2016) or < 10 years (EAU 2021 and NCCN 2021 guidelines).
2. For men with high risk N0M0 or N1M0 prostate cancer, observation is an option for the management of men with no cancer-related symptoms and with the life expectancy ≤ 5 years.
3. Men with cancer related symptoms or with metastatic prostate cancer (M1) should be treated.

Follow Up and Intervention During Watchful Waiting

1. Watchful waiting for untreated prostate cancer does not necessarily involve *routine* follow up and testing (this is determined on an individual basis). If testing is done, it may include a history and physical examination (to check for development of cancer-related symptoms), PSA, creatinine, alkaline phosphatase, bladder ultrasound to check for rising post void residual, and renal ultrasound to check for hydronephrosis. Additional prostate biopsies are typically not indicated.
2. The intent of watchful waiting is to administer palliative therapy if the patient's cancer progresses to a point where cancer-related symptoms are imminent or already present. There are no universally accepted "trigger" criteria that define when cancer-related symptoms are imminent. Some possible triggers are discussed below.
   a. PSA and PSA doubling time—the NCCN 2021 guideline suggests using PSA > 100 as a trigger. The EAU 2021 guideline suggests using PSA > 50 or PSA doubling time ≤ 12 months as triggers. The EAU recommendation is likely based on a study by Studer et al (2008), which indicated that *untreated men with stage T0-T4, N0-N1, M0 are more likely to die from prostate cancer if they have PSA > 50 or PSA doubling time ≤ 12 months (the risk increases starting in 1-2 years, with the 7-year risk of death from prostate cancer reaching 48% in men with PSA doubling time ≤ 12 months and 32% in men with PSA > 50). Therefore, men who have a life expectancy of > 1-2 years and who have a PSA doubling time ≤ 12 months or a PSA > 50 may benefit from initiating ADT before symptoms or metastases develop (although it is unclear if this improves their survival).*
   b. Asymptomatic progressive increase in post void residual that is caused by prostate cancer.
   c. Asymptomatic ureteral obstruction that is caused by prostate cancer (from the primary tumor or metastasis).

Active Surveillance for Untreated Prostate Cancer

General Information

1. Active surveillance for untreated prostate cancer involves routine follow up and testing, with the intent providing curative treatment if the cancer increases in risk. This option is typically used in men with low risk or very low risk prostate cancer whose life expectancy is > 10 years.
2. Men considering surveillance should be counseled on the risk of life threatening progression.
3. Active surveillance is different than watchful waiting (for a comparison, see page 212).

Data Used to Determine Eligibility for Active Surveillance

1. It is important to accurately characterize the patient's cancer to reduce the risk of missing aggressive features that may preclude surveillance. Besides a recent PSA, DRE, and the initial biopsy pathology, additional tests (such as those listed below) may be used to determine eligibility for surveillance.
2. Prostate mpMRI—*several guidelines recommend using prostate mpMRI to help select patients for active surveillance. Some guidelines also recommend obtaining both systemic and mpMRI guided biopsies to determine eligibility for surveillance.*
   a. AUA/SAR 2019 guideline—"...it is strongly recommended that an mpMRI be performed in men considering active surveillance..." But "evidence is inadequate to establish that mpMRI guided biopsy is a required step in the pathway for active surveillance."
   b. EAU-EANM-ESTRO-ESUR-SIOG (DETECTIVE) consensus 2019—"For inclusion [in active surveillance], all patients need mpMRI at some point...[and]...prostate biopsies should be performed by mpMRI guided targeted biospies...with systematic biopsies."
   c. NCCN 2021—"Consider confirmatory prostate biopsy with or without mpMRI...to establish candidacy for active surveillance."
3. Confirmatory biopsy—this is a second prostate biopsy (typically within one year of diagnosis) used to help detect higher grade and/or higher volume cancer that may have been missed on the initial biopsy. The results can help determine eligibility for surveillance. There is debate regarding whether a confirmatory biopsy is required for active surveillance.
   a. If the initial biopsy consisted of an adequate systematic and mpMRI guided biopsy, then a confirmation biopsy is generally unnecessary.
   b. If the initial biopsy was only a systematic biopsy, then obtain mpMRI (if not already done) and perform mpMRI guided biopsies and another set of systematic biopsies. If the confirmatory biopsy is done soon after the initial biopsy (e.g. 1-2 months later) and the initial systematic biopsy was adequate, then the additional systematic sampling can be omitted.
   c. If mpMRI is not available, perform a thorough systematic confirmatory biopsy (the technique of confirmatory biopsy is discussed below).
   d. Technique for the systematic component of the confirmatory biopsy—sampling should include at least the same number and location of cores used for the initial systematic biopsy (see page 192). However, *data suggests that it is also important to sample the anterior-apical peripheral zone and the anterior transition zone on repeat biopsy.*
      i. 25-50% of cancers have foci in both the anterior-apical PZ and other areas of the prostate. Thus, *biopsy patterns that do not sample the anterior-apical PZ will underestimate the amount of cancer in 25-50% of cases.* Anterior-apical PZ biopsies are important in men on surveillance because they improve estimation of cancer volume.

ii. In 48 men who progressed on surveillance and underwent radical prostatectomy, Duffield et al (2009) found that the dominant cancer nodule was located in the anterior prostate (especially the anterior transition zone) in 42% of cases. Thus, *surveillance biopsies should include cores from the anterior prostate (including the anterior transition zone) so that a significant cancer is not missed.*

iii. Some urologists obtain more than 10-12 cores (e.g. a saturation biopsy) when performing systematic biopsies during surveillance (to minimize the risk of underestimating the amount of cancer).

4. Molecular tests—it is not known if patient outcome can be improved by using these tests to guide clinical decisions. In men who have worse prognosis based on these tests, the clinician may consider treating the patient or performing more comprehensive and more frequent surveillance tests. Examples of these tests include Prolaris, Oncotype DX, Decipher, and Promark (see page 202 for more details on these tests).

Which Men are Eligible for Active Surveillance?

1. Men with aggressive prostate cancers (such as intraductal and cribriform) and men with non-adenocarcinoma prostate cancers should be excluded from active surveillance.

2. Very low risk and low risk prostate cancer
   a. *The NCCN, AUA, EAU, and ASCO recommend active surveillance as the preferred management for most men with life expectancy $\geq$ 10 years and either very low risk or low risk prostate cancer.*
   b. *Factors that should be considered in the decision for active surveillance include patient age, cancer volume, and ethnicity.* Men who are diagnosed at a young age and who have a long (e.g. $\geq$ 20 year) life expectancy are more likely to be affected by the cancer in their lifetime. Also men who with African ancestry or high cancer volume (e.g. > 2 positive cores on systematic biopsy) have a higher risk of progression.
   c. For men with very low risk prostate cancer and life expectancy $\geq$ 20 years, curative treatment is a reasonable alternative.
   d. For men with low risk prostate cancer and life expectancy $\geq$ 10 years, curative treatment is a reasonable alternative.
   e. Very low risk and low risk cancers have a low rate of metastasis and cancer related death for 10-15 years after diagnosis.
   f. If men with very low risk prostate cancer undergo RP, pathology shows Gleason score = 7 in 23%, Gleason score $\geq$ 8 in 1%, and local spread outside the prostate in 8% (7% have extracapsular penetration and 1% have seminal vesicle invasion). As discussed previously, adequate evaluation of the cancer before enrolling a patient in active surveillance may help ensure that these adverse pathologic findings are not missed.

3. Favorable intermediate risk prostate cancer—active surveillance is an option for select men with favorable intermediate risk prostate cancer. However, *surveillance in these men has a higher risk of metastasis than curative treatment.* The best candidates for surveillance in this group may be men with clinical stage $\leq$ T2a, PSA < 10, < 33% of cores positive, and < 10% Gleason pattern 4. Low risk on a molecular tissue test may lend support to active surveillance.

4. Active surveillance is not recommended for unfavorable intermediate risk, high risk, or metastatic (N1 or M1) prostate cancer.

Follow Up Testing During Active Surveillance

1. The goal of surveillance testing is to determine if progression of the cancer (to a more threatening state) has occurred. When progression occurs, curative therapy may be administered. The optimal surveillance protocol is unknown.

2. Active surveillance should include testing at a planned interval (routine testing), even in the absence of clinical changes. Tests should also be performed when there is a clinical change suggestive of cancer progression (testing done for clinical indication). *The recommended tests for routine monitoring are PSA, DRE, and prostate biopsies.* mpMRI may be used routinely; however, routine use of molecular tissue testing is not recommended.

3. The AUA, EAU, and NCCN all recommend performing routine PSA and DRE during active surveillance. The recommend interval for these tests are shown below.

Guideline	Routine** PSA & DRE Interval Recommended during Active Surveillance	
	PSA Interval (months)	DRE Interval (months)
AUA 2017	Not specified	Not specified
EAU 2021	6	12
NCCN 2021	≥ 6	≥ 12
ASCO 2016	3 to 6	≤ 12

PSA = prostate specific antigen; DRE = digital rectal exam
** Routine follow up is conducted at pre-specified intervals. Additional testing should be performed when there is a clinical change suggestive of cancer progression.

4. The chart below shows guideline recommendations for routine use of mpMRI and prostate biopsy during surveillance.

Guideline	Recommended Routine** Follow Up Tests During Active Surveillance for Prostate Cancer				
	Multiparametric MRI		Prostate Biopsies		Molecular Markers
	Recommended or Consider?	Interval (years)	Recommended or Consider?	Interval (years)	
AUA 2017	Consider Use	Not specified	Recommended	Not specified*	Not Recommended
EAU 2021	Not Specified†	-	Not Specified	-	Not Recommended
NCCN 2021	Recommended	≥ 1	Recommended	≥ 1	Not Specified
ASCO 2016	Not Recommended‡	-	Recommended	2 to 5	Not Recommended‡

MRI = magnetic resonance imaging.
* No specific interval was recommended, but the AUA guideline states that "intervals vary from 1-5 years."
† Routine use of mpMRI was not specified, but the guideline recommends mpMRI if the PSA rises.
‡ Although mpMRI and molecular markers were not recommended for *routine* use, the ASCO guideline states that they "...may be indicated when a patient's clinical findings are discordant with the pathologic findings and could be useful in identifying occult cancers or changes indicative of tumor progression in patients at risk."
** Routine follow up is conducted at pre-specified intervals. Additional testing should be performed when there is a clinical change suggestive of cancer progression (additional testing may include mpMRI, prostate biopsy, molecular markers, or any indicated tests).

5. Multiparametric prostate MRI
   a. Men with an abnormal prostate mpMRI have an increased risk of progression during surveillance.
   b. Men with a normal mpMRI can still have clinically significant cancer. Among men on surveillance for low risk or very low risk cancer that have a normal MRI, 10-30% will have unrecognized pT3 or Gleason $\geq$ 7 cancer (which is why mpMRI alone is not reliable enough to assess for progression in men undergoing surveillance). *mpMRI should not be used as a replacement for prostate biopsy during active surveillance.*
   c. *mpMRI can be particularly useful in men on surveillance who never had an mpMRI and whose PSA rises despite minimal cancer on prior systematic biopsy (these men may harbor an undetected higher risk cancer).*
6. Surveillance prostate biopsies—in this text, "routine surveillance biopsy" refers to a prostate biopsy that is performed at a planned interval during routine surveillance (i.e. not done for clinical changes). A "triggered surveillance biopsy" refers to a biopsy that is performed because of a change in clinical circumstances.
   a. The NCCN & EAU guidelines state that a surveillance biopsy should be considered if prostate exam changes, MRI suggests more aggressive disease, or PSA increases. The AUA 2017 guideline did not specify any triggers. It should be noted that *PSA, PSA kinetics, and prostate exam are unreliable for detecting progression of prostate cancer.*
   b. The AUA/SAR 2019 guideline states that biopsies during active surveillance should include systematic and mpMRI guided sampling.
   c. Technique for the systematic component of the surveillance biopsy— sampling should include at least the same number and location of cores used for the initial systematic biopsy (see page 192). However, data suggests that *it is important to sample the anterior-apical peripheral zone and the anterior transition zone on repeat biopsy* (see page 213).
7. The following factors increase the risk of progression during surveillance: abnormal MRI, PSA density > 0.15, higher cancer volume (e.g. > 2 positive cores on systematic biopsy), and African ancestry. PSA doubling time does not appear to predict progression in this setting.
8. Approximately 30% of men undergoing surveillance for localized prostate cancer will elect to have treatment within 5 years.
9. The optimal triggers for determining the need for curative treatment are unknown. Triggers may include the appearance of Gleason pattern 4 or 5 cancer, an increase in cancer volume (e.g. cancer found in more cores), or tumor bulging into or invading into the prostate capsule.
10. Men whose life expectancy declines to less than 5 to 10 years may be transitioned to watchful waiting.
11. *The cure rate is similar for men treated at the time of initial diagnosis and for men treated at the time of initial progression after close surveillance.*
12. There are no proven methods to prevent progression during surveillance.
    a. Diet changes and smoking cessation during surveillance have no proven benefit, but they may be reasonable.
    b. Androgen deprivation during surveillance is not recommended.
    c. 5α-reductase inhibitors (5ARI) are not recommended to prevent progression during surveillance. The randomized REDEEM trial showed that dutasteride does not prevent pathological progression during surveillance (see page 291). However, retrospective data with long term follow up suggests that 5ARI may reduce pathologic progression during surveillance.

Cryotherapy

General Information

1. Freezing of tissue creates a region of *coagulative necrosis*.
2. Freezing achieves cell kill by the following methods.
   a. Cell rupture—occurs when intracellular ice formation generates shear forces that tear the cell membrane. Cell rupture occurs during freezing.
   b. Apoptosis (genetically regulated cell death)—apoptosis is stimulated by extreme local conditions that occur after freezing (pH, osmolarity, etc.). Apoptosis usually occurs 6-12 hours after freezing.
   c. Ischemia—freezing induces thrombosis in small vessels, leading to local hypoxia. Cell death from ischemia occurs 24-48 hours after freezing.

Technique

1. Using transrectal ultrasound guidance and a brachytherapy template, cryoprobes are inserted through the perineum and into the prostate.
2. A catheter-like urethral warming device helps prevent freezing injury to the urethra and reduces postoperative urethral sloughing.
3. The freezing process is monitored by transrectal ultrasound and by percutaneous thermocouples (needle-like probes that monitor tissue temperature in real time).
   a. Ice reflects sound waves; therefore, the edge of the ice ball appears as a hyperechoic line on ultrasound and the tissue beyond this line cannot be visualized sonographically. If freezing is started at the posterior prostate, then transrectal ultrasound cannot visualize the unfrozen anterior prostate. Thus, *the prostate is frozen from anterior to posterior to permit optimal visualization of the prostate during freezing.*
   b. Thermocouples are usually placed in critical structures (such as the rectal wall and the urinary sphincter). Using thermocouples may help prevent freezing injury to these critical structures.
4. Freezing
   a. Rapid freezing is more destructive than slow freezing.
   b. The optimum freezing temperature is unknown, but data suggests that human cells cannot survive below -40° C (even with slow freezing). *To ensure cell death, urologists often freeze to a temperature of -40° C.*
   c. Two freeze-thaw cycles are recommended because 2 cycles achieve greater cell destruction than a single cycle.
   d. Prostate freezing is conducted from anterior to posterior.
   e. The temperature at the center of the ice ball is -40° C, which ensures necrosis in this region. Between the necrosis zone and the edge of the ice ball, the temperature is -40° to 0° C, thus, cells may survive (albeit injured) in this region. Notice that the necrosis zone is smaller than the frozen region revealed by ultrasound. In order to account for this, the hyperechoic edge of the ice

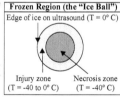

Frozen Region (the "Ice Ball")
Edge of ice on ultrasound (T = 0° C)

Injury zone (T = -40 to 0° C)   Necrosis zone (T = -40° C)

ball is often allowed to extend outside the prostate capsule to ensure adequate cell kill at the periphery of the prostate. Thermocouples can be placed at the prostate capsule to ensure that this location reaches -40° C. The width of the injury zone is dependant on the properties of the cryotherapy probe (know the properties of your probe!).
5. In most cases, the entire prostate is frozen. Partial (focal) cryotherapy is still considered investigational because long term data are lacking.
6. Cryotherapy can be performed in a minor surgical procedure in which the patient goes home within 24 hours.

Patient Selection
1. Poor candidates for cryotherapy
   a. Men who are concerned about maintaining erections—erectile dysfunction occurs in most men undergoing complete prostate freezing.
   b. Previous TURP—*men with previous TURP are at high risk for urethral necrosis and sloughing*, especially men who have an expansive cavity in the prostatic urethra (i.e. a large TURP defect).
   c. Men with large prostates—it is difficult to achieve a uniformly cold temperature during freezing of a large prostate. Before treatment, the prostate size is determined using transrectal ultrasound. Ideally prostate size should be < 40 cc. For prostates > 40 cc, androgen deprivation may be used to reduce the gland size before cryotherapy.
   d. Men with a high risk of regional lymph node metastasis—pelvic imaging and/or pelvic lymph node dissection should be considered before cryotherapy in men at risk for N1 disease.
   e. High risk localized prostate cancer—cryotherapy is not recommended for men with high risk localized prostate cancer. Cryotherapy is probably not effective for palliative treatment of urinary obstruction or bleeding caused by prostate cancer.
   f. Men who cannot have a transrectal ultrasound—probe placement and freezing are guided using transrectal ultrasound. If the patient is unable to undergo transrectal ultrasound (e.g. anal stricture or no anus from prior abdominal perineal resection), then cryotherapy is contraindicated.
2. Cryotherapy is usually restricted to men with very low, low, or intermediate risk prostate cancer who have not undergone TURP.
   a. Cryotherapy may be a reasonable alternative to radical prostatectomy in men with obesity, previous pelvic surgery, or previous pelvic radiation.
   b. Cryotherapy may be a reasonable alternative to XRT in men with rectal disorders, inflammatory bowel disease, or who had pelvic radiation.
   c. Salvage cryotherapy can be performed after XRT, brachytherapy, or cryotherapy. After brachytherapy, the seeds and the cryoprobes can have a similar ultrasonic appearance in the transverse plane (hyperechoic points), but they can easily be differentiated in the sagittal plane (seeds appear as hyperechoic points, cryoprobes appear as hyperechoic lines).

Efficacy
1. Neoadjuvant androgen deprivation does not appear to improve the cure rate, but it may be used to shrink the prostate before freezing.
2. Urethral warming prevents freezing of the prostatic urethra and reduces postoperative urethral sloughing; however, it also allows peri-urethal prostate tissue to survive. This surviving tissue continues to produce PSA (thus, PSA is rarely undetectable after cryotherapy) and it may contain cancer (35-45% of prostate cancers are within 1 mm of the urethra). Without urethral warming, total cryotherapy has a high risk of bladder outlet obstruction requiring TURP.
3. There is no universally accepted PSA cut-point that defines biochemical recurrence after cryotherapy.
   a. Men with PSA ≤ 0.4 are much less likely to develop biopsy proven recurrence.
   b. Using various definitions of recurrence, disease free survival is 65% to 92% in men with low risk or intermediate risk prostate cancer.
   c. *Local recurrence after cryotherapy tends to occur in the prostate apex.*

Side Effects

1. Cryotherapy after radiation is more likely to cause side effects than primary cryotherapy.
2. Urinary retention—caused by prostate swelling or sloughing of urethral tissue after cryotherapy. Retention often resolves in 1-2 weeks and can be managed by anti-inflammatory agents and an indwelling catheter.
3. Genital swelling—this is common, but it usually resolves in 2-8 weeks.
4. Penile paresthesia—more common after aggressive anterior freezing. It usually resolves in 2-4 months.
5. Erectile dysfunction (ED)—to ensure necrosis at the peripheral prostate, freezing is often extended beyond the prostate capsule; thus, injury to the neurovascular bundles is common. For whole gland cryotherapy, ED occurs in approximately 80-90% of men.
6. Urethral sloughing—occurs in ≤ 15%.
7. Urethral obstruction (from sloughing or stenosis)—*the risk of urinary incontinence is very high when TURP or bladder neck resection is performed after cryotherapy;* thus, aggressive resection should be avoided.
8. Rectal pain—occurs in up to 12% of men after primary cryotherapy and up to 40% of men after cryotherapy for radiation failure.
9. Urinary incontinence—long term stress incontinence is usually mild and occurs in up to 8% of men after primary cryotherapy and up to 22% of men after cryotherapy for radiation failure.
10. Fistula—urethrorectal and urethrocutaneous fistulas occur in < 1% of men after primary cryotherapy and up to 10% of men after cryotherapy for radiation failure.

Radical Prostatectomy (RP)

RP Surgical Technique

1. RP is surgical removal of the entire prostate and seminal vesicles. It may be accomplished by robotic, laparoscopic, or open technique. Open approaches include retropubic, perineal, and trans-sacral.
    a. Open and robotic techniques have a similar cure rate and a similar risk of sexual and urinary side effects.
    b. Open perineal and robotic approaches result in less blood loss than the open retropubic approach.
2. Neoadjuvant androgen deprivation (NAD) does not improve disease-free or overall survival. Thus, *NAD is not recommended before RP.*
3. Nerve sparing
    a. The *neurovascular bundles (NVB) course posterior-lateral to the prostate* and are composed of cavernous blood vessels and nerves (which promote erections). During nerve sparing, the NVB are preserved by dissecting them away from the prostate.
    b. Potency after radical prostatectomy is better when nerve sparing is performed. Bilateral nerve sparing results in a higher chance of potency than unilateral nerve sparing.
    c. In appropriately selected patients, cancer control is probably not compromised by nerve sparing. Intraoperative frozen sections of the prostate may help exclude cancer near the neurovascular bundle.
    d. The ideal candidate for nerve sparing would have clinical stage T1 or T2, PSA < 10, Gleason score ≤ 6, small volume of cancer on prostate biopsies, and good preoperative potency. These patients tend to have organ confined cancer that has not invaded the neurovascular bundle.
    e. When the NVBs are resected, nerve grafts do not help restore erections.

4. Bladder neck preservation
   a. Bladder neck preservation does not improve the final degree of urinary continence, but it may permit continence to return sooner after surgery.
   b. Bladder neck preservation reduces the risk of bladder neck contracture.
   c. Cancer control is probably not compromised. Intraoperative bladder neck biopsies can be performed to exclude residual tumor.
5. Pelvic lymph node dissection (PLND)
   a. Very low risk and low risk—PLND is optional in these men because the risk of regional node metastasis is very small. Nomograms that predict the risk of regional node metastasis can be used to help decide on whether to perform PLND in these men.
   b. Intermediate risk—the NCCN recommends PLND if a nomogram shows a $\geq$ 2% risk of lymph node metastases, whereas the EAU recommends PLND if a nomogram shows a $\geq$ 5% risk of lymph node metastases. The AUA recommends PLND in unfavorable intermediate risk, but PLND is optional in favorable intermediate risk cancer.
   c. High risk—the AUA, EAU, and NCCN recommend PLND.
   d. *The EAU and NCCN recommend performing PLND using the extended template, while the AUA mentions the extended template as an option.*
   e. Limited PLND—removal of lymphatic tissue in the area bounded by the external iliac vein anteriorly, the obturator nerve posteriorly, the origin of the internal iliac artery proximally, Cooper's ligament distally, the bladder medially, and the pelvic side wall laterally.
   f. Extended PLND—consists of a limited PLND plus removal of the lymphatic tissue posterior to the obturator nerve (the boundaries are the same as limited PLND except the posterior boundary is the floor of the pelvis). *An extended PLND will detect metastases twice as often as a limited PLND. Complications occur more often with an extended PLND.*
   g. *Removal of the lymphatic tissue anterior and lateral to the external iliac vessels increases the risk of lymphedema; therefore, dissection in this region should be avoided.*
   h. It is unknown if survival is improved by removing lymph node metastases. However, knowing if regional lymph node metastases are present can guide subsequent therapy.

Complications of PLND

1. Complications from PLND are rare. *However, the risk of complications is higher with an extended PLND.*
2. Complications of PLND include
   a. Iliac vessel injury
   b. Lymphocele—if the lymphocele is symptomatic or infected, place a percutaneous drain. Send the fluid for spot creatinine and culture. Spot creatinine will be 25-450 mg/dl for a urine leak (urinoma), but it will be similar to serum creatinine for a lymphocele (0.5-1.5 mg/dl for normal renal function). Remove the drain when output is minimal and infection has resolved. If lymph output persists, consider infusing a sclerosing agent into the lymphocele (e.g. doxycycline or dilute povidone-iodine) or performing a peritoneal window (open or laparoscopic). Consider obtaining a follow up pelvic ultrasound to rule out recurrence.
   c. Leg lymphedema—if leg swelling occurs postoperatively, obtain a lower extremity doppler to check for deep venous thrombosis. If this is negative, obtain a pelvic CT or ultrasound to check for lymphocele.
   d. Obturator nerve injury—if the nerve is severed, it can be re-approximated. Obturator nerve injury may impair leg adduction. If this symptom persists, consider obtaining a pelvic CT (a lymphocele may be compressing the nerve) and a referral to a neurologist.

Complications and Side Effects of RP

1. Sexual dysfunction
   a. Erectile dysfunction—for more details, see page 519. Postoperative rehabilitation may help recovery of erections. Postoperative potency is better when
      i. Preoperative erectile function is good.
      ii. Age is less than 60.
      iii. Nerve sparing is performed—bilateral nerve sparing results in a higher chance of potency than unilateral nerve sparing.
   b. Loss of penile length—approximately 70% of men will have a lifelong decrease in penis length (mean loss of length = 1 cm, range = 0 to 5 cm).
   c. Aspermia—men will have lifelong absence of ejaculate fluid when they have an orgasm ("dry orgasm").
   d. Urine incontinence with sexual arousal or with orgasm—more common in the first year post surgery, then tends to improve.
   e. Pain with orgasm—discomfort may occur in up to 20% of men.
2. Stress urinary incontinence (SUI)—often occurs, but usually improves during the first year after surgery. Younger men recover continence more completely than older men. Chronic severe SUI probably occurs in < 5%. *Preserving adequate urethral length during RP helps maintain urinary continence.* See Post-prostatectomy Incontinence, page 367.
3. Bladder neck/anastomotic stricture—occurs in 1-2% of cases. *Anastomotic strictures increase the risk of long term urinary incontinence.*
4. Other risks—infection, bleeding, inguinal hernia, and rectal injury (rare).

Prognostic Factors Obtained from RP Surgical Pathology

1. Positive surgical margins
   a. Men with a positive margin are more likely to recur. Approximately 50% of men with a positive margin will recur.
   b. A positive surgical margin is associated with a higher risk of death from prostate cancer and a lower overall survival.
   c. In men with a positive margin, adjuvant XRT decreases biochemical recurrence and may improve overall survival.
   d. The most common site of a positive margin is the *apex* for open and robotic retropubic prostatectomy and *anterior* for open perineal prostatectomy.
   e. Positive margins are more likely to occur with
      • Higher preoperative PSA (especially PSA > 10 ng/ml)
      • High Gleason score (especially Gleason ≥ 8)
      • High clinical tumor stage (especially T2b-T4)
      • High number of positive prostate biopsy cores
   f. *The size of a negative margin does not impact prognosis. In other words, a close margin achieves the same cure rate as an ample margin; therefore a close margin should be considered as truly negative.*
   g. *The extent of the positive margin impacts prognosis, with a higher rate of recurrence in men with a larger positive margin.*
2. Capsular penetration, Gleason score 8-10, seminal vesicle (SV) invasion, and lymph node involvement are all associated with higher risk of developing cancer recurrence, distant metastases, and death from prostate cancer.
3. Grossly positive lymph nodes appear to have a worse prognosis than lymph nodes with micrometastases.

Treatment of Positive Lymph Nodes Found During RP

1. Traditionally, RP was abandoned when positive lymph nodes were found during surgery. However, retrospective data shows that when lymph node metastases are found during pelvic lymph node dissection (PLND), RP improves overall and cancer specific survival compared to abandoning RP. *Therefore, RP should be continued when there is an incidental finding of regional lymph node metastasis during PLND.*

2. Post-RP treatment options for pN1 disease include observation, lifelong castration, or pelvic XRT with lifelong castration.

3. Observation after RP—non-randomized studies report a 10 year cancer specific survival of up to 60-70% in pN1 men who underwent RP followed by observation (with palliative ADT for clinical progression). *Observation may be most appropriate in men with ≤ 2 regional node metastases because they have a higher cancer specific survival.* For example, Shumacher et al (2008) showed that among pN1 men who underwent RP followed by observation, 10 year cancer specific survival was 78.6% in men with ≤ 2 positive nodes and 33.4% in men with ≥ 3 positive nodes.

4. Long term ADT after RP—ECOG 3886 studied men who underwent RP with PLND and who had microscopic pelvic lymph node metastasis. Men were randomized after RP to observation or lifelong castration. At a median follow up of 12 years, overall and disease-specific survival were significantly better for castration than for observation. Non-randomized studies and a meta-analysis show no survival benefit to castration in this setting. However, *immediate castration may improve survival in men with microscopic pelvic lymph node metastases who underwent RP.*

5. XRT and long term ADT after RP—in men with pN1 who underwent RP, retrospective data shows that postoperative XRT+ADT results in a higher cancer specific survival and overall survival than either postoperative ADT alone or observation alone.

6. *The NCCN guideline states that men with lymph node metastasis found at RP should be considered for immediate ADT with or without XRT.*

Radiation Therapy After RP

1. Adjuvant XRT—administered for known residual cancer after RP (postoperative PSA is detectable) or for an increased risk of possible future recurrence (postoperative PSA is undetectable, but the patient has adverse pathologic findings at RP). It is usually delivered after the patient regains adequate urinary continence (e.g. 4-6 months after RP).

2. Salvage XRT—administered for local recurrence of cancer (postoperative PSA was undetectable, but subsequently became detectable). See Salvage XRT, page 234.

3. *In the post RP setting, XRT dose to the prostatic fossa should be at least 64-65 Gy* (ASTRO/AUA 2019 guideline). The role of adding androgen deprivation to post prostatectomy XRT is unclear.

4. Decipher RP test—this molecular test is performed on cancer from the RP specimen in men who are candidates for post-RP radiation (i.e they have biochemical recurrence, seminal vesicle invasion, extraprostatic extension, or positive surgical margins). Higher Decipher scores correlate with a higher risk of developing metastasis and death from prostate cancer. Men with a low risk score have a similar risk of developing metastasis whether they are treated with adjuvant or salvage XRT; thus, these men may be more optimally managed by surveillance (with salvage XRT as needed). In men with an average or high risk score, salvage XRT was associated with a significantly higher risk of developing metastasis than adjuvant XRT; thus, these men may be more optimally manage with adjuvant XRT.

5. Adjuvant XRT versus observation—four randomized trials have evaluated adjuvant XRT versus observation after RP (SWOG 8794, EORTC 22911, ARO 96-02, FinnProstate).

   a. The sum of evidence from these trials indicates that *in N0M0 men whose RP pathology shows extracapsular extension, seminal vesicle invasion, or a positive surgical margin, adjuvant XRT reduces biochemical recurrence, local failure, and clinical progression compared to observation* (with a median follow up of 9 to 12.5 years).

   b. It is unclear if adjuvant XRT improves overall survival (SWOG 8794 showed an improved overall survival with XRT, whereas EORTC 22911, ARO 96-02, and FinnProstate did not).

   c. It is unclear if adjuvant XRT improves metastasis-free survival (SWOG 8794 showed an improved metastasis-free survival with XRT, whereas EORTC 22911, ARO 96-02, and FinnProstate were not powered to assess metastasis-free survival).

   d. *Adjuvant XRT achieves the greatest reduction in recurrence for men with a positive surgical margin.* However, men with extracapsular extension or seminal vesicle invasion still appear to benefit from adjuvant XRT.

   e. Men who receive adjuvant XRT are less likely to subsequently receive hormone therapy.

   f. The ASTRO/AUA 2019 guideline states that "Physicians should offer adjuvant radiotherapy to patients with adverse pathologic findings at prostatectomy including seminal vesicle invasion, positive surgical margins, or extraprostatic extension because of demonstrated reductions in biochemical recurrence, local recurrence, and clinical progression", but "...the impact of adjuvant radiotherapy on subsequent metastases and overall survival is less clear."

   g. Adjuvant XRT is unlikely to cause urinary incontinence, but it increases the risk of proctitis, erectile dysfunction, and urethral stricture.

6. Adjuvant versus Salvage XRT

   a. Among N0M0 men with an undetectable PSA after RP and pathologic risk(s) for recurrence, three randomized trials (RAVES, RADICALS, and GETUG-AFU17) showed no difference in biochemical progression between adjuvant XRT and salvage XRT (median follow was 5 to 6.5 years). Also, salvage XRT resulted in less grade ≥ 2 genitourinary toxicity (including lower rates of urinary incontinence and urethral stricture) and less grade ≥ 2 erectile dysfunction. In these studies, pathologic risks for recurrence were a positive surgical margin, stage pT3 (extracapsular extension and/or seminal vesicle invasion), and/or Gleason score 7-10. Salvage XRT was administered within a few months of recurrence, and recurrence was primarily defined as PSA ≥ 0.1-0.2. Only 10-20% of patients in these studies had multiple risk factors for recurrence.

   b. *When the postoperative PSA is undetectable in men with adverse pathologic findings on RP specimen, observation avoids unnecessary XRT in patients who are cured by RP alone. Furthermore, in these patients, observation with salvage XRT for a recurrence achieves equivalent cancer control and results in less severe side effects compared to adjuvant XRT.*

7. *Given the data described above, observation (with salvage XRT if local recurrence occurs) is probably the preferred option in men with an undetectable PSA after RP and __one__ pathologic risk for recurrence (positive surgical margin, pT3, or Gleason score 7-10). Adjuvant XRT may be more suitable for men with an unfavorable Decipher RP score or for men with more than one pathologic risk factor for recurrence.*

Radiation Therapy

General Information

1. Radiation therapy for prostate cancer can be dividing into 2 main categories.
   a. External beam radiation therapy (XRT)—a radiation source outside the body shoots a radiation beam into the body (i.e. radiation is delivered from the outside in).
   b Brachytherapy—radiation is delivered using radioactive implants that are placed inside the body (i.e. radiation is delivered from the inside out).
2. Depending on the clinical scenario, radiation for prostate cancer may entail brachytherapy, XRT, or a combination of both.
3. Mechanism of action—radiation damages cellular DNA, which causes cells to stop dividing or to die. Radiation can halt the growth of malignant cells, but it can also damage normal tissues (which may cause side effects).
4. Hydrogel spacer—SpaceOAR® is an absorbable liquid that is injected through the perineum and into the space between the rectum and the prostate. After injection, the hydrogel polymerizes within 10 seconds to form a soft hydrogel spacer that increases the distance between the prostate and the rectum. After approximately 3 months, the hydrogel spacer is eliminated by hydrolysis and absorption. A randomized study showed that in men with low or intermediate risk prostate cancer undergoing IMRT, hydrogel spacer significantly reduced rectal radiation exposure and reduced late rectal toxicity by 5% (less grade 1 rectal bleeding and less severe proctitis). Retrospective data shows similar results in men undergoing brachytherapy. *Hydrogel spacer should not be used in men whose prostate cancer invades the rectum or shows obvious posterior extension outside the prostate. Hydrogel spacer is injected transperineal (not transrectal).*

External Beam Radiation (XRT)

1. XRT treats cancer by shooting a beam of high energy particles into the malignant tissue.
2. Non-conformal XRT (two dimensional XRT)—in the distant past, prostate radiation was delivered by blanketing a region from a few directions (e.g. four field box technique), which resulted a high radiation dose to normal tissue. The damage to normal tissue limited the dose of radiation that could be delivered to the cancer (compromising cure rates). For prostate radiation, non-conformal XRT has been replaced by conformal XRT.
3. Conformal XRT (three dimensional conformal XRT)—narrow beams of radiation are delivered from many directions. The radiation dose is much higher where the beams intersect than in the surrounding areas. A computer is used to create pattern of beams such that the area of intersection conforms to the shape of the prostate (hence the name conformal). Therefore, higher doses can be delivered to the prostate (improving the chance of cure) while lower doses are delivered to the surrounding tissue (minimizing side effects). The initial version of conformal radiation was called three dimensional conformal radiation therapy (3D-CRT). As technology improved, XRT became even more conformal. Some studies show that newer, highly conformal techniques *(such as IMRT and VMAT)* may reduce side effects and reduce recurrence. *Therefore, IMRT and VMAT are often recommended for curative treatment of prostate cancer.*

a. Intensity modulated radiation therapy (IMRT)—compared to standard 3D-CRT, IMRT uses many more stationary beams and the dose of the beams can be changed (or modulated), which results in higher a radiation dose to the target and a lower radiation dose to surrounding normal tissues (and thus less side effects). Image guided radiation therapy (IGRT) is a form of IMRT where the prostate is tracked in real time during XRT to minimize the risk of radiating surrounding tissue.

b. Volumetric modulated arc therapy (VMAT)—this is similar to IMRT except it delivers the radiation dose as the beam continuously rotates (or arcs) around the patient (whereas IMRT uses stationary beams). VMAT and IMRT have similar efficacy and side effects, but VMAT has significantly shorter treatment times per fraction (often only 2 to 3 minutes). Rapid Arc is an example of VMAT.

4. Type of high energy particle used for prostate XRT—either protons or photons are used for prostate XRT. *Photon beam is the most common type of XRT used for prostate cancer. Protons and photons can deliver highly conformal radiotherapy, are equally effective for cancer control, and have a similar long term side effect profile. Therefore, proton beam XRT offers no advantage to photon beam XRT.*

5. Fractionation—the total dose of radiation is divided into smaller portions (called fractions) that are delivered over time. A fraction is often delivered each weekday until the total treatment dose is reached. Fractionation is utilized for several reasons:

a. It provides time for normal cells to recover from the radiation damage—this may help reduce permanent damage to normal tissues and may reduce side effects. Cancer cells are less efficient at recovering from radiation damage; thus, far fewer cancer cells recover between fractions.

b. It improves anti-cancer effects—cancer cells that are in a radiation resistant state (e.g. certain phases of the cell cycle) during one fraction have a chance to move into a radiation sensitive state for the next fraction.

6. Degrees of Fractionation

a. When the dose per fraction is higher, it takes less time to reach the total treatment dose and the duration of therapy is shorter.

b. The ASTRO/ASCO/AUA 2018 guideline proposed the following definitions for degrees of fractionation. The gaps in dose between these definitions are not well studied and remain outside the scope of the definitions.

Term	Dose of the XRT Fraction
Conventional Fractionation	1.8 to 2.0 Gy
Moderate Hypofractionation	2.4 to 3.4 Gy
Extreme Hypofractionation (Ultrahypofractionation)	> 5.0 Gy

XRT = external beam radiation

c. Moderate hypofractionation versus conventional fractionation—*moderate hypofractionation and conventional fractionation achieve similar cancer control. Hypofractionation can cause a higher rate of acute bowel side effects,* but the risk of late bowel side effects and the rate of urinary side effects (early or late) are similar. *The ASTRO/ASCO/AUA 2018 and EAU 2021 guidelines recommend either conventional fractionation or moderate hypofractionation for XRT in localized prostate cancer.*

d. Extreme hypofractionation (ultrahypofractionation)—stereotactic radiation therapy is an XRT technique that uses extreme hypofractionation. In the ASTRO/ASCO/AUA 2018 guideline, extreme hypofractionation was not recommended as a standard therapy for localized prostate cancer, but its use was conditional for low and intermediate risk patients and not recommended for high risk patients based on weak evidence. However, the results of the HYPO-RT-PC trial were reported after those guidelines were published. In the HYPO-RT-PC trial, men with intermediate or high risk localized prostate cancer were randomized to XRT using conventional fractionation or to XRT using extreme hypofractionation. At a median follow up of 5 years, failure free survival and late side effects were similar between the two groups, but extreme hypofractionation caused a higher rate of early (acute) urinary and bowel side effects. Questions remain as to whether extreme hypofractionation will have acceptable cure rates and side effects beyond 5 years. The NCCN 2021 states that ultrahypofractionation is acceptable for localized prostate cancer of any risk level. However, the EAU 2021 guideline states "it seems prudent to restrict extreme HFX to prospective clinical trials..."

7. Dose escalation—with the advent of highly conformal techniques, oncologists were able to administer a higher radiation dose to the prostate (dose escalation) without substantially worsening side effects. The higher radiation dose led to higher cure rates. For conventional fractionation, *randomized trials showed that an XRT dose of 75-80 Gy to the prostate resulted in higher cure rates compared to a dose of $\leq$ 70 Gy (without substantially increasing side effects).*

8. Androgen deprivation therapy (ADT) with XRT
   a. Low risk or very low risk—adding ADT to XRT is not beneficial.
   b. Intermediate risk—XRT with 4-6 months of androgen deprivation therapy (ADT) improves cancer specific survival and overall survival compared to XRT alone.
   c. High risk or N1—compared to XRT alone or XRT with short term ADT (4-6 months), XRT with long-term ADT (started shortly before XRT and continued for 2-3 years) achieves a higher disease-free survival and overall survival in men with Gleason score 8-10, clinical stage T3 or T4, or regional lymph node metastasis (N1).
   d. When ADT is administered with radiation, the usual regimen consists of medical castration (LHRH agonist or GnRH antagonist) with or without a first generation antiandrogen.
   e. Adjuvant ADT appears to decrease the risk of severe late gastrointestinal and genitourinary side effects from prostate XRT (i.e. grade 3 or higher toxicity occurring long after XRT).
   f. In men who undergo XRT for locally advanced prostate cancer, lengthening the duration of ADT from 4 months to 2-3 years does not increase the risk of cardiovascular mortality.

9. Hydrogel spacer—this is an absorbable injectable liquid that increases the space between the rectum and the prostate. A randomized study showed that use of hydrogel spacer significantly reduced rectal radiation exposure and reduced late rectal toxicity by 5%. For details, see page 224.

10. Contraindications to radiation therapy—see page 229.

11. After XRT without androgen deprivation, a lower PSA nadir and a longer time to achieve the PSA nadir are associated with higher disease free survival. When PSA nadir < 0.5, relapse is unlikely.

12. Side effects—see Side Effects from Radiation Therapy, page 229.

13. Common XRT regimens based on risk level.

Prostate Cancer Risk Level		Common XRT Regimens (Adapted from AUA, EAU, NCCN, & EORTC Guidelines)	
		XRT Field	**Androgen Deprivation Therapy (duration)†**
Localized (N0M0)	Very Low or Low	Prostate ± SV‡	None
	Favorable Intermediate*	Prostate ± SV± Pelvic LN‡	Optional (4-6 months)
	Unfavorable Intermediate	Prostate + SV + Pelvic LN	Recommended (4-6 months)
	High	Prostate + SV + Pelvic LN	Recommended (2-3 years)
	N1M0	Prostate + SV + Pelvic LN	Recommended (2-3 years)

XRT = external beam radiation; SV = seminal vesicles; LN = lymph nodes

† Androgen deprivation therapy using castration with or without a first generation antiandrogen, typically starting 2 months before XRT.

* If the patient is classified as favorable intermediate risk based on PSA, prostate exam, and grade group (Gleason score), but other tests (such as molecular tests) suggest a more aggressive cancer, then the patient may be treated as unfavorable intermediate risk.

‡ Nomograms that predict the risk of seminal vesicle and regional lymph node involvement can be used to help determine whether these areas should be radiated.

Temporary Brachytherapy (High Dose Rate Brachytherapy or HDR)

1. HDR can used alone or combined with 4-5 weeks of XRT.
2. HDR is delivered using Iridium 192 (Ir-192). Using transrectal ultrasound guidance, percutaneous cannulas are inserted through the perineum and into the prostate. During several sessions (over 1-2 days), the iridium is placed into each cannula for a specific duration to deliver the radiation, and then removed from the body. When the HDR is complete, the cannulas are removed.
3. Hydrogel spacer—this is an absorbable injectable liquid that increases the space between the rectum and the prostate. Retrospective data in men undergoing brachytherapy shows that hydrogel spacer significantly reduces rectal radiation exposure and may reduced rectal toxicity. For details, see page 224.
4. Contraindications and side effects of HDR are similar to permanent brachytherapy. For contraindications to radiation therapy, see page 229. For side effects of radiation therapy, page 229.
5. In 2012, the American Brachytherapy Society was unable to formulate HDR guidelines because of highly variable treatment regimens in the data (there has been no update to those guidelines at the time this book was published).

Permanent Brachytherapy (Low Dose Rate Brachytherapy; "Seeds")

1. Contraindications to radiation therapy—see page 229.
2. Permanent seed implants only (monotherapy)—radioactive pellets of Iodine 125 (I-125), Palladium 103 (Pd-103), or Cesium 131 (Cs-131) are placed through the perineum into the prostate using transrectal ultrasound guidance. This can be accomplished during a minor surgical procedure. The radioactive pellets are left inside the prostate indefinitely.

3. Comparison of radioactive implants

Seed Type	Half Life (days)	Time Needed to Deliver 90% of its Radiation Dose	Recommended Prescription Dose* for Seeds	
			Seeds Only	Seeds + XRT
I-125	60	204 days (~ 7 months)	140-160 Gy	108-110 Gy
Pd-103	17	58 days (~ 2 months)	110-125 Gy	90-100 Gy
Cs-131	9.7	33 days (~ 1 month)	115 Gy	85 Gy

* Based on the 2012 American Brachytherapy Society guidelines and the 2008 Cesium Advisory Group Recommendations.

4. For a combination of XRT and seeds, there is not enough evidence to recommend an optimal time interval between the therapies or which therapy should be applied first. However, XRT is usually performed first.

Prostate Cancer Risk Level	Common Brachytherapy Regimens (Adapted from AUA, EAU, NCCN, & ASCO Guidelines)	
	Radiation Modality	Androgen Deprivation Therapy (duration)†
Low	Brachytherapy only	None‡
Favorable Intermediate	Brachytherapy ± XRT	None‡
Unfavorable Intermediate	Brachytherapy + XRT	Optional (4-6 months)
High	Brachytherapy + XRT	Recommended (1-3 years)

† Androgen deprivation therapy using castration with or without an antiandrogen.
‡ Not recommended unless used for downsizing of the prostate before treatment.

5. After seed placement, post-implant dosimetry should be performed.
6. Hydrogel spacer—this absorbable injectable liquid increases the space between the rectum and the prostate. Retrospective data in men undergoing brachytherapy shows that hydrogel spacer significantly reduces rectal radiation and may reduced rectal toxicity. For details, see page 224.
7. With large prostates, the pubic arch may interfere with seed placement. The prostate may be down-sized with androgen deprivation to reduce pubic arch interference, but it is unknown if downsizing the prostate below 60 cc decreases the risk of urinary retention.
8. Complications
   a. Urinary incontinence—more common if TURP has been performed before or after brachytherapy ($\leq$ 7% without TURP versus 10-30% with TURP). Peripheral loading of seeds (away from the urethra) in men who had a TURP can reduce incontinence to < 5%; however, it is unknown if peripheral loading of seeds compromises cure.
   b. Urinary retention—occurs in 2-15%. The risk is higher for men with prostate size > 60 cc or with more severe baseline voiding symptoms (e.g. IPSS score > 20). Retention is initially managed by indwelling catheter or by clean intermittent catheterization. Up to 8% of men require TURP/TUIP for persistent retention; however, *the risk of urinary incontinence is higher when TURP or bladder neck resection is performed after prostate radiation.* Other treatments that may help the patient void include alpha-blockers, a course of steroids (taper dose), nonsteroidal anti-inflammatory drugs, and 5α-reductase inhibitors.
   c. *More optimal candidates for brachytherapy have no previous TURP, prostate volume < 50 cc, mild voiding symptoms (IPSS $\leq$ 12), urine flow > 15 ml/sec, and post void residual < 100 ml.*
   d. Other side effects—see Side Effects from Radiation Therapy, page 229.

Relative Contraindications to Radiation Therapy
1. Inflammatory disease of the rectum
2. Previous pelvic radiation (with near maximum dose already delivered)
3. Indwelling urethral catheter
4. Relative contraindications specific to brachytherapy
   a. Large median lobe of the prostate
   b. *Brachytherapy is usually avoided in men with prostate size > 60 g, low urine flow rate (< 10 ml/sec), high post void residual (> 100 ml), or significant voiding symptoms (IPSS > 20 or AUA score > 15) because these factors increase the risk of urinary retention.*
   c. Previous TURP—seeds should not be placed too close the urethra. An expansive cavity in the prostatic urethra (i.e. a large TURP defect) may limit seed placement and compromise radiation dosimetry.

Side Effects from Radiation Therapy
1. Erectile dysfunction—with radiation, erections are preserved initially but worsen over several years, whereas with nerve sparing RP, erections are worse initially and tend to improve over 1-4 years.
2. Bladder irritation (urgency, dysuria, etc.)—common during radiation, but severe and chronic in < 5% of cases.
3. Rectal irritation (diarrhea, rectal bleeding)—common during radiation, but severe and chronic in < 5% of cases.
4. Urine retention—up to 15% after brachytherapy. Uncommon with XRT.
5. Infertility and decreased ejaculate volume—common.
6. Hemorrhagic cystitis*—up to 8% with long-term follow up.
7. Urethral stricture*—approximately 3% with long-term follow up.
8. Urinary incontinence*—approximately 3% with long-term follow up.
9. Bowel incontinence or rectal stricture*—rare.
10. Small risk of secondary malignancy (e.g. bladder cancer)*—rare.
    * These side effects can develop even up to 15 years after radiation.

PSA Bounce after Radiation Therapy
1. PSA bounce is a temporary increase in PSA after radiation in men who are not receiving androgen deprivation. The rise in PSA may last 6-18 months.
2. PSA bounce usually occurs 1-3 years after radiation, but may occur up to 5 years after therapy. PSA bounces are usually small (e.g. 1 mg/dl), but bounces up to 16 ng/ml have been observed. Several bounces may occur.
3. 20-40% of patients have a PSA bounce after radiation.
4. PSA bounce may be caused by radiation induced inflammation and cellular damage, but it may also be caused by cancer recurrence.
5. The major concern in cases of a benign PSA bounce is that it may be confused with recurrent prostate cancer, leading to unnecessary treatment.
6. After external beam radiation—PSA bounce (especially > 1.4 ng/ml) is associated with a higher risk of biochemical recurrence.
7. After brachytherapy—PSA bounce may actually be associated with a lower risk of biochemical recurrence.

High Intensity Focused Ultrasound (HIFU)
1. High intensity focused ultrasound (HIFU) is still considered investigational; thus, its use is usually restricted to clinical trials.
2. If HIFU is utilized, it should only be used in men with very low, low, or intermediate risk prostate cancer.

Treatment of Stage N1M0 Prostate Cancer

Clinical Stage N0M0 but Pathologic N1 Found at Prostatectomy

1. Retrospective data shows that when lymph node metastases are found during pelvic lymph node dissection (PLND), RP improves overall and cancer specific survival compared to abandoning RP. *Therefore, RP should be continued when there is an incidental finding of regional lymph node metastasis during PLND.*
2. For men with clinical N0M0 prostate cancer who underwent RP+PLND and who were found to have regional lymph node metastases (pathologic N1), treatment options include observation, ADT alone, or pelvic radiation with ADT. For more details, see page 222.
3. *The NCCN guideline states that men with lymph node metastasis found at RP should be considered for immediate ADT with or without XRT.*

Clinical Stage N1M0

1. For men with clinical stage N1M0 prostate cancer and life expectancy ≤ 5 years, watchful waiting or ADT are reasonable management options.
2. For men with clinical stage N1M0 prostate cancer and life expectancy > 5 years, treatment options include RP with long term ADT (and possible postoperative XRT), XRT with long term ADT, or ADT alone. However, *data suggests that using local treatment (XRT or RP + XRT) with a long term course of ADT (2-3 years) achieves better cancer specific and overall survival compared to observation or ADT alone.*
3. For clinical stage N1M0 men undergoing XRT+long term ADT or ADT alone, the following regimens may be used for ADT: castration alone, castration with a first generation antiandrogen, or *castration with abiraterone.*
4. ADT alone—ERORTC 30891 enrolled men with clinical N1M0 prostate cancer and randomized them to immediate ADT or observation with delayed ADT for symptomatic progression. Immediate ADT resulted in a small, but statistically significant, improvement in overall survival, but no improvement in cancer specific survival.
5. RP and long term ADT (with or without pelvic XRT)
   a. Several (but not all) retrospective studies in men with pN1 prostate cancer show improved cancer specific survival and overall survival in men undergoing RP and long term ADT compared to ADT alone.
   b. Retrospective studies in men with pN1 who underwent RP show improved cancer specific survival and overall survival in men undergoing adjuvant XRT + long term ADT compared to either postoperative ADT alone or observation.
   c. *These studies suggest that men with clinically positive lymph nodes may benefit from multimodal therapy with RP + XRT + long term androgen deprivation and that multimodal treatment is better than ADT alone.*
6. XRT and long term ADT
   a. Multiple retrospective studies in men with clinical N1M0 prostate cancer show that XRT with long term ADT improves cancer specific and overall survival compared to ADT alone.
   b. Several randomized trials whose study population included some men with clinical N1M0 cancer showed that XRT with long term ADT improved disease free and overall survival compared to XRT with either short term or no ADT (e.g. RTOG 85-31, RTOG 92-02, EORTC 22961).
   c. *These studies suggest that men with clinically positive lymph nodes may benefit from multimodal therapy with XRT + long term androgen deprivation and that multimodal treatment is better than ADT alone.*

<u>Recurrence After Curative Treatment</u>

Types of Recurrence

1. Biochemical recurrence (PSA recurrence)—this is when the only sign of recurrence is elevation of PSA (i.e. the cancer is too small to be identified on imaging studies). *Relapse rarely occurs without an elevation of PSA; therefore, biochemical recurrence is almost always the first sign of relapse. Biochemical recurrence is the most common type of recurrence.*
2. Local recurrence—cancer identified within the prostate (after radiation or ablation) or near the urethral anastomosis (after radical prostatectomy).
3. Distant (systemic) recurrence—cancer identified in distant organs.
4. Clinical recurrence—either local or distant recurrence. The term clinical recurrence is often reserved for men with cancer related symptoms.

General Concepts

1. *Biochemical recurrence increases the risk of developing distant metastasis and the risk of dying from prostate cancer. On average, metastases become detectable on conventional imaging 8 years after biochemical recurrence.*
2. Risks of recurrence
   a. High pre-treatment PSA level (especially PSA $\geq$ 10 ng/ml)
   b. High grade tumor (especially Gleason score $\geq$ 7)
   c. High T stage (especially T3 or higher)
   d. Positive surgical margins (if prostatectomy was done)
   e. Positive regional lymph nodes
   f. Smoking
3. PSA doubling time (PSADT) can be used to assess prognosis in men with recurrent or advanced prostate cancer. PSADT is the number of months it takes for the PSA to double. PSADT calculation requires $\geq$ 3 PSA values measured $\geq$ 1 month apart. A short PSADT indicates worse prognosis. For more details on PSADT, see page 301.
4. *After recurrence, a PSA doubling time (PSADT) > 15 months is associated with a low risk of death from prostate cancer over 10 years.* Therefore, surveillance is a reasonable option in men with recurrent prostate cancer when PSADT is > 15 months and life expectancy is < 10 years.
5. *After recurrence, PSADT < 3 months is associated with a higher risk of death from prostate cancer.* Therefore, men with PSADT < 3 months should probably be treated aggressively.

Identifying the Location of Recurrence

1. Several criteria help predict whether biochemical recurrence is likely to be local or systemic. No single criteria is best, and a combination of criteria should probably used to help predict the location of recurrence.

Local Recurrence More Likely	Systemic Recurrence More Likely
Recurrence > 1 year after RP, or Recurrence > 1.5 years after XRT	Recurrence $\leq$ 1 year after RP, or Recurrence $\leq$ 1.5 years after XRT
Post-treatment PSADT $\geq$ 12 months	Post-treatment PSADT $\leq$ 6 months
Gleason score $\leq$ 6	Gleason score $\geq$ 8
Positive surgical margin	Negative surgical margins
No seminal vesicle invasion	Seminal vesicle invasion
No node metastasis (N0)	Node metastasis (N1)

PSADT = prostate specific antigen doubling time; RP = radical prostatectomy; XRT = external beam radiation

2. Imaging tests to determine the location of recurrence
   a. The standard imaging evaluation at the time of recurrence includes bone scan and/or abdominopelvic cross sectional imaging (CT or MRI). However, these tests are rarely positive in men with a low PSA.

    b. Men receiving androgen deprivation (ADT) for castration resistant prostate cancer (CRPC)—*perform bone scan, pelvic imaging, and chest imaging when CRPC is initially diagnosed because the risk of a positive bone scan is $\geq$ 10% (even when PSA is low and PSADT is long).*

    c. Men not receiving ADT—CT scan and bone scan are positive in only 1% of men with recurrence when PSA < 10 and PSADT > 6-9 months. With PSADT < 6-9 months (regardless of PSA), bone scan is positive in at least 10% of men; thus, *men with recurrence and not on ADT should probably undergo a metastatic evaluation when PSADT is less than 12 months even if the PSA is low.* Bone scan and CT scan should also probably be done for PSA > 10.

    d. PET/CT appears to be more sensitive than bone scan and CT scan for detecting the location of recurrence. *Some guidelines state that the clinician should consider PET scan only after bone scan and or abdominopelvic CT MRI show no metastasis. The EAU 2021 guideline recommends performing PSMA PET CT for the initial imaging of men with biochemical recurrence who are candidates for curative salvage treatment (if PSMA is not available and PSA $\leq$ 1, then choline or fluciclovine were mentioned as alternatives).* At PSA < 1, PSMA is more sensitive at detecting cancer than other types of PET scans.

3. Biopsy of the prostatic fossa—*prostate biopsy to diagnose recurrence is performed only when the patient is a candidate for curative salvage therapy.*

    a. After radiation—prostate cancer dies slowly after radiation; thus, biopsy is often avoided within 18 months of radiation. Post-radiation biopsies are difficult to interpret because the tissue may look like cancer, but it may be biologically inactive. *Men who are considering salvage cryotherapy after failing radiation should undergo seminal vesicle (SV) biopsy (in addition to prostate biopsy) because cancer in the SV occurs in up to 42% of men who recur after radiation.*

    b. After radical prostatectomy—*biopsy of the prostatic fossa is usually unnecessary after RP, even when salvage XRT is planned* because the biopsy results do not predict the outcome of salvage therapy. Transrectal biopsy of the prostatic fossa reveals prostate cancer in up to 50% of men with biochemical recurrence. A positive biopsy is more likely when the local recurrence is palpable, visible on imaging, and/or with PSA > 2.0.

    c. After cryotherapy—*local recurrence or persistence after cryotherapy tends to occur at the prostate apex. Therefore, prostate biopsy after cryotherapy should include thorough sampling of the apex.*

Post Cryotherapy Recurrence

1. Recurrence is present when any of the following criteria are found.

    a. Rising PSA—there is no universally accepted definition of biochemical recurrence after cryotherapy; however, *the serum PSA should decline to a low level after cryotherapy and should not rise on successive occasions.*

    b. A positive prostate biopsy after cryotherapy (local recurrence).

    c. A distant metastasis is detected (systemic recurrence).

2. *Before administering curative salvage therapy for cryotherapy failure, local recurrence must be confirmed by prostate biopsy. Recurrence or persistence after cryotherapy tends to occur at the prostate apex.* Curative salvage therapy may be offered when a prostate biopsy shows cancer and the cancer is localized. In this setting, treatment options include RP, XRT, brachytherapy, cryotherapy, androgen deprivation, and surveillance.

3. Salvage cryotherapy (repeat cryotherapy)—the ideal candidate has clinical stage T1-T2 N0M0, Gleason score $\leq$ 7, PSA < 4, long PSA doubling time, and life expectancy > 10 years.

4. Salvage XRT or salvage brachytherapy—data are sparse.

5. Salvage radical prostatectomy—data are sparse, but a high rate of complications is expected.
6. Salvage high intensity focused ultrasound—data are sparse.

Post Radiation Recurrence
1. General Concepts
   a. PSA can increase during radiation, but this is generally not caused by cancer progression.
   b. PSA can "bounce" up and down after radiation and this is often a benign process. See PSA Bounce after Radiation Therapy, page 229.
2. Recurrence is present when any of the following criteria are found.
   a. Rising PSA—*the 2005 RTOG-ASTRO consensus defines biochemical recurrence after radiation (with or without hormone therapy) as a rise of 2 ng/ml or more above the nadir PSA.* This definition was constructed mainly as a research tool rather than as a clinical guide for intervention. *In general, serum PSA should fall to a low level following radiation therapy and should not rise on successive occasions* (although allowances may need to be made for benign PSA bounce).
   b. Positive prostate biopsy $\geq$ 18 months after radiation (local recurrence).
   c. A distant metastasis is detected (systemic recurrence).
3. *Before administering curative salvage therapy for radiation failure, local recurrence must be confirmed by prostate biopsy. Seminal vesicle biopsy should also be performed.* Curative salvage therapy may be offered when a prostate biopsy shows cancer and the cancer is localized (see Identifying the Location of the Recurrence, page 231). In this setting, standard treatment options include radical prostatectomy, cryotherapy, brachytherapy, androgen deprivation, and surveillance.
4. Salvage radical prostatectomy
   a. Salvage RP is seldom utilized because it is technically challenging and it has a higher risk of complications than primary RP: rectal injury (6%), urinary incontinence (up to 50%; 20% require an artificial sphincter), anastomotic stenosis (20-30%), and erectile dysfunction (> 50%).
   b. The ideal candidate has clinical stage T1-T2 N0M0, Gleason score $\leq$ 7, PSA < 10, long PSA doubling time, and life expectancy > 10 years.
   c. In appropriately selected patients, 5 year disease free survival is 70%.
5. Salvage cryotherapy
   a. Salvage cryotherapy has a higher complication rate than primary cryotherapy. Long term complications after salvage cryotherapy include persistent urinary incontinence (up to 22%), erectile dysfunction (> 80%), chronic rectal pain (8-40%), and urinary fistula (up to 10%).
   b. The ideal candidate meets all of the following criteria:
      i. Clinical stage T1-T2 N0M0, Gleason score $\leq$ 7, PSA < 4, and long PSA doubling time.
      ii. Negative seminal vesicle biopsy after radiation—SV biopsy is indicated because cancer in the SV occurs in up to 42% of men who recur after radiation. Cryotherapy has not been shown to an effective treatment for cancer in the seminal vesicles.
      iii. Life expectancy > 10 years.
6. Salvage brachytherapy
   a. Salvage brachytherapy has a higher complication rate than primary brachytherapy. Long term complications include erectile dysfunction (80%), urinary incontinence (15%), urine retention (5%), rectal ulcers (4%), and rectal complications requiring colostomy (2%).
   b. In appropriately selected patients, 5 year disease free survival is 60%.
7. Salvage high intensity focused ultrasound—data are limited, but 5 year disease free rate is approximately 50%.

Post Prostatectomy Recurrence
1. Recurrence is present when any of the following criteria are found.
   a. Rising PSA—*the ASTRO AUA 2019 guideline defines biochemical recurrence as a PSA ≥ 0.2 ng ml followed by a subsequent confirmatory PSA ≥ 0.2 ng ml. The NCCN guideline defines biochemical recurrence as a detectable PSA that increases on 2 or more determinations.* The utility of using ultra-sensitive PSA (which detects PSA at 0.01 ng/ml or lower) has not been established.
   b. Positive biopsy of the urethral anastomosis region (local recurrence).
   c. A distant metastasis is detected (systemic recurrence).
2. 45% of recurrences occur within 2 years of RP, 77% within 5 years of RP, and 96% within 9 years of RP.
3. *PSA recurrence after RP is associated with a higher risk of metastasis and death from prostate cancer.* From the time of PSA recurrence, the median time to detectable metastasis (using conventional imaging) is 8 years and the median time to death from prostate cancer is 13 years. Men with a higher Gleason score and a shorter PSA doubling time tend to progress more rapidly.
4. Treatment options for local recurrence include XRT, androgen deprivation, and surveillance. Curative salvage therapy may be offered when clinical data and/or imaging suggests that the cancer is confined to the prostate fossa (see Identifying the Location of the Recurrence, page 231). *When salvage XRT is planned after RP, biopsy of the prostatic fossa is unnecessary because the biopsy results do not predict the outcome of salvage XRT.*
5. Salvage XRT
   a. Salvage XRT reduces potency; but, it usually has minimal impact on urinary continence (if administered long enough after RP).
   b. *Salvage XRT is more effective and achieves a higher disease-free survival when it is delivered at a low PSA. The ASTRO AUA 2019 guideline states that salvage XRT "...should be administered at the earliest sign of PSA recurrence and, ideally, before PSA rises to 1.0". The EAU 2021 guideline recommends offering salvage XRT when the PSA becomes detectable.*
   c. The ideal candidate meets all of the following criteria.
      i. PSA ≤ 1.0 at time of salvage XRT, long PSA doubling time, PSA recurrence > 1-2 years after prostatectomy, and life expectancy > 10 years.
      ii. Prostatectomy pathology showed Gleason score ≤ 7, uninvolved seminal vesicles, and uninvolved lymph nodes (i.e. pT1-T2, N0M0).
   d. *Salvage XRT dose to the prostatic fossa should be at least 64-65 Gy.* If possible, XRT should be administered when continence and erections have recovered after RP.
   e. The role of androgen deprivation with salvage XRT—the ASTRO/AUA 2019 guidelines states "Clinicians should offer hormone therapy to patients treated with salvage radiotherapy." The NCCN 2021 states that 6 months of castration (with or without a first generation antiandrogen) can be administered with salvage XRT. If the PSA ≥ 1.0 at the time of salvage XRT, then consider 2 years of androgen deprivation (level 1 evidence supports use of bicalutamide 150 mg po q day for 2 years in this setting, but castration may be an alternative).
   f. In appropriately selected men, 10 year cancer-specific survival is 70-83%. Retrospective data suggests that salvage XRT may improve cancer specific and overall survival.

Managing Complications of Locally Advanced Disease

1. Bladder outlet obstruction—usually treated with TURP, suprapubic tube, or urethral catheter.
2. Ureteral obstruction—treated with ureteral stents or nephrostomy tubes.
3. Persistent bleeding from the prostate—may be treated with
   a. Androgen deprivation in men who are not already on this therapy.
   b. TURP and/or transurethral cauterization.
   c. External beam radiation to the prostate in men who have not had pelvic radiation.
   d. Embolization

Treatment of Non-curable Prostate Cancer

General Information

1. Non-curable prostate cancer includes any of the following:
   a. Curative treatment has failed and no other curative options are feasible.
   b. Castration resistant prostate cancer.
   c. Metastatic prostate cancer (stage M1).
2. Treatments for non-curable prostate cancer include castration (medical or surgical), antiandrogens, inhibitors of androgen synthesis, chemotherapy, and immunotherapy. These treatments are discussed in more detail in the sections that follow.

Castration & Castration Resistance

Definitions

1. Androgen deprivation therapy (ADT)—ADT can be defined as any therapy that reduces the binding of androgens to the androgen receptor; however *ADT usually refers specifically to castration with or without concomitant use of a first generation antiandrogen.*
2. Castration—defined as treatment with surgical castration (bilateral orchiectomy) or medical castration (LHRH agonist or GnRH antagonist). Medical castration is reversible, whereas orchiectomy is irreversible. *LHRH agonists, GnRH antagonists, and orchiectomy are equally effective in controlling prostate cancer. There is limited evidence that orchiectomy and GnRH antagonists are safer than LHRH agonists because they are associated with fewer cardiac events, especially in men with known cardiovascular disease.*
3. Castration naive—defined as no previous treatment with castration.
4. Castration sensitive prostate cancer (CSPC)—defined as prostate cancer that has not been previously treated with castration (castration naive) or that is responding to castration (i.e. the PSA and cancer volume are not increasing). CSPC is also called "hormone sensitive prostate cancer."
5. Castration resistant prostate cancer (CRPC)—defined as prostate cancer that is no longer responding to castration (i.e. PSA and/or cancer volume is increasing) even though serum testosterone is < 50 ng/dl.
6. Monotherapy—defined as the use of only a one therapy for ADT.
7. Combined androgen blockade—defined as treatment with castration and a first generation nonsteroidal antiandrogen.

General Information About ADT

1. Medical castration is typically administered continuously; however, intermittent medical castration is an option for some men (see below).

2. When starting an LHRH agonist, be aware of the flare phenomenon (see page 292). If indicated, administer a first generation antiandrogen to prevent the flare. GnRH antagonists and orchiectomy do not cause a flare.

3. Combined androgen deprivation therapy (castration with a first generation antiandrogen)—studies that examined combined ADT used an LHRH agonist or orchiectomy for castration. *Combined ADT significantly improves overall survival by up to 5% after 5 years of therapy compared to castration alone*, but its use must be balanced against the greater side effects and cost. In essence, combined ADT confers a statistically significant improvement in overall survival, but its clinical benefit is questionable. Nonetheless, *combined androgen blockade should be considered in men starting androgen deprivation therapy.* There is minimal data to support the use of a first generation antiandrogen with a GnRH antagonist; thus, combined ADT is typically used only with a LHRH agonist or orchiectomy.

4. Castration is a recommended part of the initial management of metastatic (stage M1) prostate cancer (see page 252).

5. *Relugolix (a oral GnRH antagonist) should not be used with abiraterone, enzalutamide, darolutamide, or apalutamide because of potential drug interactions.* Relugolix has not been adequately studied when used in combination with chemotherapy, abiraterone, enzalutamide, darolutamide, or apalutamide.

6. *Monotherapy with either a steroidal or non-steroidal antiandrogen (instead of castration) is not recommended because it is less effective than castration.* However, it may be discussed as an alternative in men who cannot or will not undergo castration.

   a. Compared to castration, monotherapy with a first generation nonsteroidal antiandrogen results in:
      i. Lower overall survival.
      ii. Higher rate of gynecomastia and breast pain.
      iii. Less hot flashes and fatigue.
      iv. Significantly better quality of life in the domains of sexual interest and physical capacity.
      v. No impairment of libido or erections
      vi. No osteoporosis.
   b. Nonsteroidal antiandrogens are FDA approved for prostate cancer when used with castration, but they are *not* FDA approved for monotherapy.

Intermittent ADT

1. Intermittent ADT is an option for men with castration *sensitive* prostate cancer.

2. Intermittent ADT results in better sexual function, better quality of life, and less side effects (when off therapy) than continuous ADT.

3. Intermittent and continuous ADT appear to have a similar risk of progression and a similar risk of becoming castration resistant.

4. Intermittent and continuous ADT achieve a similar overall survival. In some studies, death from prostate cancer is more common on intermittent ADT, whereas death from other causes is more common on continuous ADT (these differences offset each other, so overall survival is equivalent).

5. In summary, *intermittent ADT appears to reduce ADT related side effects compared to continuous ADT without compromising cancer control or survival.*

6. Intermittent ADT can be utilized in men with metastatic (stage M1) or non-metastatic (stage M0) castration *sensitive* prostate cancer.

7. A typical protocol used in the studies: If PSA declines to < 4 and there is no clinical progression after 6-9 months of ADT, then stop ADT. If PSA rises above 10-20 or there is clinical progression, then resume ADT. In men who develop clinical progression (significant worsening of existing metastases, new metastases, or significant cancer related symptoms), stop intermittent ADT and administer continuous ADT thereafter.

8. Men who have significant ADT related side effects may benefit from intermittent ADT.

9. Continuous ADT may be better than intermittent ADT in the following scenarios (although the evidence is poor quality).

   a. Men who have minimal or non-bothersome ADT related side effects—these men are unlikely to benefit from a reduction in side effects while on intermittent ADT.

   b. Non-metastatic prostate cancer (stage M0) with grade group 4 or 5 (Gleason score 8-10)—for these men, median overall survival was 14 months longer with continuous ADT compared to intermittent ADT.

   c. Metastatic prostate cancer (stage M1) and a PSA > 4 at 7-8 months after starting ADT—for these men, continuous ADT may be best because their median overall survival is only 1.1 years.

Prognostic Indicators After Castration

1. *A PSA > 0.2 ng/ml at 7-8 months after castration is associated with a higher risk of death from prostate cancer in men with biochemical recurrence after curative therapy (M0 with rising PSA) and in men with metastatic disease (M1).* The higher the PSA at this time point, the higher the risk of mortality.

PSA (ng/ml) at 8 Months After Castration for M0 Prostate Cancer with Rising PSA after RP or XRT	7-year Prostate Cancer Specific Mortality
≤ 0.2	2%
≥ 0.2	49%

Data from J Clin Oncol, 23: 6556, 2005.

PSA (ng/ml) at 7-8 Months After Castration for M1 Prostate Cancer	Approximate Median Overall Survival
≤ 0.2	6.2 years
> 0.2 and ≤ 4.0	3.7 years
> 4.0	1 to 2 years

Data from J Clin Oncol, 24: 3984, 2006 & J Clin Oncol, 36(4): 376, 2017.

2. *A PSA doubling time (PSADT) < 3 months (at any time before or after castration) is associated with a higher risk of death from prostate cancer in men with biochemical recurrence after curative therapy (M0 with rising PSA) and in men with metastatic disease (M1).* Prognosis improves as the PSADT increases.

How Low Should Testosterone Be After Castration?

1. *Serum testosterone (T) should be < 50 ng/dl after castration.* This level was defined > 40 years ago, when testing was less accurate. With modern testing methods, some data suggest that breakthrough T > 20 ng/dl increases the risk of progressing to castration resistant prostate cancer; therefore, some clinicians use T < 20 ng/dl to delineate adequate response to medical castration.

2. See page 292 for information on castration and testosterone.

Evaluation of Rising PSA after Castration

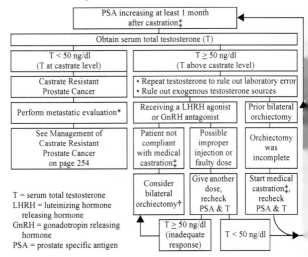

‡ Castration is defined as treatment with surgical castration (bilateral orchiectomy) or medical castration (LHRH agonist or GnRH antagonist).

† If the patient refuses orchiectomy, add a first generation antiandrogen.

* All men with CRPC should undergo bone scan, pelvic imaging, and chest imaging when castration resistance is initially diagnosed because they have ≥ 10% risk of positive bone scan (even when PSA is low and PSA doubling time is long).

Castration Resistant Prostate Cancer (CRPC)

1. CRPC is present when PSA rises after surgical castration (orchiectomy) or medical castration (LHRH agonist or GnRH antagonist), despite having a serum testosterone < 50 ng/dl (i.e the cancer grows despite castration).
   a. CRPC has also been called "hormone refractory" or "androgen independent"; however, the preferred term is castration resistant.
   b. PSA can rise when castration is not adequate; therefore, a serum testosterone (T) level must be checked when PSA rises during castration. If T > 50 ng/dl, then castration is inadequate. If T < 50 ng/dl, then the patient has CRPC.
2. *Prostate cancer responds to castration for an average of 2-3 years before CRPC develops,* but the response can range from months to > 10 years.
3. In men with CRPC, some cancer cells still respond to androgen suppression; thus, *castration should be continued while other cancer therapies are administered. Retrospective data suggests that continuing castration in CRPC improves overall survival (Taylor 1993).*
4. *All men with CRPC should undergo bone scan, pelvic imaging, and chest imaging when castration resistance is initially diagnosed because they have ≥ 10% risk of positive bone scan (even when PSA is low and PSA doubling time is long).*
5. For treatment of CRPC, see table on page 254.

<u>Androgen Synthesis Inhibitors</u>

Ketoconazole
1. This medication is not FDA approved for the treatment of prostate cancer, and it is not commonly used anymore.
2. Mechanism of action—*ketoconazole is a competitive inhibitor of several cytochrome P450 enzymes*, including 11ß hydroxylase and CYP17 (a complex that contains 17-α-hydroxylase and C17, 20-lyase).
   a. Inhibition of CYP17 *reduces synthesis of androgen in the adrenal glands and the testicles.*
   b. Inhibition of 11ß-hydroxylase reduces synthesis of aldosterone and glucocorticoid in the adrenal glands. Thus, mineralocorticoid and glucocorticoid replacement is recommended when using ketoconazole.
3. Castrate levels of testosterone may occur by 8 hours after a 400 mg oral dose. The effects are dose dependent (testosterone is diminished with 800 mg/day, and eliminated with 1600 mg/day).
4. Side effects—*hepatotoxicity*, weakness, lethargy, nausea, vomiting, decreased libido. The dose limiting side effect is nausea/vomiting.
5. Adult dose = ketoconazole 400 mg po TID [Tabs: 200 mg] with a steroid (e.g. hydrocortisone 10 mg po TID or prednisone 5 mg po BID). Side effects may be reduced by starting at 200 mg po TID and increasing the dose to 400 mg po TID as tolerated.
6. Requires stomach acid for dissolution and absorption. Therefore, give all gastric acid blockers 2 hours after the ketoconazole dose.
7. Ketoconazole decreases warfarin metabolism.
8. Avoid use with hypoglycemic agents (causes severe hypoglycemia).

Abiraterone
1. Abiraterone is FDA approved for use *with castration* for the treatment of metastatic high risk castration sensitive prostate cancer or metastatic castration resistant prostate cancer. High risk is defined in one of studies as at least 2 of the following criteria: Gleason score ≥ 8, visceral metastasis, or ≥ 3 bone metastasis.
2. Mechanism of action—*abiraterone is a selective irreversible inhibitor of CYP17* (a cytochrome P-450 enzyme complex that contains C17,20-lyase and 17-α-hydroxylase). CYP17 is required for androgen production and is present in the testis, adrenal gland, prostate, and other tissues. *By inhibiting CYP17, abiraterone reduces androgen production.* In the adrenal glands, inhibiting CYP17 reduces the synthesis of androgens and glucocorticoids, but it increases the synthesis of mineralocorticoids; thus, abiraterone can cause glucocorticoid insufficiency and mineralocorticoid excess. A steroid is administered with abiraterone to prevent glucocorticoid insufficiency.
3. Note that abiraterone and ketoconazole both inhibit CYP17; however, they differ in the following ways:
   a. Abiraterone is a selective inhibitor of CYP17, whereas ketoconazole is a nonselective inhibitor of several cytochrome complexes (including CYP17 and 11ß hydroxylase).
   b. Abiraterone is a potent inhibitor of CYP17, whereas ketoconazole is a weak inhibitor of CYP17.
   c. Abiraterone is an irreversible inhibitor, whereas ketoconazole is a reversible (competitive) inhibitor.
   d. Abiraterone increases aldosterone (because it inhibits only CYP17), whereas ketoconazole decreases aldosterone (because it also inhibits 11ß hydroxylase).

4. Background—androgens can be produced within prostate cancer cells. These intra-tumor androgens stimulate prostate cancer growth, even when circulating extra-tumor androgens are minimal. Abiraterone reduces both intra-tumor testosterone and circulating extra-tumor testosterone.

5. Dose for U.S. Brand Zytiga®—abiraterone 1000 mg po q day on an empty stomach [Tabs: 250, 500 mg] with oral prednisone.

   a. For castration *sensitive* disease, administer prednisone 5 mg po *daily.*

   b. For castration *resistant* disease, administer prednisone 5 mg po *BID.*

   c. Taking abiraterone with food can increase its absorption and increase the risk of side effects. Therefore, *Zytiga® should be taken on an empty stomach* (at least 1 hour before or 2 hours after a meal).

   d. The dose of abiraterone does not need to be adjusted for renal dysfunction, but it may need to be adjusted for liver dysfunction.

   e. A randomized phase 2 trial showed that 250 mg po q day after a low fat breakfast was non-inferior to the standard dose of 1000 mg po q day after an overnight fast. Although the lower dose is not FDA approved, it is less expensive. If side effects are problematic at the lower dose (food can increase the absorption in an unpredictable manner), then try switching to the standard dose (1000 mg on an empty stomach).

6. Dose for U.S. Brand Yonsa®—this is a fine particle formulation of abiraterone. It is important to realize that the dose per tablet and the administered dose are different from the original abiraterone formulation (U.S. Brand name Zytiga®). The dose is Yonsa® 500 mg po q day [Tabs: 125 mg] with methylprednisolone 4 mg po BID. *Yonsa® may be taken with or without food.*

7. Before starting therapy—check blood pressure, serum potassium, and liver function tests. Control hypertension and correct hypokalemia before starting abiraterone. Be cautious administering abiraterone in patients with medical conditions that can be exacerbated by its side effects, e.g. heart failure, cardiac arrhythmia, and liver dysfunction.

8. During therapy—Monitor blood pressure, serum potassium, serum phosphate, liver function tests, fluid retention, and signs of adrenocortical insufficiency (usually every 2 weeks for the initial 3 months after starting therapy, and then every month thereafter).

9. Efficacy

   a. In metastatic castration sensitive prostate cancer, abiraterone improves overall survival and progression compared to placebo.

   b. In men with metastatic CRPC (previous treated with docetaxel or not), abiraterone improves overall survival by 4-5 months and delays progression compared to placebo.

10. Side effects

    a. *Hyperaldosteronism (mineralocorticoid excess)— fluid retention or edema (27%), hypokalemia (28%), hypertension (9%)*, alkalosis.

    b. Other common side effects—fatigue, musculoskeletal pain (joint, muscle), nausea, vomiting, hot flashes, diarrhea, cough, and headache.

    c. Other less common side effects—liver dysfunction (severe in 6%), cardiac failure (2.6%), and cardiac arrhythmia (4%).

11. Men who failed ketoconazole have a higher failure rate with abiraterone, and vise versa; thus, when one of these medications fails, the other medication should be avoided.

12. *Use of abiraterone in combination with Radium-223 is not recommended because it results in a higher rate of fractures and mortality.*

Aminoglutethimide

1. This medication is largely of historical interest since it is almost never used anymore.
2. Mechanism of action—aminoglutethimide blocks the transformation of cholesterol to pregnenolone by inhibiting a cytochrome P-450 enzyme called CYP11A1 (also called P450scc), which reduces the synthesis of glucocorticoids, aldosterone, and androgens. Thus, glucocorticoid and mineralocorticoid replacement is required when using aminoglutethimide.
3. Side effects—hypotension, nausea, vomiting, fatigue, anorexia, depression, edema, skin rashes.
4. Adult dose = aminoglutethimide 250 mg po q 6 hours.

First Generation Nonsteroidal Antiandrogens

General Information

1. First generation nonsteroidal antiandrogens include bicalutamide, flutamide, and nilutamide. These medications are FDA approved for the treatment of prostate cancer when used with castration for combined androgen deprivation. *Compared to castration alone, combined androgen deprivation with a non-steroidal antiandrogen increases overall survival by up to 5% at 5 years,* but this marginal benefit must be balanced against the greater side effects and cost.
2. Mechanism of action—antiandrogens inhibit the androgen receptor (they prevent the binding of DHT and testosterone to the androgen receptor). Androgen receptors in the pituitary and hypothalamus are also blocked, which prevents androgens from engaging in negative feedback and leads to an increase in the serum level of LH. Thus, adrenal and gonadal androgen production actually increases.
3. Excess testosterone may be converted to estrogen by aromatase (which is in adipose tissue), resulting in gynecomastia.
4. Flutamide
   a. Adult dose = flutamide 250 mg po TID [Caps: 125 mg].
   b. Side effects—hepatotoxicity, gynecomastia, diarrhea, nausea, and vomiting. Gastrointestinal side effects are the dose limiting factor.
5. Bicalutamide
   a. Adult dose = bicalutamide 50 mg po q day [Tabs: 50 mg].
   b. Side effects—similar to flutamide, but has less gastrointestinal effects.
6. Nilutamide
   a. Adult dose = nilutamide 300 mg po q day for 30 days, then 150 mg po q day thereafter [Tabs: 50 mg].
   b. Side effects—visual disturbances, alcohol intolerance, rarely interstitial pneumonitis, nausea, vomiting.

Antiandrogen Withdrawal (AAW)

1. AAW is a decline in PSA (usually defined as $\geq$ 50% decrease in PSA) that occurs after stopping a first generation antiandrogen. Occasionally, AAW may also generate a clinical improvement.
2. AAW occurs in approximately 30% of patients.
3. The reduction in PSA usually lasts 3-6 months; however, it can last longer than 12 months in up to 20% of patients.
4. A longer duration of antiandrogen use appears to improve the chance of AAW.
5. When flutamide is stopped, PSA decline begins within a few days (because of its short half life).

6. When bicalutamide is stopped, PSA decline begins in 4-8 weeks (because of its long half life).
7. In addition to antiandrogens, a PSA decline after withdrawal has also been reported with megestrol acetate, diethylstilbestrol, and ketoconazole.

Second Generation Nonsteroidal Antiandrogens

Second Generation Nonsteroidal Antiandrogens
1. Second generation nonsteroidal antiandrogens include enzalutamide, apalutamide, and darolutamide.
2. Mechanism of action—these medications inhibit multiple steps in the androgen receptor (AR) signaling pathway, including inhibition of the following steps:
   a. Androgen binding to the androgen receptor.
   b. Nuclear translocation of the androgen receptor.
   c. Binding of the androgen receptor to DNA.
3. Compared to first generation antiandrogens, second generation nonsteroidal antiandrogens are considered more effective because they have *a higher affinity for the androgen receptor* and because of differences in the mechanism of action that are shown below.

Characteristic	2nd Generation Antiandrogen	1st Generation Antiandrogen
Binding of androgen to AR	Inhibits	Inhibits
Translocation of AR to nucleus	Inhibits	Promotes
Binding of AR to DNA	Inhibits	Promotes

AR = androgen receptor

4. *Second generation antiandrogens are FDA approved for use with concomitant castration.*

	FDA Approved Clinical Indications as of April 2021 For Second Generation Nonsteroidal Antiandrogens		
Medication	Non-Metastatic Castration Resistant	Metastatic Castration Sensitive	Metastatic Castration Resistant
Darolutamide	Approved	No	No
Apalutamide	Approved	Approved	No
Enzalutamide	Approved	Approved	Approved

FDA = United States Food and Drug Administration

5. Side effects
   a. These medications share some of their more frequently experienced side effects, including fatigue, hot flashes, nausea, diarrhea, hypertension, weakness (asthenia), falls, bone fracture, and musculoskeletal pain.
   b. They also share some of the more rarely experienced side effects, including seizure, mental impairment, and ischemic heart disease.
   c. Enzalutamide and apalutamide cross the blood brain barrier and inhibit GABA receptors, whereas darolutamide crosses the blood brain barrier in negligible amounts. *As a result, darolutamide appears to cause less central nervous system side effects (e.g. mental impairment).*
   d. *Apalutamide is the only medication in this class associated with an appreciable rate of hypothyroidism.*
6. Metabolism—all of these medications are metabolized by the hepatic cytochrome P450 system; therefore, other drugs that use this system can alter the circulating concentration of the antiandrogen, and vise versa.

Enzalutamide (US Brand: Xtandi®)

1. Enzalutamide is FDA approved for use *with castration* in the treatment of metastatic castration sensitive prostate cancer and castration resistant prostate cancer (metastatic or not). Its use in M0 castrate resistant prostate cancer is typically confined to men with PSA doubling time $\leq$ 10 months because men with a higher PSA doubling time have not been well studied.
2. Enzalutamide is a second generation nonsteroidal antiandrogen.
3. Properties and mechanism of action—see Second Generation Nonsteroidal Antiandrogens, page 242.
4. Dose—Enzalutamide 160 mg po q day with or without food [Caps: 40 mg].
   a. Initial dose adjustment is not required for mild to moderate renal dysfunction (e.g. creatinine clearance > 30 ml/min). Initial dose adjustment is not required for liver dysfunction. The use of enzalutamide in severe renal dysfunction has not been studied.
   b. If severe side effects occur, enzalutamide may be stopped until the symptoms improve sufficiently, and if warranted, it can be resumed at lower dose (80 mg or 120 mg).
5. Efficacy
   a. In men with non-metastatic CRPC and PSA doubling time $\leq$ 10, enzalutamide improves overall and metastasis free survival compared to placebo.
   b. In men with metastatic castration sensitive prostate cancer, enzalutamide improves overall survival and progression compared to either placebo or a first generation antiandrogen.
   c. In men with metastatic CRPC not previously treated with chemotherapy, enzalutamide significantly improves overall survival, progression free survival, and time to skeletal related event compared to placebo.
   d. In men with metastatic CRPC who had been previously treated with docetaxel, enzalutamide significantly increases mean overall survival, radiographic progression free survival, time to skeletal related event, and quality of life compared to placebo. It also reduces pain (45% of men have pain relief within 13 weeks).
   e. *When compared in randomized trials for CRPC, enzalutamide achieves significantly better progression free survival than bicalutamide.*
6. Side effects
   a. Common side effects include fatigue, hot flashes, nausea, loss of appetite, diarrhea, constipation, hypertension, dizziness, weakness (asthenia), falls, bone fracture, rash, and musculoskeletal pain.
   b. *Falls*—occurs in 11% of men, and is more common in the elderly.
   c. *Bone fractures*—occurs in 10% of men.
   d. Central nervous system (CNS) side effects
      i. *Mental impairment*—disturbance in memory, attention, or cognition occurs in up to 5% of men. *Hallucinations occur in about 1.6% of men* (mainly in men using concomitant opioids).
      ii. *Seizures occur in < 1% of men* and can occur after years of tolerating enzalutamide. In men at risk for seizure, the safety of enzalutamide is unknown because these men were excluded from the trials.
      iii. *Posterior reversible encephalopathy syndrome*—there have been a few case reports of this neurologic syndrome that can present with rapidly evolving neurological symptoms (such as seizure, headache, confusion, lethargy). Confirmation requires brain imaging.
   e. *Ischemic heart disease*—occurs in approximately 3% of patients.
   f. Neutropenia—severe in only 1%.
   g. Liver enzyme abnormalities—severe in < 1%.

Apalutamide (U.S. Brand: Erleada®)

1. Apalutamide is FDA approved for use *with castration* in the treatment of metastatic castration sensitive prostate cancer and non-metastatic castration resistant prostate cancer. Its use in M0 castrate resistant prostate cancer is typically confined to men with PSA doubling time < 10 months because men with a higher PSA doubling time have not been well studied.

2. Apalutamide is a second generation nonsteroidal antiandrogen.

3. Properties and mechanism of action—see Second Generation Nonsteroidal Antiandrogens, page 242.

4. Dose—apalutamide 240 mg po q day with or without food [Tabs: 60 mg].
   a. Initial dose adjustment is not required for mild to moderate renal dysfunction (e.g. GFR > 30 ml/min) or mild to moderate liver dysfunction. The use of apalutamide in severe renal dysfunction and in severe liver dysfunction has not been studied.
   b. If severe side effects occur, apalutamide may be stopped until the symptoms improve sufficiently, and if warranted, it can be resumed at lower dose (120 mg or 180 mg).

5. Efficacy
   a. In men with non-metastatic CRPC and PSA doubling time ≤ 10, apalutamide improves overall survival, metastasis free survival, and time to symptomatic progression compared to placebo.
   b. In men with metastatic castration sensitive prostate cancer, apalutamide improves overall survival and progression compared to placebo.

6. Side effects
   a. The most common side effects include fatigue, hot flashes, nausea, loss of appetite, diarrhea, hypertension, weakness (asthenia), falls, bone fracture, rash, and musculoskeletal pain (back, joint, or muscle). Diarrhea occurs more often with apalutamide than with enzalutamide or darolutamide (although these drugs have never been directly compared).
   b. *Hypothyroidism*—occurs in 8% of patients, but only 5% required thyroid replacement therapy.
   c. *Falls*—occurs in 16% of men, and was more common in the elderly.
   d. *Bone fractures*—occurs in ≤ 12% of men.
   e. Central nervous system (CNS) side effects
      i. *Mental impairment*—disturbance in memory, attention, or cognition occur in up to 5% of men.
      ii. *Seizures occur in < 1% of men*. Seizures can occur even after years of tolerating apalutamide. In men at risk for seizure, the safety of apalutamide is unknown because these men were excluded from the trials.
   f. *Ischemic heart disease*—occurs in approximately 4% of patients.
   g. Neutropenia—severe in approximately 1%.
   h. Liver enzyme abnormalities—severe in < 1%.

Darolutamide (U.S. Brand: Nubeqa™)
1. Darolutamide is FDA approved for use *with castration* in the treatment of non-metastatic castration resistant prostate cancer. Its use in M0 castrate resistant prostate cancer is typically confined to men with PSA doubling time < 10 months because men with a higher PSA doubling time have not been well studied.
2. Darolutamide is a second generation nonsteroidal antiandrogen.
3. Mechanism of action—see Second Generation Nonsteroidal Antiandrogens, page 242.
4. Properties—darolutamide has as similar mechanism of action as apalutamide and enzalutamide, but has several distinct properties.
   a. Darolutamide has the ability to bind to mutant androgen receptors, including receptors that generate resistance to bicalutamide, enzalutamide, and apalutamide.
   b. Darolutamide does not increase serum testosterone (whereas enzalutamide and apalutamide can).
   c. Darolutamide has a negligible penetration of the blood brain barrier compared to enzalutamide and apalutamide, which appears to result in fewer CNS side effects. The risk of CNS side effects has never been directly compared between darolutamide, apalutamide, and enzalutamide, but the risk of seizure for all 3 medications is < 1%. *Nonetheless, darolutamide had no increased incidence of seizure, mental impairment, or falls compared to placebo.*
5. Dose—darolutamide 600 mg po BID with food [Tabs: 300 mg].
   a. Initial dose adjustment is not required for mild to moderate renal dysfunction (GFR > 30 ml/min) and not required for mild hepatic dysfunction. See the full prescribing information for dose recommendation in men with several renal impairment or with moderate to severe hepatic impairment.
   b. If severe side effects occur, darolutamide may be stopped (or the dose reduced to 300 mg po BID) until the symptoms improve sufficiently. If warranted, it can be resumed at the recommended dose of 600 mg po BID (if a lower dose is required, doses of less than 300 mg po BID are not recommended).
6. Efficacy—in men with non-metastatic CRPC and PSA doubling time ≤ 10, apalutamide improves overall survival, metastasis free survival, and time to symptomatic progression compared to placebo.
7. Side effects
   a. The most common side effects include fatigue, hot flashes, nausea, diarrhea, weakness (asthenia), falls, bone fracture, rash, and musculoskeletal pain (back, joint, or muscle). *Falls, fractures, and mental impairment occurred less often with darolutamide than with enzalutamide or apalutamide (although these drugs have never been directly compared).*
   b. *Falls*—occurs in 4% of men.
   c. *Bone fractures*—occurs in 4% of men.
   d. Central nervous system (CNS) side effects
      i. *Mental impairment*—disturbance in memory, attention, or cognition occurs in < 1% of men.
      ii. *Seizures occur in < 1% of men.*
   e. *Ischemic heart disease*—occurs in approximately 3% of patients.
   f. Neutropenia—severe in approximately 4%.
   g. Liver enzyme abnormalities—severe in < 1%.

Chemotherapy

Docetaxel (Taxotere®)

1. *A docetaxel based regimen is considered first line chemotherapy because it achieves longer overall survival compared to mitoxantrone.*
2. Docetaxel is a taxane. *Taxanes are mitotic inhibitors (they prevent cell division) and were first derived from the yew tree (genus Taxus).*
3. Docetaxel (in combination with prednisone 5 mg po BID) is FDA approved for treatment of castration resistant metastatic prostate cancer.
4. Mechanism of action—*taxanes function mainly by disrupting normal microtubule function, which ultimately inhibits mitosis.* Taxanes bind to tubulin, which causes polymerization of tubulin into poorly functioning microtubules. When the microtubules are poorly functioning, the cell cannot divide (mitosis is inhibited) and the cell dies.
5. Efficacy—compared to mitoxantrone, *docetaxel increases overall survival by approximately 3 months* and is more likely to achieve $\geq$ 50% reduction in PSA. Docetaxel may also improve pain and quality of life compared to mitoxantrone.
6. Administration
   a. Docetaxel is administered intravenously every 3 weeks (the every 3 week regimen is more effective than a weekly regimen). A common treatment plan is 10 cycles (although nearly 55% of men receive fewer cycles, mainly because of disease progression).
   b. The patient is premedicated to reduce the incidence and severity of fluid retention and hypersensitivity reactions. *Premedication consists of oral corticosteroids (such as dexamethasone) starting the day before each infusion and continuing for 3 days.*
7. Side Effects
   a. *Bone marrow suppression is the major dose-limiting toxicity of docetaxel. The most common severe (grade 3 or 4) side effect is neutropenia.*
   b. Common side effects include: fatigue, neutropenia, anemia, nausea, vomiting, diarrhea, sensory neuropathy, alopecia, nail changes, change in taste (dysgeusia), stomatitis, dyspnea, peripheral edema.
8. Monitoring during therapy should include complete blood count.
9. Docetaxel is primarily metabolized by the liver (through CYP3A). Concomitant use of drugs that inhibit hepatic CYP3A (such as ketoconazole and abiraterone) should be avoided because they will likely increase serum docetaxel concentrations.

Cabazitaxel

1. Cabazitaxel is a taxane.
2. Cabazitaxel (in combination with prednisone 10 mg po daily) is FDA approved for the treatment of men with castration resistant metastatic prostate cancer that have been previously treated with a docetaxel containing chemotherapy regimen.
3. Mechanism of action—*taxanes function mainly by disrupting normal microtubule function, which ultimately inhibits mitosis.*
4. Background—P-glycoprotein 1 (also know as Multi-drug Resistance Protein 1 or MDR1) is an efflux pump that transports certain drugs out of the cell. MDR1 can generate resistance to a specific drug by pumping it out of the cell (where the drug cannot exert a therapeutic effect). MDR1 can pump docetaxel out of the cell and can create docetaxel resistance. However, cabazitaxel is not susceptible to MDR1; therefore, *cabazitaxel can have efficacy in cancers that are resistant to docetaxel.*

5. Efficacy—compared to mitoxantrone, cabazitaxel is more likely to achieve > 50% reduction in PSA and increases overall survival by approximately 2.4 months. Cabazitaxel is no better than mitoxantrone for improving pain.
6. Administration
   a. Cabazitaxel is administered intravenously every 3 weeks. A common treatment plan is 10 cycles (although 70% of men receive fewer cycles, mainly because of disease progression).
   b. To reduce fluid retention and hypersensitivity reactions, *premedicate the patient 30 minutes prior to cabazitaxel infusion with intravenous corticosteroid (e.g. dexamethasone), H1 antagonist (e.g. diphenhydramine), and H2 antagonist (e.g ranitidine).*
7. Side Effects
   a. *Bone marrow suppression is the major dose-limiting toxicity of cabazitaxel. The most common severe (grade 3 or 4) side effect is neutropenia. Cabazitaxel has a higher rate of grade 3 or 4 neutropenia than docetaxel. Thus, granulocyte colony stimulating factor (G-CSF) is often administered to help prevent neutropenia.*
   b. Common side effects: fatigue, nausea, vomiting, diarrhea, anemia, neutropenia, thrombocytopenia, sensory neuropathy, alopecia, nail changes, change in taste (dysgeusia), stomatitis, dyspnea, edema.
8. Monitoring during therapy should include complete blood count.
9. Cabazitaxel is primarily metabolized by the liver (through CYP3A). Concomitant use of drugs that inhibit hepatic CYP3A (such as ketoconazole and abiraterone) should be avoided because they will likely increase serum cabazitaxel concentrations.

Mitoxantrone

1. Mechanism of action—mitoxantrone disrupts DNA synthesis and repair by intercalating into DNA and by inhibiting topoisomerase II.
2. *Mitoxantrone does not improve survival, but it reduces cancer-related pain.* It is FDA approved to treat pain arising from advanced CRPC.
3. Mitoxantrone is inferior to docetaxel for treating metastatic CRPC; thus, a docetaxel based regimen is preferred for initial therapy in these men.
4. Mitoxantrone is indicated for treating cancer-related pain in men who are not candidates for a docetaxel based regimen or in men who failed a docetaxel based regimen.
5. Regimen—mitoxantrone IV q 3 weeks *with daily oral corticosteroids.*
6. Potential major side effects include myelosuppression (common), congestive heart failure (~3%), and secondary leukemia (1%).

	Mitoxantrone	Docetaxel	Cabazitaxel
Dose Schedule	q 3 weeks	q 3 weeks	q 3 weeks
Administered with steroids	Yes	Yes	Yes
Main toxicity	Bone marrow suppression	Bone marrow suppression	Bone marrow suppression*
Improves Overall Survival	No	Yes	Yes
Reduces Cancer Related Pain	Yes	Yes	Yes
MDR1 Susceptibility	?	Susceptible‡	Not susceptible‡
For metastatic CRPC, use is restricted to men with:	Cancer Related Pain	No Restriction	Previous docetaxel

CRPC = castration resistant prostate cancer; MDR1 = multi-drug resistance Protein 1
* Cabazitaxel has a higher rate of grade 3 or 4 neutropenia than docetaxel, so it is often administered with granulocyte colony stimulating factor.
‡ Docetaxel is susceptible to MDR1; thus, MDR1 can pump docetaxel out of the cell. Cabazitaxel is not susceptible to MDR1; therefore, cabazitaxel can have efficacy in cancers that are resistant to docetaxel.

PARP Inhibitors

General Information

1. Poly ADP-ribose polymerase (PARP) is an enzyme involved in DNA repair. Cancers that contain a mutation in the homologous recombination repair (HRR) system (such as BRCA) often rely on PARP to repair their DNA. When a PARP inhibitor is used against one of these tumors, the cells cannot repair their DNA and the cells die.
2. These agents are only effective for patients whose tumors have a mutation in the homologous recombination repair system (see page 166 for a list genes in this system).

Olaparib (U.S. Brand: Lynparza)

1. Olaparib was FDA approved in 2020 for the treatment of men with metastatic CRPC who have progressed following treatment with enzalutamide or abiraterone and who have either
   a. A suspected or known HRR germline mutation in BRCA1 or BRCA2.
   b. A suspected or known HRR somatic tumor mutation in any of 15 HRR genes.
2. Mechanism of action—PARP inhibitor.
3. Dose—olaparib 300 mg po BID with or without food [Tabs: 150, 100 mg]. See the full prescribing information for dose adjustments required in patients with renal or liver dysfunction.
4. During therapy—check complete blood count at baseline and monthly thereafter. Also, monitor for signs and symptoms of deep venous thrombosis (DVT), pulmonary embolism, and pneumonitis.
5. Efficacy—compared to treatment with enzalutamide or abiraterone, olaparib significantly improved radiographic progression-free survival by 3.8 months and overall survival by 4.4 months.
6. Side effects
   a. Common side effects—fatigue, decreased appetite, diarrhea, nausea, vomiting, dysgeusia (altered taste), dyspepsia, cough, dyspnea, abdominal pain, headache, anemia, thrombocytopenia, neutropenia.
   b Uncommon, but serious side effects
      i. Venous thrombosis—7% of patients developed venous thrombosis, including some cases of pulmonary embolism.
      ii. Myelodysplastic syndrome/acute myeloid leukemia (MDS/AML) occurred in < 1.5% of patients (and the majority of these patients died of MDS/AML). Patients previously treated with therapies that damage DNA, such as platinum containing chemotherapy, seem to be at higher risk for this syndrome.
      iii. Pneumonitis occurred in < 1% of patients.

Rucaparib (U.S. Brand: Rubraca)

1. Rucaparib was FDA approved in 2020 for the treatment of men with metastatic CRPC who have been treated with androgen receptor directed therapy (e.g. a second generation antiandrogen and/or abiraterone) and a taxane based chemotherapy and who have a BRCA germline or somatic mutation.
2. Mechanism of action—PARP inhibitor.
3. Dose—rucaparib 600 mg po BID with or without food [Tabs: 200, 250, 300 mg]. See the full prescribing information for dose adjustments required in patients with renal or liver dysfunction.
4. During therapy—check complete blood count at baseline and monthly thereafter.

5. Efficacy—FDA approval was given based on a single arm trial that showed a 44% objective response rate to rucaparib, with approximately half of these patients having a response lasting more than 6 months.
6. Side effects
   a. Common side effects—fatigue, decreased appetite, nausea, vomiting, diarrhea, constipation, rash, anemia, thrombocytopenia, increased liver function tests.
   b Uncommon, but serious side effects—myelodysplastic syndrome/acute myeloid leukemia (MDS/AML) occurred in $\leq 1.7\%$ of patients. Patients previously treated with therapies that damage DNA, such as platinum containing chemotherapy, seem to be at higher risk for this syndrome.

Immunotherapy

Sipuleucel-T (U.S. Brand: Provenge®)

1. *Sipuleucel-T is an autologous cellular immunotherapy.* Sipuleucel-T is FDA approved for the treatment of asymptomatic or minimally symptomatic metastatic castration resistant prostate cancer. Sipuleucel-T is not recommended in patients with any of the following characteristics: using opioids to control cancer related pain, visceral metastasis, rapidly progressive disease, life expectancy < 6 months, large tumor burden, ECOG performance status ≥ 2, small cell prostate cancer, or neuroendocrine prostate cancer.
2. Background
   a. Prostatic acid phosphatase (PAP) is a protein expressed by prostate cancer cells. Granulocyte macrophage colony stimulating factor (GMCSF) is an immune cell activator.
   b. During metabolism, intracellular proteins are degraded into fragments. Major histocompatibility complex (MHC) binds to these fragments, transports them to the cell membrane, and then displays them on the cell's outer surface (where T cells can examine the fragments). In an abnormal cell, some of the degraded fragments arise from a foreign or aberrant process (such as a viral infection). T cells will kill a cell that displays foreign or aberrant fragments, but will "leave alone" a cell that displays normal fragments. However, T cells can be programmed to kill a cell that displays any fragment (including a normal fragment).
   c. Antigen presenting cells (APCs) are immune cells (e.g. dendritic cells, B-lymphocytes). APCs use MHC to present antigens to T-cells. When the APC presents an antigen to a T-cell, it "programs" the T-cell to recognize and kill cells that express that antigen on their surface.
3. Preparation—leukocytes are obtained from the patient by leukapheresis. The leukocytes are centrifuged to isolate monocyte APCs. The APCs are then incubated with a PAP-GMCSF fusion protein. During incubation, APCs internalize the PAP-GMCSF protein and degrade it into fragments. These fragments are mounted onto MHC proteins, and then the MHC proteins are transported to the cell surface. Ultimately, the PAP-GMCSF fragments are presented on the APCs cell surface (the APCs are "loaded" with PAP-GMCSF). *The APCs with PAP-GMCSF fragments on their surface are the active component of sipuleucel-T.*
4. Mechanism of action—the exact mechanism of action for Sipuleucel-T is unknown; however, the following explanation is hypothesized: in vivo, the sipuleucel-T APCs "show" the PAP fragments to T-cells and "program" the T-cells to seek and destroy any other cells that express PAP fragments on their surface. Since PAP is highly expressed on the surface of prostate cancer, the "programmed" T-cells attack and lyse the prostate cancer cells.

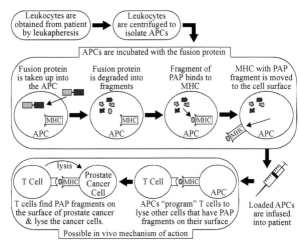

APC = antigen presenting cell; MHC = major histocompatibility complex protein
▨▬▬ = PAP-GMCSF fusion protein; ◐ = PAP fragment

5. Administration—Sipuleucel-T is administered as 3 infusions. The interval between each infusion is usually 2 weeks. 3 days before each infusion, the patient undergoes leukapheresis. The APCs obtained during leukapheresis are sent to a special laboratory, where they are loaded with PAP-GMCSF. The loaded APCs, are sent back to the clinician. 30 minutes before the infusion, administer oral acetaminophen and an oral antihistamine (such as diphenhydramine) to minimize infusion reactions. Sipuleucel-T is infused over 60 minutes. Sipuleucel-T infusion is performed without a cell filter.

6. Efficacy—Sipuleucel-T improves median overall survival by approximately 4 months compared to placebo. Post hoc analysis of a randomize study and an observational registry showed that *the overall survival benefit is greatest when Sipuleucel-T is administered at a lower PSA level*. This benefit was seen even at PSA $\leq$ 5.27 ng/ml.

7. Sipuleucel-T does not lower PSA, does not reduce measurable tumor burden, and does not improve time to progression. *So, sipuleucel-T improves overall survival, but does not alter any of the measures that are used for monitoring prostate cancer.*

8. Side effects—reactions within 24 hours of infusion are common and usually consist of mild to moderate chills, fever, fatigue, nausea, joint pain, back pain, and headache. These symptoms usually resolve within 2 days. Rare serious side effects include stroke, myocardial infarction, deep venous thrombosis, pulmonary embolism, and severe infusion reactions.

9. Timing of administration—the beneficial effect of sipuleucel-T is thought to be dependant on an intact immune system. Thus, it was assumed that sipuleucel-T would be less effective when administered with immunosuppressants (such as steroids). However, preliminary data suggests that the efficacy of sipuleucel-T may not be compromised by co-administration with steroids.

Pembrolizumab

1. The programmed death receptor-1 (PD-1) is located on lymphocytes. When certain proteins bind to PD-1, the immune system has a reduced capacity to attack normal tissues (reducing auto-immune reactions) and a reduced capacity to attack malignant tissues (hindering the body's ability to kill cancer). Tumors that have deficient DNA mismatch repair system tend to generate proteins that bind to PD-1; which means they can hinder the immune system's ability to kill cancer.

2. Mechanism of action—pembrolizumab is a therapeutic antibody that blocks the binding of proteins to PD-1, which gives the immune system a greater capacity to attack the cancer. However, the increased immune activity can also result in attacks on normal tissue (which leads to some of its side effects). Pembrolizumab is often called an immune check point inhibitor because it blocks an important regulatory component of the immune system.

3. Pembrolizumab is FDA approved for the treatment of metastatic tumors that have all of the following characteristics: microsatellite instability-high (MSI-H) or deficient DNA mismatch repair (dMMR), cancer progression after prior therapy, and no satisfactory alternative treatment options.

4. For prostate cancer, pembrolizumab is a treatment option for tumors with dMMR or MSH-H who have failed at least one therapy for metastatic CRPC.

5. For details on dMMR and MSI-H, see page 167.

6. Side effects
   a. Common side effects—fatigue, musculoskeletal pain, diarrhea, nausea, decreased appetite, rash, pruritus, fever, cough, dyspnea, constipation, abdominal pain, peripheral edema, and infusion related reactions.
   b. Less common side effects—*immune mediated side effects* (pneumonitis, colitis, hepatitis, thyroiditis, pituitary inflammation, nephritis, etc.)

7. Dose—pembrolizumab is administered intravenously. See the full prescribing information for dose and administration.

8. Monitoring during therapy—monitoring should include serum creatinine, electrolytes, glucose, liver function tests, and thyroid function tests.

Treatment for Non-curable Non-metastatic (M0) CSPC

1. Men with non-curable non-metastatic castration *sensitive* prostate cancer have a rising PSA despite having exhausted all curative treatment options.

2. Men with cancer related symptoms—*men with significant symptoms from locally advanced non-metastatic prostate cancer should be probably started on androgen deprivation therapy* (castration with or without a first generation antiandrogen). Other interventions may be necessary to relieve local symptoms (see page 235).

3. Men with no significant cancer related symptoms—the optimal treatment for these men is unknown. The preferred management options include surveillance or clinical trial. ADT is a non-preferred management option. If surveillance is chosen, ADT is started when metastasis or significant cancer related symptoms are imminent or present.
   a. The optimal time to start ADT in asymptomatic M0 prostate cancer remains unclear because of the paucity of data in these men.
   b. Duchesne et al (2016) conducted a randomized trial in men with non-curable relapse after prostatectomy or radiation. Men were randomized to immediate ADT or delayed ADT (delay was ≥ 2 years). Five year overall survival was 5% higher in the immediate ADT group

(91% versus 86%; borderline significance). The immediate ADT group also engaged in less sexual activity and had more ADT related side effects. Quality of life was similar between the two groups.

   c. Mahal et al (2018) conducted a retrospective study in men with non-curable relapse after radiation. In men with a PSA doubling time $\geq$ 6 months, the risk of dying from prostate cancer was lower when initiating ADT at PSA $\leq$ 12 compared to PSA > 12.

   d. A study by Studer et al (2008) indicated that untreated men with stage T0-T4, N0-N1, M0 and with PSA > 50 or PSA doubling time $\leq$ 12 months are more likely to die from prostate cancer (the risk becomes greater starting 1-2 years later, with the 7-year risk of death from prostate cancer reaching 48% in men with PSA doubling time $\leq$ 12 months and 32% in men with PSA > 50).

   e. *The NCCN stated "...the benefit of early ADT is uncertain" in asymptomatic non-curable M0 prostate cancer. The possible 5% overall survival benefit for immediate ADT must be balanced against the higher risk of side effects. If watchful waiting is elected, then consider starting ADT before the PSA rises above 50 and before the PSA doubling time is $\leq$ 12 months.*

4. Either intermittent or continuous ADT may be used in non-curable non-metastatic castrate sensitive prostate cancer. See page 236.

Treatment for Metastatic (M1) CSPC

1. Quantify the metastatic burden as high or low volume (see page 256).
2. *Patients with symptomatic metastases (especially bone pain) have a worse overall survival.*
3. *Medical or surgical castration is always part of the initial treatment for men with M1 CSPC.* The abbreviation ADT means castration with or without the concomitant use of a first generation antiandrogen.
4. Recommended options for treatment of men with castration *sensitive* prostate cancer (CSPC) and distant metastasis (M1) include
   a. ADT and 6 cycles of docetaxel (for men with high volume metastases)
   b. Castration and abiraterone
   c. Castration and apalutamide
   d. Castration and enzalutamide
   e. ADT and prostate XRT (for men with low volume of metastases)
5. Other treatment options include ADT alone, which may be administered intermittently or continuously (see page 236).
6. *Relugolix should not be used with abiraterone, enzalutamide, darolutamide, or apalutamide because of potential drug interactions.* Relugolix has not been adequately studied when used in combination with chemotherapy, abiraterone, enzalutamide, darolutamide, or apalutamide.
7. ADT and docetaxel—in metastatic castration sensitive prostate cancer with high volume metastases, ADT and docetaxel significantly improves overall survival and decreases progression compared to ADT alone, but the addition of docetaxel generates more severe side effects. Adding docetaxel to ADT is not beneficial for men with low volume metastasis.
8. Castration with one of the following medications: abiraterone, apalutamide, or enzalutamide—in metastatic castration sensitive prostate cancer, these combinations improve overall survival and reduce progression compared to castration alone.

9. ADT and prostate XRT—this treatment option was studied in the STAMPEDE trial. Men with untreated newly diagnosed metastatic prostate cancer were given life-long androgen deprivation (with or without up-front docetaxel chemotherapy) and randomized to either no prostate radiation or to a course of prostate radiation. Metastatic burden was classified using the CHAARTED trial definition (see definitions on page 256). *In men with low volume metastatic burden, prostate radiation improved failure-free survival and overall survival. In men with high volume metastatic burden, prostate radiation improved failure-free survival, but not overall survival.* Caveat: In this study, metastases detection was based on conventional imaging (whole body bone scintigraphy and CT/MRI). So, men with low metastatic burden on conventional imaging should not be denied prostate radiation if more sensitive techniques (e.g. PSMA PET) suggest a higher metastatic burden.

10. The diagram on page 254 shows the treatment algorithm for men with CSPC.

Treatment for Non-metastatic (M0) CRPC

1. For castration resistant prostate cancer (CRPC), *castration should be continued while other cancer therapies are administered. Retrospective data suggests that continuing castration in CRPC improves overall survival* (Taylor 1993).

2. *In M0 men with CRPC, no cancer related symptoms, and PSA doubling time ≤ 10 months, three second generation antiandrogens (apalutamide, darolutamide, and enzalutamide) all showed improved metastasis free survival and overall survival compared to placebo; therefore any one of these medications is recommended for treatment of these men.*

3. In M0 men with CRPC, no cancer related symptoms, and PSA doubling time > 10 months, no therapy has been shown to improve survival in a randomized trial. The recommended management of these men is surveillance. Alternative options include any of the therapies list below.

   a. First generation antiandrogen (flutamide, bicalutamide, or nilutamide)—starting one of these medications will reduce PSA by ≥ 50% in 30% of men. PSA reduction often lasts only a few months.

   b. Antiandrogen withdrawal—men who are already on a first generation antiandrogen may have a drop in PSA when the medication is stopped (see page 241).

   c. Change to a different first generation antiandrogen—PSA declines by ≥ 50% in 35% of men who are changed to a different first generation antiandrogen.

   d. Ketoconazole and steroids (see Ketoconazole, page 290)—PSA decreases by ≥ 50% in approximately 50% of patients, and is usually sustained for 3-8 months.

   e. Estrogens, such as diethylstilbestrol—using diethylstilbestrol 1 mg po q day, up to 43% have a PSA reduction. Other estrogenic compounds, may have similar effects (see Estrogens, page 288).

   f. Corticosteroids—see page 291.

4. In M0 men with CRPC and cancer related symptoms, the best treatment is not well defined. One of the medications listed above may be tried. Also, see Managing Complications of Locally Advanced Disease on page 235.

5. The diagram on page 254 shows the treatment algorithm for men with CRPC.

First Line Management of Prostate Cancer

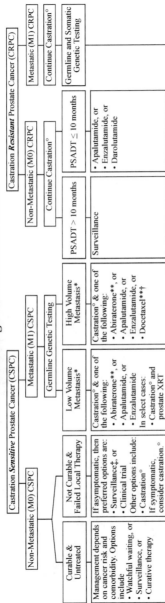

PSA = prostate specific antigen; PSADT = PSA doubling time; CSPC = castration sensitive prostate cancer;
CRPC = castration resistant prostate cancer; XRT = external beam radiation therapy

° "castration" refers to surgical castration (bilateral orchiectomy) or medical castration (with a LHRH agonist or GnRH antagonist). Relugolix should not be used with abiraterone, enzalutamide, darolutamide, or apalutamide because of potential drug interactions. Relugolix has not been adequately studied when used in combination with chemotherapy, abiraterone, enzalutamide, darolutamide, or apalutamide.

† Docetaxel improves overall survival in high volume metastatic disease, but not in low volume metastatic disease. Thus, docetaxel is not recommended for low volume metastatic disease.

* High volume metastasis is defined as having at least one visceral (non-node) metastasis and/or ≥ 4 bone metastases with at least one bone metastasis not in the vertebral bodies or pelvic bones. Low metastatic burden is defined as absence of visceral metastasis, any number of nodal metastases, and any of the following: no bone metastasis, 1 to 4 bone metastases in any distribution, or ≥ 4 bone metastases that are all confined to the vertebral bodies and pelvis.

‡ Consider starting castration before the PSA rises above 50 and before the PSA doubling time is ≤ 12 months.

** Administered with a steroid.

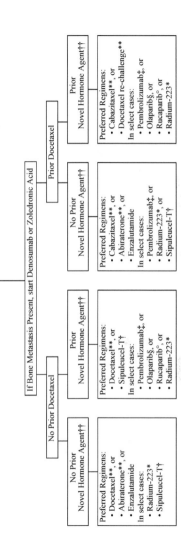

If Bone Metastasis Present, start Denosumab or Zoledronic Acid

No Prior Docetaxel

No Prior Novel Hormone Agent††

Preferred Regimens:
- Docetaxel**, or
- Abiraterone**, or
- Enzalutamide

In select cases:
- Radium-223*
- Sipuleucel-T†

Prior Novel Hormone Agent††

Preferred Regimens:
- Docetaxel**, or
- Sipuleucel-T†

In select cases:
- Pembrolizumab‡, or
- Olaparib§, or
- Rucaparib°, or
- Radium-223*

Prior Docetaxel

No Prior Novel Hormone Agent††

Preferred Regimens:
- Cabazitaxel**, or
- Abiraterone**, or
- Enzalutamide

In select cases:
- Pembrolizumab‡, or
- Radium-223* or
- Sipuleucel-T†

Prior Novel Hormone Agent††

Preferred Regimens:
- Cabazitaxel**, or
- Docetaxel re-challenge**

In select cases:
- Pembrolizumab‡, or
- Olaparib§, or
- Rucaparib°, or
- Radium-223*

* Radium-223 is indicated for men with all of the following criteria: symptomatic bone metastases, no visceral metastases, and malignant lymphadenopathy ≤3cm in size.
Radium should not be used in combination with chemotherapy (because of cumulative myelosuppression) or with abiraterone (because of increased fractures and mortality).
† Sipuleucel-T is indicated for treatment metastatic CRPC in men who have asymptomatic or minimally symptomatic metastases. Sipuleucel-T is not recommended for men with any of the following characteristics: using opioids to control cancer related pain, visceral metastasis, rapidly progressive disease, life expectancy < 6 months, large tumor burden, ECOG performance status ≥ 2, small cell prostate cancer, or neuroendocrine prostate cancer.
‡ Pembrolizumab is a PD-1 inhibitor that is indicated for treatment metastatic CRPC in men who have DNA mismatch repair (dMMR) or microsatellite instability-high (MSI-H).
§ Olaparib is a PARP inhibitor that is indicated for treatment metastatic CRPC in men who have a mutation in the homologous recombination repair (HRR) system.
° Rucaparib is a PARP inhibitor that is indicated for treatment metastatic CRPC in men who have a BRCA1 or BRCA2 mutation (germline or somatic).
** Administered with a steroid.
†† Novel hormone agents include abiraterone, apalutamide, enzalutamide, and darolutamide.

Treatment of Metastatic (M1) CRPC

Treatment Options
1. For CRPC, *castration should be continued while other cancer therapies are administered. Retrospective data suggests that continuing castration in CRPC improves overall survival* (Taylor 1993).
2. Quantify the metastatic burden.
   a. High volume metastasis—defined as having at least one visceral (non-node) metastasis and/or ≥ 4 bone metastases with at least one bone metastasis not in the vertebral bodies or pelvic bones.
   b. Low metastatic burden—defined as absence of visceral metastasis, any number of nodal metastases, and any of the following: no bone metastasis, 1 to 4 bone metastases in any distribution, or ≥ 4 bone metastasis that are all confined to the vertebral bodies and pelvis.
3. *Patients with symptomatic metastases (especially bone pain) have a worse overall survival.*
4. When bone metastases are present, consider treatment with zoledronic acid or denosumab to prevent skeletal related events (see page 257).
5. See page 254 for the treatment of metastatic CRPC.

AR-V7 (Androgen Receptor Splice Variant 7)
1. Under normal circumstances, androgenic stimulation is controlled by an androgen receptor signaling pathway (ARSP), which is triggered when androgens bind to a certain domain on the normal androgen receptor (AR).
2. Some prostate cancer treatments depend on a intact ARSP to exert their anti-cancer effect (ARSP-dependant therapies). These therapies include medications that lower androgens (such as abiraterone) and medications that inhibit the binding of androgens to the AR (such enzalutamide).
3. The AR-V7 protein is an abnormal androgen receptor. It lacks the androgen binding domain; therefore, it does not bind to androgens and does not participate in the normal ARSP. However, it still stimulates androgenic effects in the tissue (including cancer growth). Because AR-V7 is not involved in normal ARSP, it continues to stimulate cancer growth in the presence of therapies that exert their anti-cancer effect through the ASRP. In fact, *ARSP-dependant therapies (such as abiraterone and enzalutamide) are less effective in the presence of AR-V7.* Therapies that do not depend on the ARSP (such as cytotoxic chemotherapy) are generally not effected by the presence of AR-V7.
4. *When AR-V7 is positive (i.e AR-V7 is present), men treated with taxane chemotherapy have a better progression free and overall survival than men treated with enzalutamide or abiraterone.*
5. When AR-V7 is negative (i.e. AR-V7 is absent), most studies show a similar progression free and overall survival whether the patient was treated with enzalutamide, abiraterone, or taxane chemotherapy.
6. In men with metastatic CRPC, AR-V7 was present in only 3% of men who had not been treated with enzalutamide, abiraterone, or taxane chemotherapy, but was present in 19-38% of men who had already been treated with (and progressed on) either enzalutamide or abiraterone.
7. *Testing for AR-V7 may be most useful in men with metastatic CRPC who have progressed on an ARSP-dependant therapy (such as enzalutamide or abiraterone) because these men are more likely to have AR-V7. If AR-V7 is present, then chemotherapy will be more effective than switching a different ARSP-dependant therapy.*
8. Testing for an AR-V7 mutation is typically accomplished by examining circulating tumor cells.

Sequencing of Therapy for CRPC Prostate Cancer

1. For CRPC, *castration should be continued while other cancer therapies are administered. Retrospective data suggests that continuing castration in CRPC improves overall survival* (Taylor 1993).
2. When a specific therapy (other than castration) fails to control CRPC, then consider switching to a therapy that has a different mechanism of action than the previous therapies.
3. Limited data suggests that abiraterone followed by enzalutamide may result in a less PSA progression than enzalutamide followed by abiraterone.
4. Androgen synthesis inhibitors and antiandrogens are less effective in the presence of AR-V7. *If AR-V7 is present, consider using a therapy that has a different mechanism of action than the androgen synthesis inhibitors and antiandrogens, such as docetaxel.*

Treatment and Prevention of Bone Metastasis

General information

1. A skeletal related event (SRE) is usually defined as bone fracture, spinal cord compression, or a bone condition that requires radiation or surgery. *Pathologic fractures in men receiving androgen deprivation have been correlated with decreased overall survival.*
2. Approximately 50% of men with CRPC and untreated bone metastases will develop a SRE within 2 years. The incidence of SREs in this population can be reduced significantly by treating with an osteoclast inhibitor (e.g. zoledronic acid or denosumab).
3. Bone resorption is the process by which osteoclasts catabolize bone and release minerals (including calcium) into to the blood.
4. Under normal conditions, bone is constantly remodeled through a balance of bone formation (by osteoblasts) and bone resorption (by osteoclasts).
5. RANK (receptor activator of nuclear factor-κB) is a receptor on the surface of osteoclasts. RANK ligand, a protein produced by osteoblasts, is one of the key regulators of remodeling. When RANK ligand binds to the RANK receptor, osteoclasts are stimulated to resorb (break down) bone.
6. When cancer metastasizes to bone, the cancer often secretes mediators that alter the balance of local bone remodeling. For example, cancer can stimulate an increase in RANK ligand production. This increase in RANK ligand causes osteoclast overactivity, resulting in excessive bone resorption. Excessive bone resorption releases growth factors that stimulate cancer growth. Cancer growth further stimulates RANK ligand production. This endless cycle of tumor growth and bone resorption weakens the bone and increases the risk of skeletal related events.
7. *Denosumab and bisphosphonates (such as zoledronic acid) are both osteoclast inhibitors;* however, the mechanism by which they inhibit the osteoclast is different.

Treatment of Bone Metastases

1. For bone metastasis with castration sensitive metastatic prostate cancer
   a. Start androgen deprivation with medical or surgical castration.
   b. Start zoledronic acid or denosumab to prevent or delay SREs.
2. For bone metastasis with castration resistant metastatic prostate cancer
   a. Continue castration.
   b. Start zoledronic acid or denosumab to prevent or delay SREs.

3. Painful bone metastasis
   a. Focal bone metastases—may be treated with external beam radiation, which eliminates bone pain in 25-40% of cases and improves bone pain in 80% of cases. For non-vertebral bone metastases, the dose is 8 Gy per lesion (delivered in a single fraction).
   b. Diffuse bone metastases—may be treated with chemotherapy or bone seeking radionucleotides.
4. Significant threat of fracture in a weight bearing bone—usually requires orthopedic surgery.
5. Pathologic fracture—usually requires orthopedic surgery.

Zoledronic Acid (Zometa[8])

1. Zoledronic acid is a bisphosphonate (a compound that has 2 phosphonate groups). Bisphosphonates bind to calcium. Since the largest store of calcium is in the skeleton, bisphosphonates concentrate in bone.
2. Mechanism of action—*zoledronic acid prevents bone resorption (break down of bones) by inhibiting osteoclast activity.*
3. Zoledronic acid is FDA approved to prevent SREs in patients with CRPC and bone metastases.
4. In men with CRPC and bone metastasis, *zoledronic acid significantly reduces SREs and delays the onset of SREs by nearly 6 months compared to placebo, but it does not improve overall survival.* It significantly reduces pathologic fractures. It may reduce spinal cord compression and the need for bone radiation, but these trends did not reach statistical significance.
5. Prior to therapy—perform routine oral examination. Consider obtaining a dental examination and preventative dentistry for patients with poor oral hygiene, periodontal disease, dental implants, oral trauma (e.g. poorly fitting dentures), recent dental/oral surgery (e.g. dental extraction), steroid use, or other risk factors that may increase osteonecrosis the jaw.
6. Dose—in men with creatinine clearance (CrCl) > 60 ml/min: zoledronic acid 4 mg IV (infused over no less than 15 minutes) every 3-4 weeks. For use in men with CrCl = ≤ 60 ml/min see the prescribing information.
   a. During therapy, administer at least 500 mg calcium and 400 IU vitamin D3 orally each day.
   b. The optimal duration of therapy is not known, but mean duration of treatment in studies is approximately 9 months.
7. Side effects—the most common side effects are anemia, dyspnea, flu-like symptoms (fever, chills, fatigue, weakness), arthralgia, bone pain, and gastrointestinal symptoms (nausea, vomiting, constipation, diarrhea).
   a. Zoledronic acid can cause renal insufficiency (17%), anemia (33%), neutropenia (12%), thrombocytopenia (10%), hypocalcemia (1%), hypophosphatemia (<12%) and hypomagnesemia (1%).
   b. Other rare side effects reported with bisphosphonates
      i. Osteonecrosis of the jaw.
      ii. Severe bone, joint, or muscle pain (relieved by stopping therapy).
      iii. Atypical subtrochanteric and diaphyseal femoral fractures.
      iv. Ocular inflammation (uveitis, scleritis).
8. During therapy—obtain serum creatinine before each dose. Monitor calcium, phosphate, magnesium, and creatinine during therapy. It may also be prudent to monitor complete blood count.
   a. Monitor for symptoms of osteonecrosis of the jaw (pain, numbness, or jaw/mouth swelling) and femoral fracture (thigh or groin pain)
   b. Maintenance of good oral hygiene and preventative dentistry are recommended during therapy. Invasive dental procedures should be avoided during treatment.

Denosumab 120 mg (Xgeva®)

1. Denosumab 120 mg subcutaneous injection every 4 weeks is FDA approved to prevent SREs in patients with bone metastases from solid tumors (including prostate cancer). At a lower dose and frequency (60 mg subcutaneous injection every 6 months), it is FDA approved to increase bone mass in men at high risk for fracture who are receiving androgen deprivation for *non-metastatic* prostate cancer (see page 296).

2. Mechanism of action—*denosumab is a monoclonal antibody that binds to RANK ligand and prevents it from activating the RANK receptor; therefore, denosumab prevents bone resorption by inhibiting osteoclast activity.*

3. In men with CRPC and bone metastasis, Denosumab 120 mg reduces SREs and delays the onset of SREs.

4. In men with CRPC and no bone metastases, *denosumab 120 mg delays the development of bone metastases but does not improve overall survival.* Smith et al (2011) randomized men with non-metastatic CRPC who had PSA ≥ 8 ng/ml and/or PSA doubling time ≤ 10 months to placebo or denosumab 120 mg subcutaneous injection every 4 weeks. Denosumab 120 mg significantly delayed the onset of bone metastases by a median of 4.2 months compared to placebo. Both groups had a similar overall survival. So far, the FDA has not approved denosumab for prevention of bone metastasis.

5. A randomized trial comparing zoledronic acid and denosumab in men with CRPC and bone metastases showed the following results.
   a. Time to SRE was significantly longer for denosumab (by a median of 3.6 months) compared to zoledronic acid, but the rate of various SREs were similar. In other words, SREs were equally likely to occur, but the onset of the SRE was later in men receiving denosumab.
   b. Hypocalcemia occurred significantly more often with denosumab (13% vs. 6%).
   c. Osteonecrosis of the jaw was slightly more common with denosumab (2% vs. 1%), although this difference was not statistically significant.
   d. Denosumab caused less acute phase reactions than zoledronic acid. Acute phase reactions produce flu-like symptoms (such as fever, chills, arthralgia, bone pain, fatigue), typically within 3 days of treatment.
   e. *There was no difference in overall survival or progression free survival between denosumab and zoledronic acid.*

6. Other differences between denosumab and zoledronic acid
   a. Denosumab is a subcutaneous injection, whereas zoledronic acid is an intravenous injection.
   b. Denosumab is not eliminated by the kidneys and it is not nephrotoxic; thus, it does not require monitoring of renal function or dose adjustment for renal insufficiency. Zoledronic acid is eliminated by the kidneys and can be nephrotoxic; thus, it requires monitoring of renal function and dose adjustment for renal insufficiency.

7. Prior to treatment
   a. Check calcium level and correct hypocalcemia.
   b. Perform routine oral examination. Dental examination and appropriate preventative dentistry should be considered in patients with poor oral hygiene, periodontal disease, dental implants, oral trauma (such as from poorly fitting dentures), recent dental/oral surgery (such as dental extraction), steroid use, or other risk factors that may increase osteonecrosis of the jaw.

8. Dose to prevent skeletal related events in patients with bone metastases from solid tumors—denosumab 120 mg subcutaneous injection (in upper thigh, upper arm, or abdomen) every 4 weeks, with oral administration of calcium (e.g. 1000 mg daily) and vitamin D3 (e.g. $\geq$ 400 IU daily).

9. Side effects
   a. The most common side effects were fatigue, weakness (asthenia), nausea, and hypophosphatemia.
   b. Denosumab (120 mg dose) causes severe hypocalcemia in 3% of patients. Patients on dialysis or with creatinine clearance < 30 ml/min may have a higher risk of hypocalcemia.
   c. Denosumab (120 mg dose) causes severe hypophosphatemia in 15% of patients.
   d. Denosumab (120 mg dose) rarely causes osteonecrosis of the jaw, but the risk of increases with duration of therapy (risk is 1.1% during the first year, 3-4% during the second year, and 4-7% per year thereafter).

10. During therapy
   a. Monitor calcium and phosphate levels in all patients. In addition, consider monitoring magnesium in patients with renal insufficiency.
   b. Monitor for symptoms of osteonecrosis of the jaw (pain, numbness, or swelling in the jaw or inside the mouth).
   c. Maintenance of good oral hygiene and preventative dentistry are recommended during therapy. Invasive dental procedures should be avoided during treatment with denosumab 120 mg.

Bone Seeking Radionuclides: β-particle Emitters

1. β-particle emitters (β-emitters) deliver radiation to bone metastases, resulting in a reduction in cancer-related bone pain.
2. These agents are used mainly for men with painful bone metastases that are numerous enough to make external beam radiation impractical.
3. Examples of β-emitters include strontium and samarium.
4. β-emitters improve cancer-related bone pain in approximately 50% of men, and eliminate bone pain in 10% of men. However, up to 25% of men will have a initial increase in pain (a pain flare).
5. β-emitters do not improve survival or reduce skeletal related events.
6. *Bone marrow suppression is the major dose-limiting toxicity. The most common side effect is thrombocytopenia.*

Bone Seeking Radionuclides: α-particle Emitters [Radium-223 (Xofigo™)]

1. Radium-223 is a radioactive, α-particle emitting element that kills tumor cells by creating double strand breaks in DNA. Radium-223 has several properties that make it particularly suitable for treating bone metastases.
   a. Radium-223 mimics calcium—radium and calcium have a similar chemical behavior because they are in the same group of elements on the periodic table. *Like calcium, radium is taken up into areas of increased bone metabolism* (thus, Radium is most effective in osteoblastic lesions).
   b. α-particle emitter—α-particle radiation travels a very short distance (< 100 microns); therefore, it can kill the nearby cancer cells with minimal damage to surrounding normal tissue.
2. Radium-223 is FDA approved for the treatment of men with castration resistant prostate cancer and symptomatic bone metastases, but without visceral metastases. Patients with malignant lymphadenopathy $\geq$ 3 cm in size were excluded from the trials; thus, Radium-223 is not recommended in men with malignant lymphadenopathy $\geq$ 3 cm in size.
3. *Radium is the only bone targeted therapy that improves overall survival in men with metastatic CRPC.* Radium usually does not reduce PSA.

4. The ALSYMPCA trial randomized 921 men with CRPC, no visceral metastases, and ≥ 2 bone metastases to placebo or Radium-223. Radium significantly improved median overall survival by 3.6 months, delayed the onset of SREs by a median of approximately 5 months (including pathologic fracture, spinal cord compression, and need for bone radiation), improved quality of life, and reduced bone pain. Side effects were similar between Radium and placebo.
5. Common side effects include nausea, vomiting, diarrhea, and peripheral edema. Radium rarely causes significant thrombocytopenia, neutropenia, or anemia. Obtain complete blood count before each dose. If significant myelosuppression is present, radium should be discontinued.
6. Dose: Radium-223 55 kBq per kg body mass IV q 4 weeks for 6 doses.
7. *Do not co-administer Radium with chemotherapy (because of cumulative myelosuppression) or with abiraterone (because of increased fractures and mortality).* Castration, bisphosphonates, and denosumab can be co-administered with Radium and do not reduce the efficacy of Radium.

Comparison of Treatments for Bone Metastases in Men with CRPC

Statistically Significant Clinical Effect	Zoledronic Acid	Denosumab 120 mg	Beta-Emitters	Radium-223
Reduces SREs	Yes	Yes	No	Yes
Delays onset of SREs	Yes	Yes	No	Yes
Delays pathologic bone fracture	Yes	?	No	Yes
Delays spinal cord compression	No*	?	No	Yes
Delays need for bone radiation	No*	?	No	Yes
Delays ECOG PS deterioration	No	?	?	Yes
Reduces bone pain	Yes	Yes	Yes	Yes
Improves quality of life	No	Maybe	Maybe	Yes
Improves overall survival	No	No	No	*Yes*

ECOG PS = ECOG performance status (see page 31)
SREs = skeletal related events; ? = unknown, no data published.
* A delay was observed, but it did not reach statistical significance.

Acute Spinal Cord Compression from Metastasis
1. Symptoms from acute spinal cord compression depend on the level and degree of compression. Metastases from prostate cancer often occur in the lumbar spine, which corresponds to the sacral spinal cord and cauda equina. Therefore, neurologic symptoms tend to involve the lower extremities, bowel, and bladder. Symptoms may include weakness or paresis below the level of injury, sensation loss below the level of injury, urinary/fecal incontinence or retention, and back pain.
2. Start intravenous steroids—a commonly used dose is dexamethasone 100 mg IV bolus, followed by dexamethasone 25 mg po QID x 3 days. Thereafter, the dose is tapered.
3. Start immediate androgen deprivation by one of the following methods:
   a. Bilateral orchiectomy—testosterone reaches castrate level in 2-12 hours.
   b. Start ketoconazole 400 mg po q 8 hours—castrate testosterone levels are often reached 8 hours after a 400 mg oral dose (See page 290).
   c. GnRH antagonists—these agents do not cause flare. *Do not give LHRH agonists* because the flare can make spinal compression acutely worse.
4. Plain spine x-rays may be obtained. However, it probably better to obtain an MRI of the entire spine (this will identify not only symptomatic lesions, but also lesions that may cause impending problems).

5. Surgical decompression may be indicated in any of the following cases.
   • Failure of androgen deprivation and radiation.
   • Spinal instability from vertebral body collapse.
   • Recurrent spine compression in an area of previous radiation therapy.
   • Bone protrusion into the spinal cord.
   • Neurologic compromise from spinal metastasis.
6. External beam radiation therapy to the spinal metastases should be instituted immediately if surgical therapy is not indicated.
7. Neurosurgery, radiation oncology, and medical oncology consults may be helpful in managing patients with cord compression.

REFERENCES

General (including cancer statistics)

ASCO—Chen RC, et al: Active surveillance for the management of localized prostate cancer (Cancer Care Ontario Guideline): American Society of Clinical Oncology clinical practice guideline endorsement. J Urol, 34(18): 2182, 2016.

AUA—Carroll, P, et al: PSA testing for the pretreatment staging and posttreatment management of prostate cancer. AUA Inc., 2013. (www.auanet.org).

AUA/ASTRO/SUO—Lowrance W, et al: Advanced prostate cancer: AUA/ASTRO/SUO guideline 2020. AUA Inc., 2020. (www.auanet.org).

AUA/ASTRO/SUO—Sanda MG, et al: Clinically localized prostate cancer: AUA/ASTRO/SUO guideline. AUA, Inc., 2017. (www.auanet.org).

EAU—Mottet N, et al: EAU-EANM-ESTRO-ESUR-ISUP-SIOG guidelines on prostate cancer. European Association of Urology, 2021. (www.uroweb.org).

National Cancer Institute: Surveillance, Epidemiology, and End Results (SEER) program. Table 1.18: Lifetime risk of dying from cancer by site & race, http://seer.cancer.gov/csr/1975_2016/results_merged/topic_lifetime_risk.pdf

NCCN—National Comprehensive Cancer Network clinical practice guidelines in oncology: Prostate cancer. V.2.2021, 2021 (www.nccn.org).

Risk Factors For Prostate Cancer: Family History & Ethnicity

Brandt A, et al: Age-specific risk of incident prostate cancer and risk of death from prostate cancer defined by the number of affected family members. Eur Urol, 58(2): 275, 2010.

Brandt A, et al: Risk for incident and fatal prostate cancer in men with a family history of any incident and fatal cancer. Ann Oncol, 23(1): 251, 2012.

Bruner DW, et al: Relative risk of prostate cancer for men with affected relatives: systematic review and meta-analysis. Int J Cancer, 107: 797, 2003.

Lloyd T, et al: Lifetime risk of being diagnosed with, or dying from, prostate cancer by major ethnic group in England 2008-2010. BMC Medicine, 13: 171, 2015.

Risk Factors For Prostate Cancer: Mutations & Genetics

Bottcher R, et al: Cribriform and intraductal prostate cancer are associated with increased genomic instability and distinct genomic alternations. BMC Cancer, 18(1): 8, 2018.

Castro E, et al. PROREPAIR-B: a prospective cohort study of the impact of germline DNA repair mutations on the outcomes of patients with metastatic castration-resistant prostate cancer. J Clin Oncol, 37: 490, 2019.

Pritchard CC, et al: Inherited DNA-repair gene mutations in men with metastatic prostate cancer. N Engl J Med, 375: 443, 2016.

Struewing JP, et al: The risk of cancer associated with specific mutations of BRCA1 and BRCA2 among Ashkenazi Jews. N Engl J Med, 336(20): 1401, 1997.

Screening PSA to Predict Future Risk of Metastasis and Death

Bul M, et al: Prostate cancer incidence and disease specific survival of men with initial prostate specific antigen less than 3.0 ng/ml who are participating in ERSPC Rotterdam. Eur Urol, 59: 498, 2011.

Carlsson S, et al: Influence of blood prostate specific antigen levels at age 60 on benefits and harms of prostate cancer screening: population based cohort study. BMJ, 348: g2296, 2014.

Vickers AJ, et al: Prostate specific antigen concentration at age 60 and death or metastasis from prostate cancer: case control study. BMJ, 341: c4521, 2010.

Vickers AJ, et al: Strategy for detection of prostate cancer based on relation between prostate specific antigen at age 40-55 and long term risk of metastasis: case control study. BMJ, 346: f2023, 2013.

Smoking and Prostate Cancer

Kenfield SA, et al: Smoking and prostate cancer survival and recurrence. JAMA, 305(24): 2548, 2011.

Moreira DM, et al: Cigarette smoking is associated with and increased risk of biochemical disease recurrence, metastasis, castration resistant prostate cancer and mortality after radical prostatectomy. Cancer, 120(2): 197, 2014.

Prevention - 5α-reductase Inhibitors

Azzouni F, et al: Role of 5α-reductase inhibitors in prostate cancer prevention and treatment. Urology, 79(6): 1197, 2012.

Bonde TM, et al: 5α-reductase inhibitors and risk of prostate cancer death. J Urol, 204(4): 714, 2020.

PCPT—Thompson IM, et al: The influence of finasteride on the development of prostate cancer. N Engl J Med, 349: 213, 2003.

PCPT—Thompson IM, et al: Long term survival of participants in the prostate cancer prevention trial. N Engl J Med, 369(7): 603, 2013. Also see N Engl J Med, 369(20): 1967, 2013 for additional info in letter to editor.

Pinsky, PF, et al: Projecting prostate cancer mortality in the PCPT and REDUCE chemoprevention trials. Cancer, 119: 593, 2013.

REDUCE—Andriole GL et al: Effect of dutasteride on the risk of prostate cancer. N Engl J Med, 362(13): 1192, 2010.

Van Rompay, MI, et al: Impact of 5α-reductase inhibitor and α-blocker therapy for benign prostatic hyperplasia on prostate cancer incidence and mortality. BJU Int, 123: 511, 2019.

Theoret MR, et al: The risks and benefits of 5α-reductase inhibitors for prostate cancer prevention. N Engl J Med, 365(2): 97, 2011.

US Food and Drug Administration: December 1, 2010 Meeting of the Oncologic Drugs Advisory Committee. [www.fda.gov/downloads/ AdvisoryCommittees/CommitteesMeetingMaterials/Drugs/ OncologicDrugsAdvisoryCommittee/UCM236786.pdf]

Wilt TJ, et al: 5-α reductase inhibitors for prostate cancer chemoprevention: an updated Cochrane systematic review. BJU Int, 106: 1444, 2010.

Prevention - Green Tea

Bettuzzi S, et al: Chemoprevention of human prostate cancer by oral administration of green tea catechins in volunteers with high grade prostate intraepithelial neoplasia. Cancer Res, 66(2): 2006.

Brausi M, et al: Chemoprevention of human prostate cancer by green tea catechins: two years later. A follow-up update. Eur Urol, 54: 472, 2008.

Cui K, et al: Chemoprevention of prostate cancer in men with high grade prostatic intraepithelial neoplasia (HGPIN): a systematic review and adjusted indirect treatment comparison. Oncotarget, 8(22): 36676, 2017.

Gontero P, et al: A randomized double blind placebo controlled phase I-II study on clinical and molecular effects of dietary supplements in men with precancerous prostate lesions. Prostate, 75(11): 1177, 2015.

Kumar NB, et al: Randomized, placebo controlled trial of green tea catechins for prostate cancer prevention. Cancer Prev Res, 8(10): 879, 2015.

Micali S, et al: Effect of green tea catechins in patients with high grade prostatic intraepithelial neoplasia: results of a short term double blind placebo controlled phase II clinical trial. Arch Ital Urol Androl, 89(3): 197, 2017.

Perletti G, et al: Green tea catechins for chemoprevention of prostate cancer in patients with histologically proven HG-PIN or ASAP. Concise review and meta-analysis. Arch Ital Urol Androl, 91(3): 153, 2019.

Prevention - Lycopene

Etminan M, et al: The role of tomato products and lycopene in the prevention of prostate cancer: a meta-analysis of observational studies. Cancer Epidemiol Biomarkers Prev, 13(3): 340, 2004.

Gontero P, et al: A randomized phase I-II study on clinical and molecular effects of dietary supplements in men with precancerous prostate lesions. Prostate, 75(11): 1177, 2015.

Ilic D, et al: Lycopene for the prevention and treatment of benign prostatic hyperplasia and prostate cancer. Maturitas, 72: 269, 2012.

Kristal AR, et al: Serum lycopene concentration and prostate cancer risk: results from the prostate cancer prevention trial. Cancer Epidemiol Biomarkers Prev, 20(4): 638, 2011.\

Morgia G, et al: Association between selenium and lycopene supplementation and the incidence of prostate cancer: results from the post hoc analysis of the procomb trial. Phytomedicine, 34: 1, 2017.

Prevention - Vitamins and Selenium

Dimitrakopoulou VL, et al: Circulating vitamin D concentration and risk of seven cancers: Mendelian randomization study. BMJ, 359: j4761, 2017.

Fleshner NE, et al: Progression from high grade prostatic intraepithelial neoplasia to cancer: a randomized trial of combination vitamin E, soy, and selenium. J Clin Oncol, 29(17): 2386, 2011.

Gontero P, et al: A randomized double blind placebo controlled phase I-II study on clinical and molecular effects of dietary supplements in men with precancerous prostate lesions. Prostate, 75(11): 1177, 2015.

HOPE—Lonn E, et al: Effect of long term vitamin E supplementation on cardiovascular events and cancer. JAMA, 293(11): 1338, 2005.

Morgia G, et al: Association between selenium and lycopene supplementation and the incidence of prostate cancer: results from the post hoc analysis of the procomb trial. Phytomedicine, 34: 1, 2017.

NBT—Algotar AM, et al: Phase 3 clinical trial investigating the effect of selenium supplementation in men at high risk for prostate cancer. Prostate, 73(3): 328, 2013.

NHANES III—Freedman DM, et al: Prospective study of serum vitamin D and cancer mortality in the United States. J Natl Cancer Inst, 99: 1594, 2007.

NHANES III—Freedman DM, et al: Serum 25-hydroxyvitamin D and cancer mortality in the NHANES III study. Cancer Res, 70(21): 8587, 2010.

PHS II—Gaziano JM, et al: Vitamins E and C in the prevention of prostate and total cancer in men. JAMA, 301(1): 52, 2009.

PHS II—Gaziano JM, et al: Multivitamins in the prevention of cancer in men. JAMA, 308(18): 1871, 2012.

PHS II—Wang L, et al: Vitamin E and C supplementation and risk of cancer in men: post trial follow up in the Physicians' Health Study II randomized trial. Am J Clin Nutr, 100(3): 915, 2014.

PROtEus—Parent ME, et al: Vitamin C intake and risk of prostate cancer: the Montreal PROtEus study. Front Physiol, 9: 1218, 2018.

SELECT—Klein EA et al: Vitamin E and the risk of prostate cancer: the Selenium and vitamin E cancer prevention trial (SELECT). JAMA, 306(14):1549, 2011 [update of JAMA, 301(1): 39, 2009].

Travis RC, et al: A collaborative analysis of individual participant data from 19 prospective studies assesses circulating vitamin D and prostate cancer risk. Cancer Res, 79(1): 274, 2019.

VITAL—Manson JE, et al: Vitamin D supplements and prevention of cancer and cardiovascular disease. N Engl J Med, 380(1): 33, 2019.

Prevention - Soy protein

Bosland MC, et al: Effect of soy protein isolate supplementation on biochemical recurrence of prostate cancer after radical prostatectomy: a randomized trial. JAMA, 310(2); 170, 2013.

Fleshner NE, et al: Progression from high grade prostatic intraepithelial neoplasia to cancer: a randomized trial of combination vitamin E, soy, and selenium. J Clin Oncol, 29(17): 2386, 2011.

Prevention - Other Dietary Modifications

Castello A, et al: Mediterranean dietary pattern is associated with low risk of aggressive prostate cancer: MCC-Spain study. J Urol, 199: 430, 2018.

VITAL—Manson JE, et al: Marine n-3 fatty acids and prevention of cardiovascular disease and cancer. N Engl J Med, 380(1): 23, 2019.

Prevention - Metformin

Dell'Atti L, et al: The impact of metformin use on the risk of prostate cancer after prostate biopsy in patients with high grade intraepithelial neoplasia. Int Braz J Urol, 44(1): 69, 2018.

Feng Y, et al: Metformin use and risk of prostate cancer: results from the REDUCE study. Cancer Prev Res (Phila), 8(11): 1055, 2015.

Ghiasi B, et al: The relationship between prostate cancer and metformin consumption: a systematic review and meta-analysis study. Curr Pharm Des, 25(9): 1021, 2019.

Preston MA, et al: Metformin use and prostate cancer risk. Eur Urol, 66(6): 1012, 2014.

Ruiter R, et al: Lower risk of cancer in patients on metformin in comparison with those on sulfonylurea derivatives: results from a large population based follow up study. Diabetes Care, 35(1): 119, 2012.

Tsilidis KK, et al: Metformin does not affect cancer risk: a cohort study in the U.K. clinical practice research datalink analyzed like an intention to treat trial. Diabetes Care, 37(9): 2522, 2014.

Wright JL, et al: Metformin use and prostate cancer in Caucasian men: results from a population based case control study. Cancer Causes Control, 20(9): 1617, 2009.

Prevention - Statins

Freedland S, et al: Statin use and risk of prostate cancer and high grade prostate cancer: results from the REDUCE study. Prostate Cancer Prostatic Dis, 16(3): 254, 2013.

Platz EA, et al: Statin drug use is not associated with prostate cancer risk in men who are regularly screened. J Urol, 192(2): 379, 2014.

Screening Guidelines

ACS—American Cancer Society Recommendations for prostate cancer early detection: www.cancer.org/cancer/prostate-cancer/detection-diagnosis-staging/acs-recommendations.html (revised April 2021).

AUA—Carter HB, et al: Early detection of prostate cancer: AUA guideline. AUA Education and Research, Inc., 2018. (www.auanet.org/guidelines).

CUA—Rendon RA, et al: Canadian Urological Association recommendations on prostate cancer screening and early diagnosis. Can Urol Assoc J, 11(10): 298, 2017.

EAU—Mottet N, et al: EAU-EANM-ESTRO-ESUR-ISUP-SIOG guidelines on prostate cancer. European Association of Urology, 2021. (www.uroweb.org).

NCCN—National Comprehensive Cancer Network (NCCN) clinical practice guidelines: Prostate cancer early detection, V.1.2021, 2021. (www.nccn.org).

PCFA—Prostate Cancer Foundation of Australia and Cancer Council of Australia: PSA testing and early management of test detected prostate cancer, 2016. (https://www.prostate.org.au/media/612113/PSA-Testing-Guidelines.pdf)

U.S. Preventative Services Task Force: Screening for prostate cancer: U.S. Preventative Services Task Force recommendation statement. JAMA, 319(18): 1901, 2018.

Screening Studies

CAP—Martin RM, et al: Effect of a low-intensity PSA-based screening intervention on prostate cancer mortality. JAMA, 319(9): 883, 2018.

ERSPC—Beemsterboer PMM, et al: Prostate specific antigen testing and digital rectal examination before and during a randomized trial of screening for prostate cancer. J Urol, 164: 1216, 2000.

ERSPC—Bokhorst LP, et al: Prostate specific antigen based prostate cancer screening: reduction of prostate cancer mortality after correction for nonattendance and contamination in the Rotterdam section of the European randomized study of screening for prostate cancer. Eur Urol, 65: 329, 2014.

ERSPC—Hugosson J, et al: A 16-yr follow up of the European Randomized study of Screening for Prostate Cancer. Eur Urol, 76: 43, 2019.

ERSPC—Roobol MJ, et al: Prostate cancer mortality reduction by prostate specific antigen based screening adjusted for non-attendance and contamination in the ERSPC. Eur Urol, 56: 584, 2009.

ERSPC—Schroder FH, et al: Screening for prostate cancer decreases the risk of metastatic disease: findings from the ERSPC. Eur Urol, 62: 745, 2012.

Goteborg—Hugosson J, et al: 18-yr follow-up of the Goteborg randomized population-based prostate cancer screening trial. Scand J Urol, 52: 27, 2018.

Greiman A, et al: Six weeks of fluoroquinolone antibiotic therapy for patients with elevated serum prostate specific antigen is not clinically beneficial: a randomized controlled trial. Urology, 90: 32, 2016.

Labrie F, et al: Screening decreases prostate cancer mortality: 11-year follow-up of the 1988 Quebec prospective randomized controlled trial. Prostate, 59: 311, 2004. [update of Prostate, 38: 83, 1999].

PLCO—Crawford ED, et al: Comorbidity and mortality results from a randomized prostate cancer screening trial. J Clin Oncol, 29:355, 2011.

PLCO—Grubb RL, et al: Prostate cancer screening in the Prostate, Lung, Colorectal and Ovarian cancer screening trial. BJU Int, 102: 1524, 2008.

PLCO—Pinsky PF, et al: Extended mortality results for prostate cancer screening in the PLCO trial with median follow-up of 15 years. Cancer, 123: 592, 2017.

PLCO—Pinsky PF, et al: Extended follow up for prostate cancer incidence and mortality among participants in the PLCO randomized cancer screening trial. BJU Int, 123(5): 854, 2019.

Tsodikov A, et al: Reconciling the effects of screening on prostate cancer mortality in the ERSPC and PLCO trials. Ann Intern Med, 167: 449, 2017.

Elevated Screening PSA Returns to Normal When Rechecked

Boddy JL, et al: An elevated PSA, which normalizes, does not exclude the presence of prostate cancer. Prostate Cancer Prostatic Dis, 8(4): 349, 2005.

De Nunzio C, et al: Repeat prostate specific antigen (PSA) test before prostate biopsy: a 20% decrease in PSA values is associated with a reduced risk of prostate cancer and particularly of high grade cancer. BJU Int, 122: 83, 2018.

Eastham JA, et al: Variation of serum prostate specific antigen levels: an evaluation of year to year fluctuations. JAMA, 289(20): 2695, 2003.

Lavallee LT, et al: Reducing the harm of prostate cancer screening: repeated prostate specific antigen testing. Mayo Clin Proc, 91(1): 17, 2016.

Singh R, et al: Repeating the measurement of prostate specific antigen in symptomatic men can avoid unnecessary prostatic biopsy. BJU Int, 92: 932, 2003.

Risk of Prostate Cancer & Death from Prostate Cancer Based on PSA and DRE

Carter HB, et al: Detection of life threatening prostate cancer with prostate specific antigen velocity during a window of curability. J Natl Cancer Inst, 98(21): 1521, 2006.

Catalona WJ, et al: Comparison of digital rectal examination and serum prostate specific antigen in the early detection of prostate cancer: results of a multicenter clinical trial of 6630 men. J Urol, 151: 1283, 1994.

Flanigan RC, et al: Accuracy of digital rectal examination and transrectal ultrasonography in localizing prostate cancer. J Urol, 152: 1506, 1994.

Thompson IM, et al: Prevalence of prostate cancer among men with a prostate specific antigen level ≤ 4.0 ng per milliliter. N Engl J Med, 350: 2239, 2004.

Schroder FH, et al: Evaluation of digital rectal examination as a screening test for prostate cancer. J Natl Cancer Inst, 90: 1817, 1998.

SelectMdx

Haese A, et al: Multicenter optimization and validation of a 2-gene mRNA urine test for detection of clinically significant prostate cancer before initial prostate biopsy. J Urol, 202(2): 256, 2019.

Van Neste L, et al: Detection of high grade prostate cancer using a urinary molecular biomarker based risk score. Eur Urol, 70: 740, 2016.

ConfirmMdx

Partin AW, et al: Clinical validation of an epigenetic assay to predict negative histopathological results in repeat prostate biopsy. J Urol, 192: 1081, 2014.

Stewart GD, et al: Clinical utility of an epigenetic assay to detect occult prostate cancer in histopathologically negative biopsies: results of the MATLOC study. J Urol, 189(3): 1110, 2013.

4Kscore

Sjoberg DD, et al: Twenty year risk of prostate cancer death by mid-life prostate specific antigen and a panel of 4 kallikrein markers in a large population based cohort of healthy men. Eur Urol, 73(6): 941, 2018.

Stattin P, et al: Improving the specificity of screening for lethal prostate cancer using prostate specific antigen and a panel of kallikrein markers: a nested case control study. Eur Urol, 68: 207, 2015.

PCA3

Aubin SMJ, et al: Prostate cancer gene 3 score predicts prostate biopsy outcome in men receiving dutasteride for prevention of cancer: results from the REDUCE trial. Urology, 78(2): 380, 2011.

Gen-Probe®, Inc.: PROGENSA® PCA3 Assay package insert. (accessed 1/2013): http://gen-probe.com/pdfs/pi/501377RevB.pdf

Haese A, et al: Clinical utility of the PCA3 urine assay in European men scheduled for repeat biopsy. Eur Urol, 54(5): 1081, 2008.

Marks LS, et al: PCA3 molecular urine assay for prostate cancer in men undergoing repeat biopsy. Urology, 69: 532, 2007.

Nakanishi H, et al: PCA3 molecular urine assay correlates with prostate cancer tumor volume: implication in selecting candidates for active surveillance. J Urol, 179(5): 1804, 2008.

Ploussard G, et al: Prostate cancer antigen 3 score accurately predicts tumor volume and might help in selecting prostate cancer patients for active surveillance. Eur Urol, 59(3): 422, 2011.

Tosoian JJ, et al: Accuracy of PCA3 measurement in predicting short term biopsy progression in an active surveillance program. J Urol, 183: 534, 2010.

van Poppel H, et al: The relationship between Prostate CAncer gene 3 (PCA3) and prostate cancer significance. BJU Int, 109(3): 360, 2012.

Whitman EJ, et al: PCA3 score before radical prostatectomy predicts extracapsular extension and tumor volume. J Urol, 180: 1975, 2008.

Prostate Health Index (PHI)

Catalona WJ, et al: A multicenter study of [-2]pro-prostate specific antigen combined with prostate specific antigen and free prostate specific antigen for prostate cancer detection in the 2.0 to 10.0 ng/ml prostate specific antigen range. J Urol, 185(5): 1650, 2011.

Loeb S, et al: The Prostate Health Index selectively identifies clinically significant prostate cancer. J Urol, 193: 1163, 2015.

Prostate Biopsy

AUA—Liss MA, et al: The prevention and treatment of the more common complications related to prostate biopsy update. White Paper. AUA, Inc., 2016. (www.auanet.org/guidelines).

AUA—Taneja SS, et al: Optimal techniques of prostate biopsy and specimen handling. White Paper. AUA, Inc., 2015 (www.auanet.org).

Bjurlin MA, et al: Optimization of initial prostate biopsy in clinical practice: sampling, labeling, and specimen processing. J Urol, 189(6): 2039, 2013.

Bott SRJ, et al: Anterior prostate cancer: is it more difficult to diagnose? BJU Int, 89: 886, 2002.

Chen ME, et al: Comparison of prostate biopsy schemes by computer simulation. Urology, 53(5): 951, 1999.

Chen ME, et al: Detailed mapping of prostate carcinoma foci: biopsy strategy implications. Cancer, 89(8): 1800, 2000.

Demura T, et al: Differences in tumor core distribution between palpable and non-palpable prostate tumors in patients diagnosed using extensive transperineal ultrasound guided template prostate biopsy. Cancer, 103(9): 1826, 2005.

Fainberg J, et al: Erectile dysfunction is a transient complication of prostate biopsy: a systematic review and meta-analysis. J Urol, 205(3): 664, 2021.

Kawakami S, et al: Transrectal ultrasound guided transperineal 14-core systematic biopsy detects apico-anterior cancer foci of T1c prostate cancer. Int J Urol, 11(8):613, 2004.

Matlaga BR, et al: Prostate biopsy: indications and technique. J Urol, 169: 12, 2003.

Matsumoto K, et al: Computer simulated additional deep apical biopsy enhances cancer detection in palpably benign prostate gland. Int J Urol, 13: 1290, 2006.

Meng M, et al: The utility of anterior apical horn biopsies in prostate cancer. Urol Oncol, 21(5): 361, 2003.

Moussa AS, et al: Importance of additional "extreme" anterior apical needle biopsies in the initial detection of prostate cancer. Urology, 75: 1034, 2010.

Noguchi M, et al: An analysis of 148 consecutive transition zone cancers: clinical and histological characteristics. J Urol, 163: 1751, 2000.

Orikasa K, et al: Anterior apical biopsy: is it useful for prostate cancer detection? Int J Urol, 15: 900, 2008.

Pradere B, et al: Nonantibiotic strategies for the prevention of infectious complications following prostate biopsy: a systematic review and meta-analysis. J Urol, 205(3): 653, 2021.

Rodriguez LV, Terris MK: Risks and complications of transrectal ultrasound guided prostate needle biopsy: a prospective study and review of the literature. J Urol, 160: 2115, 1998.

Sato T, et al: Cancer core distribution in patients diagnosed by extended transperineal prostate biopsy. Urology, 66(1): 114, 2005.

Takashima R, et al: Anterior distribution of stage T1c non-palpable tumors in radical prostatectomy specimens. Urology, 59(5): 692, 2002.

Volanis D, et al: Incidence of needle tract seeding following prostate biopsy for suspected cancer: a review of the literature. BJU Int, 115: 698, 2015.

Wright JL, et al: Improved prostate cancer detection with anterior apical prostate biopsies. Urol Oncol, 24(6): 492, 2006.

Prostate MRI Before Prostate Biopsy and For Guiding Prostate Biopsy

ACR—American College of Radiology: PI-RADS prostate imaging reporting and data system 2015 version 2. ACR, 2015 (https://www.acr.org/-/media/ACR/Files/RADS/Pi-RADS/PIRADS-V2.pdf)

AUA/SAR—Collaborative Initiative of the American Urological Association and the Society of Abdominal Radiology's Prostate Cancer Disease Focused Panel: Standard operating procedure for multiparametric magnetic resonance imaging in the diagnosis, staging, and treatment of prostate cancer. AUA, Inc., 2019. (https://www.auanet.org/guidelines).

AUA/SAR—Collaborative Initiative of the American Urological Association and the Society of Abdominal Radiology's Prostate Cancer Disease Focused Panel: Prostate MRI and MRI targeted biopsy in patients with prior negative biopsy. AUA, Inc., 2016. (https://www.auanet.org/guidelines).

4M trial—van der Leest M, et al: Head to head comparison of transrectal ultrasound guided prostate biopsy versus multiparametric prostate resonance imaging with subsequent magnetic resonance guided biopsy in biopsy naive men with elevated prostate specific antigen: a large prospective multicenter clinical study. Eur Urol, 75: 570, 2019.

Gordetsky JNB, et al: Histologic findings associated with false positive multiparametric MRI performed for prostate cancer detection. Human Pathol, 83: 159, 2019.

Meng X, et al: Follow up of men with PIRADS 4 or 5 abnormality on prostate magnetic resonance imaging and nonmalignant pathological findings on initial targeted prostate biopsy. J Urol, 205(3): 748, 2021.

MRI-FIRST trial—Rouviere O, et al: Use of prostate systematic and targeted biopsy on the basis of multiparametric MRI in biopsy naive patients (MRI-FIRST): a prospective, multicenter, paired diagnostic study. Lancet Oncol, 20(1): 100, 2019

Ploussard G, et al: Assessment of the minimal targeted biopsy core number per MRI lesion for improving prostate cancer grading prediction. J Clin Med, 9: 225, 2020.

PROMIS—Ahmed HU, et al: Diagnostic accuracy of multiparametric MRI and TRU biopsy in prostate cancer (PROMIS): a paired validating confirmatory study. Lancet, 389: 815, 2017.

PRECISION trial—Kasivisvanathan V, et al: MRI targeted or standard biopsy for prostate cancer diagnosis. N Engl J Med, 378(19): 1767, 2018.

Siddiqui MM, et al: Comparison of MRI/Ultrasound fusion guided biopsy with ultrasound guided biopsy for the diagnosis of prostate cancer. JAMA, 313(4): 390, 2015.

Wegelin O, et al: The FUTURE trial: a multicenter randomized controlled trial on the target biopsy techniques based on magnetic resonance imaging in the diagnosis of prostate cancer in patients with prior negative biopsies. Eur Urol, 75(4): 582, 2019.

Seminal Vesicle Biopsy and Seminal Vesicle Ultrasound

Guillonneau B, et al: Indications for preoperative seminal vesicle biopsies in staging of clinically localized prostatic cancer. Eur Urol, 32(2): 160, 1997.

Koh H, et al: A nomogram to predict seminal vesicle invasion by the extent and location of cancer in systematic biopsy results. J Urol, 170(4): 1203, 2003.

Korman HJ, et al: Radical prostatectomy: is complete resection of the seminal vesicles really necessary? J Urol, 156(3): 1081, 1996.

Ohori M, et al: Ultrasonic detection of non-palpable seminal vesicle invasion: a clinicopathological study. Br J Urol, 72: 799, 1993.

Samaratunga H, et al: Distal seminal vesicle invasion by prostate adenocarcinoma does not occur in isolation of proximal seminal vesicle invasion or lymphovascular infiltration. Pathology, 42(4): 330, 2010.

Terris MK, et al: Efficacy of transrectal ultrasound guided seminal vesicle biopsies in the detection of prostate cancer. J Urol, 149: 1035, 1993.

Terris MK, et al: Invasion of the seminal vesicles by prostatic cancer: detection with transrectal sonography. AJR Am J Roentgenol, 155(4): 811, 1990.

Prostate Pathology: PIN, AAH, ASAP, Cancer, & Cancer Grading

Abdel-Khalek M, et al: Predictors of prostate cancer on extended biopsy in patients with high grade prostate intraepithelial neoplasia: a multivariate analysis model. BJU Int, 94: 528, 2004.

Epstein JI, et al: A contemporary prostate grading system: a validated alternative to the Gleason score. Eur Urol, 69(3): 428, 2016.

Epstein JI, et al: The pathologic interpretation and significance of prostate needle biopsy findings: implications and controversies. J Urol, 166: 402, 2001.

Fine SW, et al: A contemporary update on pathology reporting for prostate cancer: biopsy and radical prostatectomy specimens. Eur Urol, 62: 20, 2012.

Humphrey, PA: Atypical adenomatous hyperplasia (adenosis) of the prostate. J Urol, 188(6, part 1): 2371, 2012.

Klink JC, et al: High grade prostatic intraepithelial neoplasia. Korean J Urol, 53: 297, 2012.

Merrimen JL, et al: Multifocal high grade prostate intraepithelial neoplasia is a significant risk factor for prostate adenocarcinoma. J Urol, 182: 485, 2009.

Warlick C, et al: Rate of Gleason 7 or higher prostate cancer on repeat biopsy after a diagnosis of atypical small acinar proliferation. Prostate Cancer Prostatic Dis, 18(3): 255, 2015.

Prostate Pathology: Intraductal & Ductal Cancers

Bottcher R, et al: Cribriform and intraductal prostate cancer are associated with increased genomic instability and distinct genomic alternations. BMC Cancer, 18(1): 8, 2018.

Cohen RJ, et al: A proposal of the identification, histologic reporting, and implications of intraductal prostatic carcinoma. Arch Pathol Lab Med, 131: 1103, 2007.

Magers M, et al: Intraductal carcinoma of the prostate. Arch Pathol Lab Med, 139: 1234, 2015.

Morgan TM, et al: Ductal adenocarcinoma of the prostate: increased mortality and decreased serum prostate specific antigen. J Urol, 184(6): 2303, 2010.

Incidental Prostate Cancer

Abbas F, et al: Incidental prostatic adenocarcinoma in patients undergoing radical cystoprostatectomy for bladder cancer. Eur Urol, 30: 322, 1996.

Thompson IM, et al: Prevalence of prostate cancer among men with a prostate specific antigen level < 4.0 ng/ml. N Engl J Med, 350: 2239, 2004.

Surveillance & Watchful Waiting (also see Comparison of Treatments)

ASCO—Chen RC, et al: Active surveillance for the management of localized prostate cancer (Cancer Care Ontario Guideline): American Society of Clinical Oncology clinical practice guideline endorsement. J Urol, 34(18): 2182, 2016.

Albertsen PC, et al: 20-year outcomes following conservative management of clinically localized prostate cancer. JAMA, 293(17): 2095, 2005.

Carter CA, et al: Temporarily deferred therapy for men younger than 70 years and with low-risk localized prostate cancer in the prostate specific antigen era. J Clin Oncol, 21: 4001, 2003.

DETECTIVE consensus—Lam TBL, et al: EAU-EANM-ESTRO-ESUR-SIOG prostate cancer guideline panel consensus statement for deferred treatment with curative intent for localized prostate cancer from an international collaborative study (DETECTIVE study). Eur Urol, 76: 790, 2019.

Duffield AS, et al: Radical prostatectomy findings in patients in whom active surveillance of prostate cancer fails. J Urol, 182: 2274, 2009.

Epstein JI, et al: Pathologic and clinical findings to predict tumor extent of nonpalpable (stage T1c) prostate cancer. JAMA, 271(5): 368, 1994.

Iremashvili V, et al: Pathologic prostate cancer characteristics in patients eligible for active surveillance: a head to head comparison of contemporary protocols. Eur Urol, 62: 462, 2012.

Johansson JE, et al: Natural history of early, localized prostate cancer. JAMA, 291(22): 2713, 2004.

Lu-Yao GL, et al: Outcomes of localized prostate cancer following conservative management. JAMA, 302(11): 1202, 2009.

Patel MI, et al: An analysis of men with clinically localized prostate cancer who deferred definitive therapy. J Urol, 171: 1520, 2004.

Tewari A, et al: Long-term survival probability in men with clinically localized prostate cancer treated either conservatively or with definitive treatment (radiotherapy or radical prostatectomy). Urology, 68(6): 1268, 2006.

Tosoian JJ, et al: Active surveillance program for prostate cancer: an update of the Johns Hopkins experience. J Clin Oncol, 29(16): 2185, 2011.

Warlick C, et al: Delayed versus immediate surgical intervention and prostate cancer outcome. J Natl Cancer Inst, 98(5): 355, 2006.

5-α-reductase Inhibitors During Surveillance

Fleshner NE, et al: Dutasteride in localized prostate cancer management: the REDEEM randomized, double blind, placebo controlled trial. Lancet, 379: 1103, 2012.

Ashrafi AN, et al: Five alpha reductase inhibitors in men undergoing active surveillance for prostate cancer: impact on treatment and reclassification after 6 years of follow up. World J Urol, 2021 [e-published ahead of print] (https://doi.org/10.1007/s00345-021-03644-2)

Prostate MRI for Surveillance

AUA/SAR—Collaborative Initiative of the American Urological Association and the Society of Abdominal Radiology's Prostate Cancer Disease Focused Panel: Standard operating procedure for multiparametric magnetic resonance imaging in the diagnosis, staging, and treatment of prostate cancer. AUA, Inc., 2019. (https://www.auanet.org/guidelines).

Cerantola Y, et al: Can 3T multiparametric magnetic resonance imaging accurately detect prostate cancer extracapsular extension? Can Urol Assoc J, 7(11-12): e699, 2013.

Lawrentschuk N, et al: 'Prostatic evasive anterior tumors': the role of magnetic resonance imaging. BJU Int, 105(9): 1231, 2010.

Lee HD, et al: Low risk prostate cancer patients without visible tumor on multiparametric MRI could qualify for active surveillance. Jpn J Clin Oncol,43(5): 553, 2013.

Margel D, et al: Impact of multiparametric endorectal coil prostate magnetic resonance imaging on disease reclassification among active surveillance candidates: a prospective cohort study. J Urol, 187(4): 1247, 2012.

Somford DM, et al: The predictive value of endorectal 3 Tesla multiparametric magnetic resonance imaging for extraprostatic extension in patients with low, intermediate, and high risk prostate cancer. J Urol, 190(5): 1728, 2013.

Vargas HA, et al: Magnetic resonance imaging for predicting prostate biopsy findings in patients considered for active surveillance of clinically low risk prostate cancer. J Urol, 188(5): 1732, 2012.

Molecular Tests on Prostate Tissue

ConfirmMDx™—Partin AW, et al: Clinical validation of an epigenetic assay to predict negative histopathological results in repeat prostate biopsies. J Urol, 192(4): 1081, 2014.

ConfirmMDx™—Stewart GD, et al: Clinical utility of an epigenetic assay to detect occult prostate cancer in histopathologically negative biopsies: results of the MATLOC study. J Urol, 189(3): 1110, 2013.

OncotypeDx®—Klein EA, et al: a 17 gene assay to predict prostate cancer aggressiveness in the context of Gleason grade heterogeneity, tumor multifocality, and biopsy undersampling. Eur Urol, 66(3): 550, 2014.

Prolaris®—Cuzick J, et al: Prognostic value of a cell cycle progression signature for prostate cancer death in a conservatively managed needle biopsy cohort. Br J Cancer, 106: 1095, 2012.

Prolaris®—Cuzick J, et al: Prognostic value of an RNA expression signature derived from cell cycle proliferation genes for recurrence and death from prostate cancer: A retrospective study in two cohorts. Lancet Oncol, 12(3): 245, 2011.

Primary Androgen Deprivation for Localized Prostate Cancer

AstraZeneca Canada Inc.: Health Canada important drug safety information - Casodex® 150 mg, 2003.

Iversen P, et al: Antiandrogen monotherapy in patients with localized or locally advanced prostate cancer: final results from the bicalutamide early prostate cancer program at a median follow up of 9.7 years. BJU Int, 105: 1074, 2010.

Lu-Yao GL, et al: Survival following primary androgen deprivation therapy among men with localized prostate cancer. JAMA, 300(2): 173, 2008.

Lu-Yao GL, et al: Does primary androgen deprivation therapy delay the receipt of secondary cancer therapy for localized prostate cancer? Eur Urol, 62(6): 966, 2012.

Lu-Yao GL, et al: Fifteen year survival outcomes following primary androgen deprivation therapy for localized prostate cancer. JAMA Intern Med, 174(9): 1460, 2014.

Potosky AL, et al: Effectiveness of primary androgen deprivation therapy for clinically localized prostate cancer. J Clin Oncol, 32(12): 1324, 2014.

Cryotherapy (also see Comparison of Treatments)

AUA—Babaian RJ, et al: Best practice policy statement on cryosurgery for the treatment of localized prostate cancer. AUA Education and Research, Inc., 2008. (www.auanet.org).

Gould R: Total cryosurgery of the prostate versus standard cryosurgery versus radical prostatectomy: comparison of early results and the role of transurethral resection in cryosurgery. J Urol, 162: 1653, 1999.

Leibovich BC, et al: Proximity for prostate cancer to the urethra: implications for minimally invasive ablative therapies. Urology, 56: 726, 2000.

Perrotte P, et al: Quality of life after salvage cryotherapy: the impact of treatment parameters. J Urol, 162(2): 398, 1999.

Shinohara K, et al: Cryotherapy for prostate cancer. Campbell's Urology. 8th Ed. Ed. PC Walsh, et al. Philadelphia: W. B. Sanders Co., 2002, pp 3171-3181.

Shinohara K, et al: Cryosurgical ablation of prostate cancer: patterns of cancer recurrence. J Urol, 158: 2206, 1997.

Wieder J, et al: Transrectal ultrasound guided transperineal cryoablation in the treatment of prostate carcinoma: preliminary results. J Urol, 154: 435, 1995.

Radical Prostatectomy (also see Comparison of Treatments)

Marcq G, et al: Risk of biochemical recurrence based on extent and location of positive surgical margins after robot assisted laparoscopic radical prostatectomy. BMC Cancer, 18(1): 1291, 2018.

Patel VR, et al: Positive surgical margins after robotic assisted radical prostatectomy: a multi-institutional study. J Urol, 186: 511, 2011.

Wieder JA, Soloway M: Incidence, etiology, location, prevention, and treatment of positive surgical margins after prostatectomy for prostate cancer. J Urol, 160: 299, 1998.

Treatment of Pelvic Lymph Nodes Metastasis

Abdollah F, et al: Selecting the optimal candidate for adjuvant radiotherapy after radical prostatectomy for prostate cancer: a long term survival analysis. Eur Urol, 63(6): 998, 2013.

Abdollah F, et al: Impact of adjuvant radiotherapy on survival of patients with node positive prostate cancer. J Clin Oncol, 32(35): 3939, 2014.

ASCO—Loblaw DA, et al: Initial hormone management of androgen sensitive metastatic, recurrent, or progressive prostate cancer: 2007 update of an American Society of Clinical Oncology practice guideline. J Clin Oncol, 25(12) 1596, 2007.

Bader P, et al: Disease progression and survival of patients with positive lymph nodes after radical prostatectomy. Is there a chance of cure? J Urol, 169: 849, 2003.

Bhindi B, et al: Impact of radical prostatectomy on long term oncologic outcomes in a matched cohort of men with pathological node positive prostate cancer managed by castration. J Urol, 198: 86, 2017.

Briganti A, et al: Combination of adjuvant hormonal and radiation therapy significantly prolongs survival of patients with pT2-4 pN+ prostate cancer: results of a matched analysis. Eur Urol, 59(5): 832, 2011.

Da Pozzo LF, et al: Long term follow up of patients with prostate cancer and nodal metastasis treated by pelvic lymphadenectomy and radical prostatectomy: the positive impact of adjuvant radiotherapy. Eur Urol, 55(5): 1003, 2009.

Engel J, et al: Survival benefit of radical prostatectomy in lymph node positive patients with prostate cancer. Eur Urol, 57: 754, 2010.

ECOG 3886—Messing EM, et al: Immediate versus deferred androgen deprivation treatment in patients with node-positive prostate cancer after radical prostatectomy and pelvic lymphadenectomy. Lancet Oncol, 7(6): 472, 2006.

EORTC 30846—Schroder FH, et al: Early versus delayed endocrine treatment of T2-3 pN1-3 M0 prostate cancer without local treatment of the primary tumor: final results of the EORTC protocol 30846 after 13 years of follow up. Eur Urol, 55(1): 14, 2009.

EORTC 30891—Studer UE, et al: Immediate or deferred androgen deprivation for patients with prostate cancer not suitable for local treatment with curative intent: European Organization for Research and Treatment of Cancer (EORTC) trial 30891. J Clin Oncol. 24(12): 1868, 2006.

Ghavamian R, et al: Radical retropubic prostatectomy plus orchiectomy versus orchiectomy alone for pTxN+ prostate cancer. J Urol, 161: 1223, 1999.

Grimm MO, et al: Clinical outcome of patients with lymph node positive prostate cancer after radical prostatectomy versus androgen deprivation. Eur Urol, 41(6): 628, 2002.

James ND, et al: Failure free survival and radiotherapy in patients with newly diagnosed non metastatic prostate cancer: data from patients in the control arm of the STAMPEDE trial. JAMA Oncol, 2(3): 348, 2016.

Lin CC, et al: Androgen deprivation with or without radiation therapy for clinically node positive prostate cancer. J Natl Cancer Inst, 107(7): djv119, 2015 (https://doi.org/10.1093/jnci/djv119).

Schmeller N, et al: Early endocrine therapy versus radical prostatectomy combined with early endocrine therapy for stage D1 prostate cancer. Br J Urol, 79(2): 226, 1997.

Schumacher MC, et al: Good outcomes for patients with few lymph node metastases after radical retropubic prostatectomy. Eur Urol, 54: 344, 2008.

Seisen T, et al: Efficacy of local treatment in prostate cancer patients with clinically node positive disease at initial diagnosis. Eur Urol, 73(3): 452, 2018.

Steuber T, et al: Radical prostatectomy improves progression free and cancer specific survival in men with lymph node positive prostate cancer in the prostate specific antigen era: a confirmatory study. BJU Int, 107: 1755, 2010.

Touijer KA, et al: Long term outcomes of patients with lymph node metastasis treated with radical prostatectomy without adjuvant androgen deprivation therapy. Eur Urol, 65(1): 20, 2014.

Touijer KA, et al: Survival outcomes of men with lymph node positive prostate cancer after radical prostatectomy: a comparative analysis of different postoperative management strategies. Eur Urol, 73(6): 890, 2018.

Ventimiglia E, et al: A systematic review of the role of definitive local treatment in patients with clinically lymph node positive prostate cancer. Eur Urol Oncol, 2(3): 294, 2019.

Wong YN, et al: Role of androgen deprivation therapy for node positive prostate cancer. J Clin Oncol, 27(1): 100, 2009.

Zagars GK, et al: Addition of radiation therapy to androgen ablation improves outcome for subclinically node positive prostate cancer. Urology, 58(2): 233, 2001.

Neoadjuvant Androgen Deprivation with Radical Prostatectomy

Klotz LH, et al: Long term follow-up of a randomized trial of 0 versus 3 months of neoadjuvant androgen ablation before radical prostatectomy. J Urol, 170(3): 791, 2003.

Soloway MS, et al: Neoadjuvant androgen ablation before radical prostatectomy in cT2bNxM0 prostate cancer: 5 year results. J Urol: 167: 112, 2002.

Wieder JA, Soloway M: Neoadjuvant androgen deprivation before radical prostatectomy for prostate adenocarcinoma. Prostate Cancer: Principles and Practice. Ed. PW Kantoff, P Carroll, A D'Amico. Philadelphia: Lippincott Williams and Wilkins, 2002, pp 425-437.

Yee DS, et al: Long term follow up of 3 month neoadjuvant hormone therapy before radical prostatectomy in a randomized trial. BJU Int: 105(2): 185, 2010.

XRT after Radical Prostatectomy & Decipher RP test

ARO 96-02—Wiegel, et al: Adjuvant radiotherapy versus wait and see after radical prostatectomy: 10 year follow up of the ARO 96-02/AUO AP 09/95 Trial. Eur Urol, 66(2): 243, 2014.

ASTRO/AUA—Thompson IM, et al: Adjuvant and salvage radiotherapy after prostatectomy: ASTRO/AUA guideline. AUA Education and Research, Inc., 2019. (https://www.auanet.org/guidelines).

Den RB, at al: Genomic classifier identifies men with adverse pathology after radical prostatectomy who benefit from adjuvant radiation therapy. J Clin Oncol, 33(8): 944, 2015.

EORTC 22911—Bolla M, et al: Postoperative radiotherapy after radical prostatectomy for high risk prostate cancer: long term results of a randomized controlled trial (EORTC 22911). Lancet, 380(9858): 2018, 2012.

EORTC 22911—Van Cangh PJ et al: Adjuvant radiation therapy does not cause urinary incontinence after radical prostatectomy: results of a prospective randomized study. J Urol, 159: 164, 1998.

EORTC 22911—Van der Kwast TH, et al: Identification of patients with prostate cancer who benefit from immediate postoperative radiotherapy: EORTC 22911. J Clin Oncol, 25(27):4178, 2007.

FinnProstate—Hackman G, et al: Randomized trial of adjuvant radiotherapy following radical prostatectomy versus radical prostatectomy alone in prostate cancer patients with positive margins or extracapsular extension. Eur Urol, 76(5): 586, 2019.

Freedland SJ, et al: Utilization of a genomic classifier for prediction of metastasis following salvage radiation therapy after radical prostatectomy. Eur Urol, 70(4): 588, 2016.

GETUG-AFU 17—Sargos P, et al: Adjuvant radiotherapy versus early salvage radiotherapy plus short term androgen deprivation therapy in men with localised prostate cancer after radical prostatectomy (GETUG-AFU 17): a randomized phase 3 trial. Lancet Oncol, 21(10): 1341, 2020.

Porter CR, et al: Adjuvant radiotherapy after radical prostatectomy shows no ability to improve rates of overall and cancer specific survival in a matched case control study. BJU Int, 103: 597, 2008.

RADICALS—Parker CC, et al: Timing of radiotherapy after radical prostatectomy (RADICALS-RT): a randomised, controlled phase 3 trial. Lancet, 396: 1413, 2020.

RAVES—Kneebone A, et al: Adjuvant radiotherapy versus salvage radiotherapy following radical prostatectomy (TROG 08.03/ANZUP RAVES): a randomized, controlled, phase 3 non-inferiority trial. Lancet Oncol, 21(10): 1331, 2020.

Shipley WU, et al: Radiation with or without antiandrogen therapy in recurrent prostate cancer. N Engl J Med, 376(5): 417, 2017.

Sidhom, MA, et al: Post-prostatectomy radiation therapy: consensus guidelines of the Australian and New Zealand Radiation Oncology Genito-urinary Group. Radiother Oncol, 88: 10, 2008.

Spiotto MT, et al: Radiotherapy after prostatectomy: improved biochemical relapse free survival with whole pelvic compared with prostate bed only for high risk patients. Int J Radiat Oncol Biol Phys, 69(1): 54, 2007.

Spratt DE, et al: Individual patient level meta-analysis of the performance of the Decipher genomic classifier in high risk men after prostatectomy to predict development of metastatic disease. J Clin Oncol, 35(18): 1991, 2017.

Stephenson AJ, et al: Postoperative radiation therapy of pathologically advanced prostate cancer after radical prostatectomy. Eur Urol, 61: 443, 2012.

Stephensen AJ, et al: Predicting the outcome of salvage radiation therapy for recurrent prostate cancer after radical prostatectomy. J Clin Oncol, 25(15): 2035, 2007.

SWOG 8794—Swanson GP, et al: Predominant treatment failure in postprostatectomy patients is local: analysis of patterns of treatment failure in SWOG 8794. J Clin Oncol, 25(16): 2225, 2007.

SWOG 8794—Swanson GP, et al: The prognostic impact of seminal vesicle involvement found at prostatectomy and the effects of adjuvant radiation. J Urol, 180(6): 2453, 2008.

SWOG 8794—Thompson IM, et al: Adjuvant radiotherapy for pathological T3N0M0 prostate cancer significantly reduces risk of metastases and improves survival. Long term follow up of a randomized clinical trial. J Urol, 181(3): 956, 2009. [Update of JAMA, 296: 2329, 2006].

Trock BJ, et al: Prostate cancer specific survival following salvage radiotherapy vs. observation in men with biochemical recurrence after radical prostatectomy. JAMA 299(23): 2760, 2008.

Vale CL, et al: Adjuvant or early salvage radiotherapy for the treatment of localised and locally advanced prostate cancer: a prospectively planned systematic review and meta-analysis of aggregate data. Lancet, 396: 1422, 2020.

External Beam Radiation: General (also see Comparison of Treatments).

ASTRO/ASCO/AUA—Morgan SC, et al: Hypofractionated radiation therapy of localized prostate cancer: executive summary of the ASTRO, ASCO, and AUA evidence based guideline (2018). J Clin Oncol, 36(34): 3411, 2018 (also available at https://www.auanet.org/guidelines).

EORTC—Boehmer D, et al: Guidelines for primary radiotherapy of patients with prostate cancer. Radiother Oncol, 79(3): 259, 2006.

Gardner BG, et al: Late normal tissue sequela in the second decade after high dose radiation therapy with combined photons and conformal protons for locally advanced prostate cancer. J Urol, 167: 123, 2002.

HYPO-RT-PC—Widmark A, et al: Ultra-hypofractionated versus conventionally fractionated radiotherapy for prostate cancer: 5 year outcomes of the HYPO-RT-PC randomized non-inferiority phase 3 trial. Lancet, 394(10196): 385, 2019.

Ray M, et al: PSA nadir predicts biochemical and distant failures after external beam radiotherapy. Int J Radiat Oncol Biol Phys, 64(4): 1140, 2006.

External Beam Radiation: Higher versus Lower Dose (also see Comparison of Treatments)

Al-mamgani A, et al: Update of Dutch multicenter dose escalation trial of radiotherapy for localized prostate cancer. Int J Radiat Oncol Biol Phys, 72(4): 980, 2008 [update of Int J Radiat Oncol Biol Phys, 61(4): 1019, 2005]

Beckendorf V, et al: 70 Gy versus 80 Gy in localized prostate cancer: 5-year results of GETUG 06 Randomized trial. Int J Radiat Oncol Biol Phys, 80(4): 1056, 2011.

Dearnaley DP, et al: Escalated dose versus standard dose conformal radiotherapy in prostate cancer: results from MRC RT01. Lancet Oncol, 8(6): 475, 2007.

Kuban DA: Long term results of the MD Anderson randomized dose escalation trial for prostate cancer.Int J Radiat Oncol Biol Phys, 70(1): 67, 2008 [update of Int J Radiat Oncol Biol Phys, 53(5): 1097, 2002].

Syndikus I, et al: Late gastrointestinal toxicity after dose escalated conformal radiotherapy for early prostate cancer: results from the MRC RT01 trial. Int J Radiat Oncol Biol Phys, 77(3, part 2): 773, 2010.

Zietman AL, et al: Randomized trial comparing conventional dose with high dose conformal radiation therapy in early stage adenocarcinoma of the prostate. J Clin Oncol, 28: 1106, 2010.

Radiation Therapy: Hydrogel Spacer

Chao M, et al: Improving rectal dosimetry for patients with intermediate and high risk prostate cancer undergoing combined high dose rate brachytherapy and external beam radiotherapy with hydrogel space.
J Contemp Brachytherapy, 11(1): 8, 2019.

Mariados N, et al: Hydrogel spacer prospective multicenter randomized controlled pivotal trial: dosimetric and clinical effects of perirectal spacer application in men undergoing prostate image guided intensity modulated radiation therapy. Int J Radiat Oncol Biol Phys, 92(5): 971, 2015.

Pieczonka CM, et al: Hydrogel spacer application technique, patient tolerance and impact on prostate intensity modulated radiating therapy: results from a prospective randomized multicenter pivotal randomized controlled trial. Urology Practice, 3(2): 141, 2016.

Wu SY, et al: Improved rectal dosimetry with the use of SpaceOAR during high dose rate brachytherapy. Brachytherapy, 17(2): 259, 2018.

Brachytherapy (also see Comparison of Treatments)

ASCO/CCO—Chin J, et al: Brachytherapy for patients with prostate cancer: American Society of Clinical Oncology/Cancer Care Ontario joint guideline update. J Clin Oncol, 35(15): 1737, 2017.

Bice WS, et al: Recommendations for permanent prostate brachytherapy with ^{131}Cs: a consensus report from the Cesium Advisory Group. Brachytherapy, 7(4): 290, 2008.

D'Amico AV, et al: Risk of death from prostate cancer after brachytherapy alone or with radiation, androgen suppression therapy, or both in men with high risk disease. J Clin Oncol, 27(24): 3923, 2009.

Davis BJ, et al: American Brachytherapy Society consensus guidelines for transrectal ultrasound guided permanent prostate brachytherapy. Brachytherapy 11: 6, 2012 [update of Int J Radiat Oncol Biol Phys, 44(4): 789, 1999 and Int J Radiat Oncol Biol Phys, 47(2): 273, 2000].

Keyes M, et al: **American Brachytherapy Society Task Force Group report: use of androgen deprivation therapy with prostate brachytherapy - a systematic literature review. Brachytherapy, 16(2): 245, 2017.**

Merrick GS, et al: Androgen deprivation therapy does not impact cause specific or overall survival in high risk prostate cancer managed with brachytherapy and supplemental external beam. Int J Radiat Oncol Biol Phys, 68: 34, 2007.

Terek MD, et al: Identification of patients at increased risk for prolonged urinary retention following radioactive seed implantation. J Urol, 160: 1379, 1998.

Wang H, et al: Transperineal brachytherapy in patients with large prostate glands. Int J Cancer (Radiat Oncol Invest): 90, 199, 2000.

Yamada Y, et al: **American Brachytherapy Society consensus guidelines for high dose rate prostate brachytherapy. Brachytherapy 11: 20, 2012.**

PSA Bounce after Radiation

Ciezki JP, et al: PSA kinetics after prostate brachytherapy: PSA bounce phenomenon and its implications for PSA doubling time. Int J Radiat Oncol Biol Phys, 62(2): 512, 2006.

Critz FA, Williams WH, et al: Prostate specific antigen bounce after radioactive seed implantation followed by external beam radiation for prostate cancer. J Urol, 163: 1085, 2000.

Feigenberg SJ, et al: A prostate specific antigen bounce greater than 1.4 ng/ml is clinically significant after external beam radiotherapy for prostate cancer. Am J Clin Oncol, 29: 458, 2006.

Hanlon AL, et al: Patterns and fate of PSA bouncing following 3D-CRT. Int J Radiat Oncol Biol Phys, 50: 845, 2001.

Horwitz EM, et al: Biochemical and clinical significance of the post-treatment prostate specific antigen bounce for prostate cancer patients treated with external beam radiation therapy alone. Cancer, 107: 1496, 2006.

Patel C, et al: PSA bounce predicts early success in patients with permanent iodine-125 prostate implant. Urology 63(1): 110, 2004.

Rosser CJ, et al: Prostate specific antigen bounce after external beam radiation for clinically localized prostate cancer. J Urol, 168: 2001, 2002.

Hormone Therapy with Radiation

Crook J, et al: Final report of multicenter Canadian Phase III randomized trial of 3 versus 8 months of neoadjuvant androgen deprivation therapy before conventional dose radiotherapy for clinically localized prostate cancer. Int J Radiat Oncol Biol Phys, 73(2): 327, 2009.

D'Amico AV, et al: Androgen suppression and radiation vs. radiation alone for prostate cancer. JAMA, 299: 289, 2008 [Update of JAMA, 292: 821, 2004].

Efstathiou JA, et al: Cardiovascular mortality and duration of androgen deprivation for locally advanced prostate cancer: analysis of RTOG 92-02. Eur Urol, 54(4): 816, 2008.

EORTC 22863—Bolla M, et al: External irradiation with or without long term androgen suppression for prostate cancer with high metastatic risk: 10 year results. Lancet Oncol, 11: 1066, 2010.

EORTC 22961—Bolla M, et al: Duration of androgen suppression in the treatment of prostate cancer. N Engl J Med, 360(24): 2516, 2009.

GETUG-01—Pommier P, et al: Is there a role for pelvic irradiation in localized prostate adenocarcinoma? Preliminary results of GETUG-01. J Clin Oncol, 25(34): 5366, 2007.

Horwitz EM, Winter K, et al: Subset analysis of RTOG 85-31 and 86-10 indicates an advantage for long term vs. short term adjuvant hormones for patients with locally advanced non-metastatic prostate cancer treated with radiation therapy. Int J Radiat Oncol Biol Phys, 49: 947, 2001.

Jones CU, et al: Radiotherapy and short term androgen deprivation for localized prostate cancer. N Engl J Med, 365(2): 107, 2011.

Lawton CA, et al: Long-term treatment sequela after external beam irradiation with or without hormonal manipulation for adenocarcinoma of the prostate: analysis of RTOG 85-31,86-10, and 92-02. Int J Radiat Oncol Biol Phys, 70(2): 437, 2008.

RTOG 85-31—Pilepich MV et al: Androgen suppression adjuvant to definitive radiotherapy in prostate adenocarcinoma - long term results of phase III RTOG 85-31. Int J Radiat Oncol Biol Phys, 61: 1285, 2005.

RTOG 86-10—Roach M, et al: Short term neoadjuvant androgen deprivation therapy and external beam radiotherapy for locally advanced prostate cancer: long term results of RTOG 8610. J Clin Oncol, 26(4) 585, 2008.

RTOG 92-02—Lawton CAF, et al: Duration of androgen deprivation in locally advanced prostate cancer: long term update of NRG Oncology RTOG 9202. Int J Radiat Oncol Biol Phys, 92(2): 296, 2017 [update of J Clin Oncol, 26(15): 2497, 2008 & J Clin Oncol, 21: 3972, 2003].

RTOG 94-13—Lawton CA, et al: An update of the phase III trial comparing whole pelvic to prostate only radiotherapy and neoadjuvant to adjuvant total androgen suppression. Int J Radiat Oncol Biol Phys, 69(3): 646, 2007.

Comparison of Treatments: Non-randomized Trials

Abdel-Rahman O, et al: Outcomes of prostatectomy versus radiation therapy in the management of clinically localized prostate cancer patients within the PLCO trial. Clin Genitourin Cancer, 17(2): e329, 2019.

Amini A, et al: Survival outcomes of dose escalated external beam radiotherapy versus combined brachytherapy for intermediate and high risk prostate cancer using the National Cancer Database. J Urol, 195(5): 1453, 2016.

Aus G, et al: Survival in prostate carcinoma - outcomes from a prospective population based cohort of 8887 men with up to 15 years of follow up. Cancer, 103(5): 943, 2005.

Barry MJ, et al: Outcomes for men with clinically non-metastatic prostate carcinoma managed with radical prostatectomy, external beam radiotherapy, or expectant management. Cancer, 91(12): 2302, 2001.

Beesley LJ, et al: Individual and population comparisons of surgery and radiotherapy outcomes in prostate cancer using Bayesian multistate models. JAMA Network Open, 2(2): e187765, 2019.

Cooperberg MR et al: Comparative risk-adjusted mortality outcomes after primary surgery, radiotherapy, or androgen deprivation therapy for localized prostate cancer. Cancer, 116: 5226, 2010.

D'Amico AV, et al: Biochemical outcome after radical prostatectomy or external beam radiation therapy for patients with clinically localized prostate carcinoma in the PSA era. Cancer, 95(2): 281, 2002.

Huang H, et al: Evaluation of prostate cancer specific mortality with surgery versus radiation as primary therapy for localized high grade prostate cancer in men younger than 60 years. J Urol, 201: 120, 2019.

Liu L, et al: Long term survival after radical prostatectomy compared to other treatments in older men with local/regional prostate cancer. J Surg Oncol, 97(7): 583, 2008.

Muralidhar V, et al: Combined external beam radiation therapy and brachytherapy versus radical prostatectomy with adjuvant radiation therapy for Gleason 9-10 prostate cancer. J Urol, 202(5): 973, 2019.

Oake JD, et al: The comparative outcomes of radical prostatectomy versus radiotherapy for non-metastatic prostate cancer: a longitudinal population based analysis. J Urol, 2020 (https://doi.org/10.1097/JU.0000000000000805)

Pokala N, Menon M: Long term outcome following no definitive therapy, radiation and surgery for loco-regional prostate cancer in patients less than 50 years of age - analysis of 6906 patients. J Urol, 181(4, suppl): 60 (abstract 164), 2009.

Robinson D, et al: Prostate cancer death after radiotherapy or radical prostatectomy: a nationwide population based observational study. Eur Urol, 73: 502, 2018.

Shen X, et al: The impact of brachytherapy on prostate cancer specific mortality for definitive radiation therapy of high grade prostate cancer: a population based analysis. Int J Radiat Oncol Biol Phys, 83(4): 1154, 2012.

Tewari A, et al: Long term survival probability in men with clinically localized prostate cancer treated either conservatively or with definitive treatment (radiotherapy or radical prostatectomy). Urology, 68(6): 1268, 2006.

Wallis CJD, et al: Surgery versus radiotherapy for clinically localized prostate cancer: a systematic review and meta-analysis. Eur Urol, 70: 21, 2016.

Westover K, et al: Radical prostatectomy vs radiation therapy and androgen suppression therapy in high risk prostate cancer. BJU Int, 110: 1116, 2012.

Comparison of Treatments: Randomized Trials: XRT vs. Cryotherapy

Chin JL, et al: Extended follow up oncologic outcome of randomized trial between cryoablation and external beam therapy for locally advanced prostate cancer (T2c-T3b). J Urol, 188(4, part 1): 1170, 2012 [Update of Prostate Cancer Prostatic Dis, 11(1): 40, 2008].

Donnelly BJ, et al: A randomized trial of external beam radiotherapy versus cryoablation in patients with localized prostate cancer. Cancer, 116: 323, 2010.

Robinson JW, et al: A randomized trial of external beam radiotherapy versus cryoablation in patients with localized prostate cancer. Cancer, 115: 4695, 2009.

Comparison of Treatments: Randomized Trials: RP vs. XRT

Akakura K, et al: A randomized trial comparing radical prostatectomy plus endocrine therapy versus external beam radiotherapy plus endocrine therapy for locally advanced prostate cancer: results at median follow up of 102 months. Jpn J Clin Oncol, 36(12): 789, 2006.

Lennernas B, et al: Radical prostatectomy versus high dose irradiation in localized/locally advanced prostate cancer: a Swedish multicenter randomized trial with patient reported outcomes. Acta Oncologica, 54: 875, 2015.

Paulson DF, et al: Radical surgery versus radiotherapy for adenocarcinoma of the prostate. J Urol, 128: 502, 1982.

PROTECT—Donovan JL, et al: Patient reported outcomes after monitoring, surgery, or radiotherapy for prostate cancer. N Engl J Med, 375(15): 1425, 2016.

PROTECT—Hamdy FC, et al: 10-year outcomes after monitoring, surgery, or radiotherapy for localized prostate cancer. N Engl J Med, 375(15): 1425, 2016.

PROTECT—Neal DE, et al: Ten year mortality, disease progression, and treatment related side effects in men with localized prostate cancer from the ProtecT randomised controlled trial according to treatment received. Eur Urol, 77: 320, 2020.

Stranne J, et al: SPCG-15: a prospective randomized study comparing primary radical prostatectomy and primary radiotherapy plus androgen deprivation therapy for locally advanced prostate cancer. Scand J Urol, 52(5-6): 313, 2018.

Comparison of Treatments: Randomized Trials: RP vs. Brachytherapy

Crook JM, et al: Comparison of health related quality of life 5 years after SPIRIT: surgical prostatectomy versus interstitial radiation intervention trial. J Clin Oncol, 29(4): 362, 2011.

Giberti C, et al: Radical prostatectomy versus brachytherapy for low-risk prostate cancer: a prospective study. World J Urol, 27: 607, 2009.

Giberti C, et al: Robotic prostatectomy versus brachytherapy for the treatment of low risk prostate cancer. Can J Urol, 24(2): 8728, 2017.

Comparison of Treatments: Randomized Trials: Treatment vs. Surveillance

Iversen P, et al: Radical prostatectomy versus expectant treatment for early carcinoma of the prostate: twenty three year follow up of a prospective randomized study. Scan J Urol Nephrol Suppl, 172: 65, 1995.

PIVOT trial—Wilt TJ et al: Radical prostatectomy or observation for clinically localized prostate cancer: extended follow up of the Prostate Cancer Intervention Versus Observation Trial. Eur Urology, 77(6): 713, 2020.

PROTECT—Donovan JL, et al: Patient reported outcomes after monitoring, surgery, or radiotherapy for prostate cancer. N Engl J Med, 375(15): 1425, 2016.

PROTECT—Hamdy FC, et al: 10-year outcomes after monitoring, surgery, or radiotherapy for localized prostate cancer. N Engl J Med, 375(15): 1425, 2016.

PROTECT—Neal DE, et al: Ten year mortality, disease progression, and treatment related side effects in men with localized prostate cancer from the ProtecT randomised controlled trial according to treatment received. Eur Urol, 77: 320, 2020.

SPCG-4—Bill-Axelson A, et al: Radical prostatectomy or watchful waiting in prostate cancer – 29 year follow up. N Engl J Med, 379: 2319, 2018.

SPCG-4—Johansson E, et al: Long term quality of life outcomes after radical prostatectomy or watchful waiting. Lancet Oncol, 12(9): 891, 2011.

VACURG—Graversen PH, et al: Radical prostatectomy versus expectant primary treatment in stages I and II prostate cancer: a fifteen year follow up. Urology, 36(6): 493, 1990.

Widmark A, et al: Prospective randomized trial comparing external beam radiotherapy versus watchful waiting in early prostate cancer. Late breaking abstract presented at 53rd Annual ASTRO meeting Oct, 2011. (http://oncolink.org/print/pdf/14196?print_14196.pdf)

Comparison of Treatments: Randomized Trials: XRT + Brachytherapy vs. XRT

Dayes IS, et al: Long term results of a randomized trial comparing Iridium implant plus external beam radiation therapy with external beam radiation therapy alone in node negative locally advanced cancer of the prostate. Int J Radiat Oncol Biol Phys, 99(1): 90, 2017.

Hoskin PJ, et al: Randomized trial of external beam radiotherapy alone or combined with high dose rate brachytherapy boost for localized prostate cancer. Radiother Oncol, 103: 217, 2012.

Morris WJ, et al: Androgen suppression combine with elective nodal and dose escalated radiation therapy (the ASCENDE-RT trial): An analysis of survival endpoints for a randomized trial comparing a low dose rate brachytherapy boost to a dose escalated external beam boost for high and intermediate risk prostate cancer. Int J Radiat Oncol Biol Phys, 98(2): 275, 2017.

RTOG 0232—Prestidge BR, et al: Initial Report of NRG Oncology/RTOG 0232: A Phase 3 Study Comparing Combined External Beam Radiation and Transperineal Interstitial Permanent Brachytherapy With Brachytherapy Alone for Selected Patients With Intermediate-Risk Prostatic Carcinoma. Int J Radiat Oncol Biol Phys, 96(2, supplement): S4(#7), 2016.

Comparison of Treatments: Randomized Trials: XRT + ADT vs. ADT

Warde P, et al: Combined androgen deprivation therapy and radiation therapy for locally advanced prostate cancer. Lancet, 378: 2104, 2011.

SPCG-7—Fossa SD, et al: Ten and 15 year prostate cancer specific mortality in patients with non-metastatic locally advanced or aggressive intermediate prostate cancer, randomized to lifelong endocrine treatment alone or combined with radiotherapy: final results of the Scandinavian Prostate Cancer Gourp-7. Eur Urol, 70(4): 684, 2016.

Recurrence - Imaging to Detect Metastasis

ASCO—Trabulsi EJ, et al: Optimum imaging strategies for advanced prostate cancer: ASCO guideline. J Clin Oncol, 38(17): 1963, 2020.

Cher ML, et al: Limited role of radionuclide bone scintigraphy in patients with prostate specific antigen elevations after radical prostatectomy. J Urol, 160: 1387, 1998.

Dotan ZA, et al: Pattern of prostate specific antigen failure dictates the probability of a positive bone scan in patients with an increasing PSA after radical prostatectomy. J Clin Oncol, 23(9): 1962, 2005.

Moreira DM et al: Predicting bone scan positivity after biochemical recurrence following radical prostatectomy in both hormone naive men and patients receiving androgen deprivation therapy: the results from the SEARCH database. Prostate Cancer Prostatic Dis, 17: 91, 2014.

Okotie OT, Aronson WJ, Wieder JA, et al: Predictors of metastatic disease among men with biochemical failure following radical prostatectomy. J Urol, 171: 2260, 2004.

Recurrence and Salvage Therapy (see also XRT after Radical Prostatectomy)

ASTRO Consensus Panel: Consensus statements on radiation therapy of prostate cancer: guidelines for prostate re-biopsy after radiation and for radiation therapy with rising prostate-specific antigen levels after radical prostatectomy. J Clin Oncol, 17: 1155, 1999.

Amling CL, et al: Defining prostate specific antigen progression after radical prostatectomy: What is the appropriate cut point? J Urol, 165: 1146, 2001.

Chade DC, et al: Cancer control and functional outcomes of salvage radical prostatectomy for radiation recurrent prostate cancer: a systematic review of the literature. Eur Urol, 61(5): 961, 2012.

Han M, et al: Biochemical (prostate specific antigen) recurrence probability following radical prostatectomy for clinically localized prostate cancer. J Urol, 169: 517, 2003.

Kattan MW, et al: Pretreatment nomogram for predicting freedom from recurrence after permanent prostate brachytherapy in prostate cancer. Urology, 58(3): 393, 2001.

Neulander EZ, Soloway MS: Failure after radical prostatectomy. Urology, 61: 30, 2003.

Pound CR, Partin AW, et al: Natural history of progression after PSA elevation following radical prostatectomy. JAMA, 281: 1591, 1999.

Roach M, et al: Defining biochemical failure following radiotherapy with or without hormonal therapy in men with clinically localized prostate cancer: recommendations of the RTOG-ASTRO Phoenix consensus conference. Int J Radiat Oncol Biol Phys, 65(4): 965, 2006.

Stephenson AJ, et al: Preoperative nomogram predicting the 10-year probability of prostate cancer recurrence after radical prostatectomy. J Natl Cancer Inst, 98(10), 715, 2006.

Stephenson AJ, et al: Postoperative nomogram predicting the 10-year probability of prostate cancer recurrence after radical prostatectomy. J Clin Oncol, 23(28): 7005, 2005.

Advanced/Metastatic Prostate Cancer: Castration Naive

ASCO—Morris MJ, et al: Optimizing anticancer therapy in metastatic non castrate resistant prostate cancer: an American Society of Clinical Oncology clinical practice guideline. J Clin Oncol, 36(15): 1521, 2018.

STAMPEDE—Parker CC, et al: Radiotherapy to the primary tumor for newly diagnosed, metastatic prostate cancer (STAMPEDE): a randomised controlled phase 3 trial. Lancet, 392: 2353, 2018.

Castration and Combined Androgen Deprivation

Albertsen PC, et al: Cardiovascular morbidity associated with gonadotropin releasing hormone agonists and an antagonist. Eur Urol, 65(3): 565, 2014.

Duchesne GM, et al: Timing of androgen deprivation therapy in patients with prostate cancer with a rising PSA (TROG 03.06 and VCOG PR 01-03 [TOAD]): a randomized multicenter non-blinded phase 3 trial. Lancet Oncol, 17(6): 727, 2016.

Mahal BA, et al: Early versus delayed initiation of salvage androgen deprivation therapy and risk of prostate cancer specific mortality. J Natl Compr Canc Netw, 16(6): 727, 2018.

Margel D, et al: Cardiovascular morbidity in a randomized trial comparing GnRH agonist and GnRH antagonist among patients with advanced prostate cancer and preexisting cardiovascular disease. J Urol, 202(6): 1199, 2019.

Prostate Cancer Trialists' Collaborative Group: Maximum androgen blockade in advanced prostate cancer: an overview on the randomized trials. Lancet, 355: 1491, 2000.

Saad F, et al: Testosterone breakthrough rates during androgen deprivation therapy for castration sensitive prostate cancer. J Urol, 204(3): 416, 2020.

Samson DJ, et al: Systematic review and meta-analysis of monotherapy compared with combined androgen blockade for patients with advanced prostate cancer. Cancer, 95: 361, 2002.

Schroder FH, et al: Early versus delayed endocrine treatment of T2-3 pN1-3 M0 prostate cancer without local treatment of the primary tumor: final results of the EORTC protocol 30846 after 13 years of follow up. Eur Urol, 55(1): 14, 2009.

Scailteux LM, et al: Androgen deprivation therapy and cardiovascular risk: no meaningful difference between GnRH antagonist and agonist - a nationwide population based cohort study based on 2010-2013 French health insurance data. Eur J Cancer, 77: 99, 2017.

Studer UE, et al: Immediate versus deferred hormonal treatment for patients with prostate cancer who are not suitable for curative local treatment: results of the randomized trial SAKK 08/88. J Clin Oncol, 22(20): 4109, 2004.

Studer UE, et al: Using PSA to guide timing of androgen deprivation in patients with T0-4 N0-2 M0 prostate cancer not suitable for local curative treatment (EORTC 30891). Eur Urol, 53: 941, 2008.

Sun M, et al: Comparison of gonadotropin releasing hormone agonists and orchiectomy: effects of androgen deprivation therapy. JAMA Oncol, 2(4): 500, 2016.

Taylor CD, et al: Importance of continued testicular suppression in hormone refractory prostate cancer. J Clin Oncol, 11(11): 2167, 1993.

Intermittent Androgen Deprivation

Botrel TE, et al: Intermittent versus continuous androgen deprivation for locally advanced recurrent or metastatic prostate cancer: a systematic review and meta-analysis. BMC Urol, 14: 9, 2014.

Conti PD, et al: Intermittent versus continuous androgen suppression for prostate cancer. Cochrane Database Syst Rev, Issue 4: CD005009, 2007.

Crook JM, et al: Intermittent androgen suppression for rising PSA level after radiotherapy. N Engl J Med, 367: 895, 2012.

de Leval J, et al: Intermittent versus continuous total androgen blockade in the treatment of patients with advanced hormone-naive prostate cancer. Clin Prostate Cancer, 1(3): 163, 2002.

Dong Z, et al: Intermittent hormone therapy versus continuous hormone therapy for locally advanced prostate cancer: a meta-analysis. Aging Male, 18(4): 233, 2015.

Hershman DL, et al: Averse health events following intermittent and continuous androgen deprivation in patients with metastatic prostate cancer. JAMA Oncol, 2: 453, 2016.

Hussain M, et al: Intermittent versus continuous androgen deprivation in prostate cancer. N Engl J Med, 368(14): 1314, 2013.

Magnan S, et al: Intermittent vs continuous androgen deprivation therapy for prostate cancer: a systematic review and meta-analysis. JAMA Oncol, 1(9): 1261, 2015.

Miller K, et al: Randomized prospective study of intermittent versus continuous androgen suppression in advanced prostate cancer. J Clin Oncol, 25 (18, suppl): abstract # 5015, 2007.

Mottet N, et al: Intermittent hormonal therapy in the treatment of metastatic prostate cancer: a randomized trial. BJU Int, 110: 1262, 2012.

Niraula S, et al: Treatment of prostate cancer with intermittent versus continuous androgen deprivation: a systematic review of randomized trials. J Clin Oncol, 31(16): 2029, 2013.

Organ M, et al: Intermittent LHRH therapy in the management of castration resistant prostate cancer: results of a multi-institutional randomized prospective clinical trial. Am J Clin Oncol, 36(6): 601, 2013.

SEUG 9401—Calais da Silva FEC, et al: Intermittent androgen deprivation for locally advanced and metastatic prostate cancer: results from a randomized phase 3 study of the South European Uroncological Group. Eur Urol, 55: 1269, 2009.

Salonen AJ, et al: The Finn Prostate Study VII: Intermittent versus continuous androgen deprivation in patients with advanced prostate cancer. J Urol, 187: 2074, 2012.

Schulman C, et al: Intermittent versus continuous androgen deprivation therapy in patients with relapsing or locally advanced prostate cancer: a phase 3b randomized study (ICLAND). Eur Urol, 69(4): 720, 2016.

Tsai HT, et al: Efficacy of intermittent androgen deprivation therapy vs conventional continuous androgen deprivation therapy for advanced prostate cancer. Urology, 82(2): 327, 2013.

Tunn UW, et al: Intermittent androgen deprivation in patients with PSA relapse after radical prostatectomy. J Urol, 177(4, suppl): 201 (abstract #600), 2007.

Castration Level of Testosterone

Morote J, et al: Refining clinically significant castration levels in patients with prostate cancer receiving continuous androgen deprivation therapy. J Urol, 178(4): 1290, 2007.

Oefelein MG, et al: Reassessment of the definition of castrate levels of testosterone: implications for clinical decision making. Urology, 56: 1021, 2000.

Tombal B: Appropriate castration with luteinizing hormone releasing hormone agonist: what is the optimal level of testosterone. Eur Urol, 4 (suppl): 14, 2005.

Castration Resistant Prostate Cancer (CRPC)

ASCO/CCO—Basch E, et al: Systemic therapy in men with metastatic castration resistant prostate cancer: American Society of Clinical Oncology and Cancer Care Ontario clinical practice guideline. J Clin Oncol, 32(30): 2014.

AUA—Cookson MS, et al: Castration resistant prostate cancer: AUA guideline. AUA Education and Research, Inc., 2014. (www.auanet.org).

Sciarra A, et al: Androgen receptor variant 7 (AR-V7) in sequencing therapeutic agents for castration resistant prostate cancer: a critical review. Medicine (Baltimore), 98(19): e15608, 2019.

SUO—Chang SS, et al: Society of Urologic Oncology position statement: redefining the management of hormone refractory prostate carcinoma. Cancer, 103(1): 11, 2004.

Taylor CD, et al: Importance of continued testicular suppression in hormone refractory prostate cancer. J Clin Oncol, 11(11): 2167, 1993.

Nonsteroidal Antiandrogens

Armstrong AJ, et al: ARCHES: a randomized phase III study of androgen deprivation therapy with enzalutamide or placebo in men with metastatic hormone sensitive prostate cancer. J Clin Oncol, 37: 2974, 2019.

Beer TM, et al: Enzalutamide in metastatic prostate cancer before chemotherapy. N Engl J Med, 371(5): 424, 2014.

Beer TM, et al: Enzalutamide in men with chemotherapy naive metastatic castration resistant prostate cancer: extended analysis of the phase 3 PREVAIL study. Eur Urol, 71(2): 151, 2017.

Chi KN, et al: Apalutamide in patients with metastatic castration sensitive prostate cancer: final survival analysis of the randomized double blind phase III TITAN study. J Clin Oncol: e-published ahead of print (https://ascopubs.org/doi/abs/10.1200/JCO.20.03488) [Update of N Engl J Med, 381(1): 13, 2019].

Davis ID, et al: Enzalutamide with standard first line therapy in metastatic prostate cancer. N Engl J Med, 381: 121, 2019.

Fizazi K, et al: Darolutamide in non metastatic castration resistant prostate cancer. N Engl J Med, 380: 1235, 2019.

Fizazi K, et al: Nonmetastatic, castration resistant prostate cancer and survival with darolutamide. N Engl J Med, 383: 1040, 2020.

Fizazi K, et al: Effect of enzalutamide on time to first skeletal related event, pain, and quality of life in men with castration resistant prostate cancer: results from the randomized phase 3 AFFIRM trial. Lancet Oncol, 15: 1147, 2014.

Hussain M, et al: Enzalutamide in men with non metastatic, castration resistant prostate cancer. N Engl J Med, 378(26): 2465, 2018.

Iversen P, et al: Bicalutamide monotherapy compared with castration in patients with non-metastatic locally advanced prostate cancer: 6.3 years of follow up. J Urol, 164: 1579, 2000.

Scher HI, et al: Increased survival with enzalutamide in prostate cancer after chemotherapy. N Engl J Med, 367(13): 1187, 2012.

Seidenfeld J, et al: Single-therapy androgen suppression in men with advanced prostate cancer: a systematic review and meta-analysis: Ann Intern Med, 132: 566, 2000.

Small EJ, et al: Apalutamide and overall survival in non-metastatic castration resistant prostate cancer. Ann Oncol, 30(11): 1813, 2019.

Smith MR, et al: Apalutamide treatment and metastasis free survival in prostate cancer. N Engl J Med, 378(15): 1408, 2018.

Smith MR, et al: Apalutamide and over survival in prostate cancer. Eur Urol, 79(1): 150, 2021.

Smith MR, et al: Bicalutamide monotherapy versus leuprolide monotherapy for prostate cancer: effects on bone mineral density and body composition. J Clin Oncol, 22(13): 2546, 2004.

Sternberg CN, et al: Enzalutamide and survival in non-metastatic castration resistant prostate cancer. N Engl J Med, 382: 2917, 2020.

Suzuki H, et al: Alternative nonsteroidal antiandrogen therapy for advanced prostate cancer that relapsed after initial maximum androgen blockade. J Urol, 180(3): 921,2008.

Sydes MR, et al: Adding abiraterone or docetaxel to long term hormone therapy for prostate cancer: directly randomized data from the STAMPEDE multi-arm multi-stage platform protocol. Ann Oncol, 29: 1235, 2018.

Antiandrogen Withdrawal

Sartor AO, et al: Antiandrogen withdrawal in castrate refractory prostate cancer: (SWOG 9426). Cancer, 112(11): 2393, 2008.

Schellhammer PF, Venner P, Haas GP, et al: Prostate specific antigen decreases after withdrawal of antiandrogen therapy with bicalutamide or flutamide in patients receiving combined androgen blockade. J Urol, 157: 1731, 1997.

Androgen Synthesis Inhibitors

de Bono JS, et al: Abiraterone and increased survival in metastatic prostate cancer. N Engl J Med, 364: 1995, 2011.

Fizazi K, et al: Abiraterone acetate plus prednisone in patients with newly diagnosed high risk metastatic castration sensitive prostate cancer (LATITUDE): final overall survival analysis of a randomized double blind phase 3 trial. Lancet Oncol, 20(5): 686, 2019.

Pont A: Long-term experience with high dose ketoconazole therapy in patients with D2 prostate carcinoma. J Urol, 137: 902, 1987.

Ryan CJ, et al: Abiraterone in metastatic prostate cancer without previous chemotherapy. N Engl J Med, 368(2): 138, 2013.

Ryan CJ, et al: Abiraterone acetate plus prednisone versus placebo plus prednisone in chemotherapy naive men with metastatic castration resistant prostate cancer. Lancet Oncol, 16(2): 152, 2015.

Trachtenberg J: Ketoconazole therapy in advanced prostate cancer. J Urol, 132: 61, 1984.

Chemotherapy

Bahl A, et al: Impact of cabazitaxel on 2-year survival and palliation of tumor related pain in men with metastatic castration resistant prostate cancer treated in the TROPIC trial. Ann Oncol, 24(9): 2402, 2013.

Berry W, et al: Phase III study of mitoxantrone plus low dose prednisone versus low dose prednisone alone in patients with asymptomatic hormone refractory prostate cancer. J Urol, 168(6): 2439, 2002.

de Bono JS, et al: Prednisone plus cabazitaxel or mitoxantrone for metastatic castration resistant prostate cancer progressing after docetaxel treatment. Lancet, 376: 1147, 2010.

Gravis G, et al: Androgen deprivation therapy alone or with docetaxel in non castrate metastatic prostate cancer (GETUG-AFU 15): a randomized open label phase 3 trial. Lancet Oncol, 14(2): 149, 2013.

James ND, et al: Additions of docetaxel, zoledronic acid, or both to first line long term hormone therapy in prostate cancer (STAMPEDE): survival results from an adaptive multi arm multistage platform randomized controlled trial. Lancet, 387: 1163, 2016.

Kantoff PW, et al: Hydrocortisone with or without mitoxantrone in men with hormone-refractory prostate cancer: results of the Cancer and Leukemia Group B 9182 study. J Clin Oncol, 17(8): 2506, 1999.

Kyriakopoulos CE, et al: Chemohormonal therapy in metastatic hormone sensitive prostate cancer: long term survival analysis of the randomized phase III E3805 CHARTED trial. J Clin Oncol, 36(11): 1080, 2018.

Sweeney CJ, et al: Chemohormonal therapy in metastatic hormone sensitive prostate cancer. N Engl J Med, 373: 737, 2015.

SWOG 9916—Petrylak DP, et al: Docetaxel and estramustine compared with mitoxantrone and prednisone for advanced refractory prostate cancer. N Engl J Med, 351: 1513, 2004.

SWOG 9916—Berry DL, et al: Quality of life and pain in advanced stage prostate cancer: a SWOG randomized trial comparing docetaxel and estramustine to mitoxantrone and prednisone. J Clin Oncol, 24: 2828, 2006.

Tannock IF, et al: Chemotherapy with mitoxantrone plus prednisone or prednisone alone for symptomatic hormone-resistant prostate cancer. J Clin Oncol, 14(6): 1756, 1996.

TAX 327—Berthold DR, et al: Docetaxel plus prednisone or mitoxantrone plus prednisone for advanced prostate cancer: updated survival in the TAX 327 study. J Clin Oncol, 26: 242, 2008.

Sydes MR, et al: Adding abiraterone or docetaxel to long term hormone therapy for prostate cancer: directly randomized data from the STAMPEDE multi-arm multi-stage platform protocol. Ann Oncol, 29: 1235, 2018.

Immunotherapy
Higano CS, et al: Real world outcomes of sipuleucel-T treatment in PROCEED, a prospective registry of men with metastatic prostate castration resistant prostate cancer. Cancer, 125: 4172, 2019.
Kantoff PW, et al: Sipuleucel-T immunotherapy for castration resistant prostate cancer. N Engl J Med, 363: 411, 2010.
Schellhammer PF, et al: Lower baseline prostate specific antigen is associated with a greater overall survival benefit from sipuleucel-T in the immunotherapy for prostate adenocarcinoma treatment (IMPACT) trial. Urology, 81(6): 1297, 2013.

PARP Inhibitors
Abida W, et al: Preliminary results from the TRITON2 study rucaparib in patients with DNA damage repair (DDR) deficient metastatic castration resistant prostate cancer (mCRPC): updated analysis. Ann Oncol, 30(5 suppl), v327 (abstract 846PD), 2019.
(https://doi.org/10.1093/annonc/mdz248.003).
de Bono J, et al: Olaparib for metastatic castration resistant prostate cancer. N Engl J Med, 382(22): 2091, 2020.

Bone Metastasis and SREs
Abraham JL, ACP-ASIM End-of-Life Care Consensus Panel: Management of pain and spinal cord compression in patients with advanced cancer. Ann Intern Med, 131: 37, 1999.
Fizazi K, et al: Denosumab versus zoledronic acid for the treatment of bone metastases in men with castration resistant prostate cancer: a randomized, double blind study. Lancet 377(9768): 813, 2011.
Hahn SM, et al: Oncologic emergencies. Cecil Textbook of Medicine. 19th ed, Ed. Wyngaarden, et al. Philadelphia: W. B. Sanders, 1992, pp 1067-1071.
Janjan N, et al: Therapeutic guidelines for the treatment of bone metastasis: a report from the American College of Radiology Appropriateness Criteria Expert Panel on Radiation Oncology. J Palliat Med, 12(5): 417, 2009.
Parker C, et al: Alpha emitter Radium-223 and survival in metastatic prostate cancer. N Engl J Med, 369(3): 213, 2013.
Saad F, Gleason DM, et al: A randomized, placebo controlled trial of zoledronic acid in patients with hormone refractory metastatic prostate cancer. J Natl Cancer Inst, 94(19): 1458, 2002.
Saad F, et al: Long term efficacy of zoledronic acid for the prevention of skeletal complications in patients with metastatic hormone refractory prostate cancer. J Natl Cancer Inst, 96(11): 879, 2004.
Smith MR, et al: Denosumab and bone metastasis free survival in men with castration resistant prostate cancer. Lancet, 379(9810): 39, 2012.
van der Poel, HG: Radionuclide treatment in metastasized prostate cancer. EAU-EBU Update series, 5: 113, 2007.

Diet Modification
MEAL trial—Parsons JK, et al: Effect of a behavioral intervention to increase vegetable consumption on cancer progression among men with early stage prostate cancer: the MEAL randomized clinical trial. JAMA, 323(2): 140, 2020.
Moyad MA, Pienta KJ: Complementary medicine for prostatic diseases: a primer for clinicians. Urology, 59 (suppl 4a), 2002.

PSA Kinetics/PSA Doubling time/PSA Velocity in Prostate Cancer
For references, see page 302.

ANDROGEN DEPRIVATION

Androgens
1. Sources of androgens in men
   a. Testes—produce 90-95% of circulating androgens in the form of testosterone. Luteinizing hormone (LH) stimulates testosterone production in the testicular Leydig cells.
   b. Adrenal glands—produce ≤ 10% of circulating androgens in the form of androstenedione and dehydroepiandrosterone (DHEA).
2. In most reproductive tissues, testosterone is converted by 5α-reductase to dihydrotestosterone (DHT), which has a higher affinity for the androgen receptor than testosterone.

Prolactin
1. Prolactin decreases testosterone by inhibiting gonadotropin releasing hormone (GnRH) secretion from the hypothalamus. Even though prolactin reduces testosterone, it may accelerate the growth of prostate cancer by directly stimulating prostate tissue.
2. Conditions that increase prolactin—prolactinoma, hypothyroidism, stress, chronic renal failure, and certain medications (e.g. phenothiazines).

Definitions
1. Androgen deprivation therapy (ADT)—ADT can be defined as any therapy that reduces the ability of androgens to activate the androgen receptor; however, ADT usually refers specifically to castration with or without concomitant use of a first generation antiandrogen.
2. Castration—defined as treatment with surgical castration (bilateral orchiectomy) or medical castration (LHRH agonist or GnRH antagonist). Medical castration is reversible, whereas orchiectomy is irreversible. LHRH agonists, GnRH antagonists, and orchiectomy are equally effective in controlling prostate cancer. There is limited evidence that orchiectomy and GnRH antagonists are safer than LHRH agonists because they are associated with fewer cardiac events, especially in men with known cardiovascular disease.
3. Combined androgen blockade—defined as treatment with castration and a first generation nonsteroidal antiandrogen. Combined androgen blockade provides limited benefit over castration alone (see page 236).
4. Monotherapy—defined as the use of only a one medication for ADT.
5. Neoadjuvant—before curative therapy.
6. Adjuvant—after curative therapy.
7. Castration naive—defined as no previous treatment with castration.
8. Castration sensitive prostate cancer (CSPC)—defined as prostate cancer that has not been previously treated with castration (castration naive) or that is responding to castration (i.e. the PSA and cancer volume are not increasing). CSPC is also called "hormone sensitive prostate cancer."
9. Castration resistant prostate cancer (CRPC)—defined as prostate cancer that is no longer responding to castration (i.e. PSA and/or cancer volume is increasing) even though serum testosterone is < 50 ng/dl.

Summary of Androgen Deprivation
1. Surgical
   a. Bilateral orchiectomy
   b. Hypophysectomy
   c. Bilateral adrenalectomy
2. Pharmacological
   a. Estrogens
   b. Progestins
   c. Prolactin antagonists
   d. LHRH agonists
   e. GnRH antagonists
   f. Inhibitors of androgen synthesis
   g. Anti-androgens—non-steroidal or steroidal
   h. 5α-reductase inhibitors

Surgical Androgen Deprivation

Bilateral Orchiectomy (Surgical Castration)
1. Orchiectomy is the gold standard for androgen deprivation. Castrate testosterone levels occur 2-12 hours postoperatively.
2. Mechanism of action—removes the testis as a source of testosterone.
3. Orchiectomy eliminates ≥ 90% of circulating androgens (the remaining androgens arise from the adrenal gland).
4. Advantages—low cost, does not require compliance with medication to maintain castration.
5. *Orchiectomy does not cause a testosterone flare or microsurges.*
6. Side effects—see page 293.

Hypophysectomy (Ablation of the Pituitary)
1. Mechanism of action—the source of LH and ACTH is removed; therefore, testicular *and* adrenal androgen production is inhibited.
2. Not used anymore—pharmaceuticals are now used instead.

Bilateral Adrenalectomy
1. Mechanism of action—removes the adrenals as a source of androgen.
2. Not used anymore—pharmaceuticals are now used instead.

Pharmacological Androgen Deprivation

Estrogens
1. Mechanism of action—inhibits the hypothalamic-pituitary axis, which decreases luteinizing hormone (LH) secretion and, therefore, decreases testosterone production. *Estrogens increase serum prolactin, but they do not cause a testosterone flare.* Testosterone reaches castrate levels in approximately 10-14 days (range =10-60 days).
2. Examples—diethylstilbestrol (DES), Premarin®, estradiol.
3. Side effects—embolic (pulmonary embolism, deep venous thrombosis, stroke), cardiac (myocardial infarction), peripheral edema, painful gynecomastia, erectile dysfunction, weight gain, and altered fat distribution. *Estrogens do not cause hot flashes or osteoporosis.*
4. When using estrogens, consider prescribing an anticoagulant (such as aspirin or coumadin) to reduce the potential for embolic complications.
5. DES 3-5 mg/day has significant cardiovascular risk. DES 1 mg/day delays the progression of advanced prostate cancer, but has a much lower cardiovascular risk. However, castrate testosterone levels are not reliably reached with 1 mg per day. DES may also be given IV.

Progestins

1. Mechanism of action—inhibits the hypothalamic-pituitary axis, which decreases LH secretion and, therefore, decreases testosterone production. Progestins do *not* increase serum prolactin.
2. Progestins cause a transient reduction in serum testosterone, but then there is a gradual rise in testosterone (i.e. there is an *escape phenomenon*). Thus, they are usually not used alone to treat prostate cancer.
3. These agents do not cause hot flashes.
4. Examples—megestrol acetate (Megace®), cyproterone acetate (cyproterone is not available in the United States).

Luteinizing Hormone Releasing Hormone (LHRH) Agonists

1. Mechanism of action—stimulation of LHRH receptors in the pituitary produces an initial increase in LH and FSH, which causes an initial increase in testosterone ("testosterone flare", see page 292). Further LHRH agonism suppresses LH and FSH secretion, resulting in a decrease in testosterone. Testosterone reaches castrate levels within 30 days. Stimulation of the LHRH receptor with subsequent doses causes a testosterone microsurge in approximately 10% of cases.
2. Examples—leuprolide (Lupron®, Eligard™), histrelin (Vantas™), goserelin (Zoladex®), triptorelin (Trelstar®). For dosing, see page 746.
3. Testosterone flare can make tumor-related symptoms worse. See page 292.
4. Side effects—see Morbidity From Medical or Surgical Castration, page 293.
5. When stopping an LHRH agonist, the time it takes for testosterone to normalize is longer in men who are older and in men who undergo a long duration of LHRH agonist therapy. In men who stop an LHRH agonist after 2 years of use, the testosterone returns to normal or to baseline in only 72% of men by 3 years after the last dose (with a median time to recovery of 22 months).

Gonadotropin Releasing Hormone (GnRH) Antagonists

1. Mechanism of action—blocking GnRH receptors in the pituitary decreases LH, FSH, and testosterone. *GnRH antagonists do not cause a flare or microsurges. They also achieve a castrate level of testosterone faster than LHRH agonists.*
2. Examples—degarelix, relugolix, abarelix.
   a. Degarelix (Firmagon®)—degarelix achieves a castrate level of testosterone in > 95% of men by 3 days after the initial injection without causing a testosterone flare. At one year, degarelix and an LHRH agonist are equally effective. Injection site irritation is more common with degarelix than with LHRH agonists (40% versus < 3%). For dosing, see page 748.
   b. Relugolix (Orgovyx™)—relugolix achieves a castrate level of testosterone in > 95% of men by 15 days after the initial injection without causing a testosterone flare. Relugolix is the only oral agent that is used for medical castration. For dosing, see page 750. Relugolix can have drug interactions with abiraterone and antiandrogens.
   c. Abarelix is no longer available in the United States. Abarelix has a cumulative risk of systemic allergic reaction, and 30-40% of men stop responding to abarelix by the end of the first year of treatment.
3. Side effects—see page 293.
4. There is limited evidence that orchiectomy and GnRH antagonists are safer than LHRH agonists because they are associated with fewer cardiac events, especially in men with known cardiovascular disease.

Inhibitors of Androgen Synthesis

1. Ketoconazole
   a. Mechanism of action—*ketoconazole is a competitive inhibitor of several cytochrome P450 enzymes*, including 11ß hydroxylase and CYP 17 (a complex that contains 17-α-hydroxylase and C17, 20-lyase).
      i. Inhibition of CYP17 *reduces synthesis of androgen in the adrenal glands and the testicles.*
      ii. Inhibition of 11ß-hydroxylase reduces synthesis of aldosterone and glucocorticoid in the adrenal glands. Thus, glucocorticoid and mineralocorticoid replacement is recommended when using ketoconazole.
   b. Castrate levels of testosterone may occur by 8 hours after a 400 mg oral dose. The effects are dose dependent (testosterone is diminished with 800 mg/day, and eliminated with 1600 mg/day).
   c. Side effects—*hepatotoxicity*, weakness, lethargy, nausea, vomiting, decreased libido. The dose limiting side effect is nausea/vomiting.
   d. Adult dose = ketoconazole 400 mg po TID [Tabs: 200 mg] with a steroid (e.g. hydrocortisone 10 mg po TID or prednisone 5 mg po BID). Side effects may be reduced by starting ketoconazole at 200 mg po TID and increasing the dose to 400 mg po TID as tolerated.
   e. Requires stomach acid for dissolution and absorption. Therefore, give all gastric acid blockers 2 hours after the ketoconazole dose.
   f. Ketoconazole decreases warfarin metabolism.
   g. Avoid use with hypoglycemic agents (causes severe hypoglycemia).

2. Abiraterone (Zytiga®)
   a. Both abiraterone and ketoconazole inhibit CYP17; however, they differ in the following ways:
      i. Abiraterone is a selective inhibitor of CYP17, whereas ketoconazole is a nonselective inhibitor of several cytochrome complexes (including CYP17 and 11ß hydroxylase).
      ii. Abiraterone is a potent inhibitor of CYP17, whereas ketoconazole is a weak inhibitor of CYP17.
      iii. Abiraterone is an irreversible inhibitor, whereas ketoconazole is a reversible competitive inhibitor.
      iv. Abiraterone increases aldosterone (because it inhibits only CYP17), whereas ketoconazole decreases aldosterone (because it also inhibits 11ß hydroxylase).
   b. For details on Abiraterone, see page 239.

3. Aminoglutethimide
   a. Mechanism of action—aminoglutethimide blocks the transformation of cholesterol to pregnenolone by inhibiting a cytochrome P-450 enzyme called CYP11A1 (also called P450scc), which reduces the synthesis of glucocorticoids, aldosterone, and androgens. Thus, glucocorticoid and mineralocorticoid replacement is required when using aminoglutethimide. *This medication is largely of historical interest is typically not used anymore.*
   b. Side effects—hypotension, nausea, vomiting, fatigue, anorexia, depression, edema, skin rashes.
   c. Adult dose = aminoglutethimide 250 mg po q 6 hours.

Prolactin Antagonists

1. Mechanism of action—blocks prolactin secretion by the pituitary.
2. In those who are no longer responsive to standard hormone therapy, these agents can relieve symptoms, especially bone pain.
3. Examples—bromocriptine, levodopa.

5-α-reductase Inhibitors (5ARIs)

1. For treatment of prostate cancer, the NCCN guideline states that there is no proven benefit to adding a 5α-reductase inhibitor to standard androgen deprivation.

2. In general, the use of 5ARIs to prevent progression during surveillance of prostate cancer is not recommended. The REDEEM trial randomized men with low risk prostate cancer (cT1-T2a, Gleason score = 5 or 6, and PSA ≤ 11) to placebo or dutasteride 0.5 mg po q day. Follow up 12-core prostate biopsies were performed at 18 and 36 months. After 3 years, dutasteride did *not* alter progression to Gleason grade 4 or to cancer comprising > 50% of the tissue in a positive core. Dutasteride appeared to reduce the risk of having ≥ 4 cores involved with cancer, but the difference was not statistically significant. This study was underpowered and could not adequately assess pathological endpoints. However, retrospective data with long term follow up suggests that 5ARI may reduce pathologic progression during surveillance.

3. For details on 5α-reductase inhibitors, see page 318.

Nonsteroidal Antiandrogens

1. Mechanism of action—antiandrogens inhibit the androgen receptor (they prevent the binding of DHT and testosterone to the androgen receptor). Androgen receptors in the pituitary and hypothalamus are also blocked, which prevents androgens from engaging in negative feedback and leads to an increase in the serum level of LH. Thus, adrenal and gonadal androgen production actually increases.

2. Libido and potency are preserved because testosterone is not reduced.

3. Excess testosterone may be converted to estrogen by aromatase (which is in adipose tissue), resulting in gynecomastia.

4. First generation antiandrogens (flutamide, bicalutamide, nilutamide)—for more details, see page 241.

   a. Flutamide (Eulexin®)
      - Flutamide half life = 6-8 hours.
      - Adult dose = flutamide 250 mg po TID [Caps: 125 mg].
      - Side effects—hepatotoxicity, gynecomastia, diarrhea, nausea, and vomiting. Gastrointestinal side effects are the dose limiting factor.

   b. Bicalutamide (Casodex®)
      - Bicalutamide half life = approximately 5.8 days.
      - Adult dose = bicalutamide 50 mg po q day [Tabs: 50 mg].
      - Side effects–similar to flutamide but less gastrointestinal effects.

   c. Nilutamide (Nilandron™)
      - Nilutamide half life = approximately 45 hours.
      - Adult dose = nilutamide 300 mg po q day for 30 days, then 150 mg po q day thereafter [Tabs: 50 mg].
      - Side effects—visual disturbances, alcohol intolerance, rarely interstitial pneumonitis, nausea, vomiting.

5. Second generation antiandrogens (enzalutamide, apalutamide, darolutamide)—see page 242.

Steroidal Antiandrogens

1. Mechanism of action—inhibits binding of DHT and testosterone to the nuclear androgen receptors, inhibits 5α-reductase, and has negative feedback on the hypothalamic-pituitary axis.

2. Side effects—include weight gain.

3. Examples—megestrol acetate (Megace®), cyproterone acetate (cyproterone is not available in the United States).

Impact of Castration on Prostate Tissue and Testosterone

Testosterone Flare and Clinical Flare

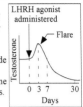

1. *Flare is caused by LHRH agonists.* When an LHRH agonist is started, testosterone increases temporarily ("testosterone flare"), which can worsen cancer related signs and symptoms ("clinical flare"). Symptoms that may occur during clinical flare include bone pain, spinal cord compression, and urinary obstruction. The increase in testosterone over baseline peaks in 3-4 days and lasts for approximately 7 days.

2. Flare is *not* caused by orchiectomy, antiandrogens, GnRH antagonists, or estrogens.

3. Flare can be prevented by using one of the following options.
   a. Use orchiectomy or a GnRH antagonist instead of an LHRH agonist.
   b. Start an antiandrogen before the LHRH agonist—antiandrogens prevent *clinical flare* by blocking the androgen receptor, but they do not prevent the testosterone flare. Most commonly the antiandrogen is started either 7 days before or at the same time as the LHRH agonist, and then continued for 4 weeks. Theoretically, it may be beneficial to achieve a steady state antiandrogen level, which can be achieved by starting the antiandrogen 4 half lives before starting the LHRH agonist.
      • Start flutamide $\geq$ *32 hours* before the LHRH agonist ($T_{1/2}$ = 6-8 hours)
      • Start nilutamide $\geq$ *8 days* before the LHRH agonist ($T_{1/2}$ = 45 hours)
      • Start bicalutamide $\geq$ *24 days* before the LHRH agonist ($T_{1/2}$ = 6 days)
   c. Start ketoconazole before the LHRH agonist—since ketoconazole may take up to 72 hours to maximally block testosterone production, consider starting it at least 3 days before the LHRH agonist.

Testosterone Level During Androgen Deprivation Therapy

1. Chance of achieving castrate testosterone
   a. Orchiectomy—usually achieves and sustains T $\leq$ 20 ng/dl.
   b. LHRH agonists—7% of men fail to achieve nadir T < 20 ng/dl and 1% fail to achieve a nadir T < 50 ng/dl.
   c. GnRH antagonists—failure to achieve nadir T < 50 ng/dl is < 1%.

2. Testosterone microsurge (breakthrough)—a temporary increase in testosterone that occurs immediately after a scheduled non-initial dose of LHRH agonist during continuous ADT. Testosterone microsurges occur in 10% of men receiving a LHRH agonist.
   a. Retrospective data suggests that men with a microsurge T > 20 ng/dl have a higher risk of progressing to castration resistant prostate cancer.
   b. Microsurges do not occur with GnRH antagonists or orchiectomy.

Therapy for Prostate Cancer	Initial Dose: T Flare	Subsequent Doses: T Microsurge§	Usual Time to Castrate T (range)°
Orchiectomy	No	No	3 hours (2-12 hours)
Ketoconazole†	No	Unknown	8 hours (8-72 hours)
LHRH agonists	Yes	Yes (~10% of the time)	30 days
GnRH antagonists	No	No	Degarelix: 3 days, Relugolix: 15 days
Intravenous DES‡	No	Unknown	*
Oral DES	No	Unknown	(10-60 days)

T = testosterone; DES = diethylstilbestrol
† At a dose of 400 mg po q 8 hours.   § Microsurge is defined as T > 50 ng/dl.
‡ At a dose of 1 gram IV q 24 hours.   ° Castrate T is defined as T < 50 ng/dl.
* Produces approximately 50% decrease in T within 24 hours.

Pathologic Changes in the Prostate From Androgen Deprivation
1. The most common pathological changes include:
   a. Atrophy of the glands—this compresses the basal cells closer so they look multi-layer (i.e. basal cell prominence).
   b. Decreased gland density.
   c. Increased fibromuscular stroma.
2. Other changes that can also be seen—apoptosis (cell death), nuclear pyknosis (dense nuclei), intracytoplasmic vacuolization, inflammation.
3. *Necrosis is rarely seen.*

Morbidity From Medical or Surgical Castration

General Information
1. The side effects from castration increase with the duration of treatment.
2. Androgen deprivation with castration may increase the risk of
   a. Changes in body habitus—including gynecomastia (see page 294), testicular atrophy, loss of muscle mass (decreased lean body weight), weight gain (obesity), and increased subcutaneous fat.
   b. Adverse lipid profile—elevated total cholesterol, LDL, triglycerides, and HDL. Most lipid changes occur within 3 months of castration.
   c. Diabetes (insulin resistance)—castration can increase fasting insulin level and generate a small increase in glycosylated hemoglobin. The risk increases within 4 months of castration, but does not appear to progressively increase with a longer duration of therapy.
   d. Cardiovascular disease—cardiovascular risk may arise from castration induced hyperlipidemia, insulin resistance, and obesity. The AHA/ACS/AUA advisory states "whether an association (or an actual cause-and-effect relationship) between ADT use and cardiovascular events and mortality exists remains controversial".
      i. LHRH agonists and bilateral orchiectomy may increase the risk of coronary artery disease, heart attack, prolonged QT interval, sudden cardiac death, and death from cardiovascular causes.
      ii. *The risk of cardiac mortality from ADT may be highest in men with a history of congestive heart failure or myocardial infarction caused by coronary artery disease.*
      iii. There is limited evidence that orchiectomy and GnRH antagonists are safer than LHRH agonists because they are associated with fewer cardiac events, especially in men with known cardiovascular disease.
   e. Anemia—normocytic anemia (normal MCV). Hemoglobin may decline within the first month after castration and often reaches its nadir by 6 months after castration. This anemia can be corrected by either stopping androgen deprivation or by administering erythropoietin.
   f. Fatigue—may be caused by anemia or low testosterone.
   g. Osteoporosis—see page 295.
   h. Periodontal disease—no increase in cavities, but there is a higher risk of plaque, gingival recession, and other indicators of periodontal disease.
   i. Sexual dysfunction—decreased libido and erectile dysfunction.
   j. Infertility
   k. Hot flashes—hot flashes can be frequent and bothersome.
   l. Cognitive deficits—recent data suggests that androgen deprivation may cause cognitive deficits such as impaired memory.
3. Long term castration may reduce the risk death from prostate cancer, but it may increase the risk of death from other causes (such as cardiovascular disease). Thus, long term androgen deprivation may not improve overall survival.

Testing for Side Effects in Men Receiving Androgen Deprivation
1. Cardiovascular risk factors—the AHA/ACS/AUA advisory recommends periodic follow up including blood pressure, lipid profile, and blood glucose. Because metabolic changes tend to occur within the first 3 months after castration, it is reasonable to conduct the initial evaluation starting 3-6 months after castration. The interval of subsequent evaluations is at the discretion of the physician.
2. Osteoporosis—the NOF recommends a DEXA scan at the time of castration and at least every 2 years thereafter to assess bone mineral density (see page 295).
3. Anemia—it may be prudent to monitor the blood count for anemia.

Hot Flashes
1. Hot flashes can be caused by LHRH agonists, GnRH antagonists, bilateral orchiectomy, and nonsteroidal antiandrogens.
2. Estrogens and progesterones do not cause hot flashes. In fact, they are used to prevent hot flashes.
3. Preventing hot flashes
   a. Progesterone—megestrol acetate 20 mg po BID is one of the most effective regimens, and has the least side effects. Titrate the dose as necessary. Weight gain is common.
   b. Estrogen—estrogens may cause painful gynecomastia, thrombosis, and cardiac side effects. Examples include: transdermal estradiol 0.05-0.10 mg patch applied twice a week; diethylstilbestrol 0.5 mg po q day.
   c. Clonidine—venlafaxine appears to be more effective.
   d. Venlafaxine—starting dose is often 37.5 mg/day. If necessary, it can be titrated up to 75 mg/day. Other serotonin reuptake inhibitors (such as paroxetine, sertraline, and fluoxetine) have also been used.
   e. Vitamin E 800 IU po q day—long-term use (> 1 year) of more than 400 IU per day may increase the risk of heart failure and mortality.
   f. Gabapentin
   g. Acupuncture

Gynecomastia from Androgen Deprivation
1. Gynecomastia (GM) is enlargement of the breasts. GM can be painful.
2. GM can be caused by medical castration, surgical castration, antiandrogens, 5α-reductase inhibitors, and estrogens.
3. GM is more common with estrogens and antiandrogens than with medical or surgical castration. 5α-reductase inhibitors rarely cause GM.
4. GM may resolve after stopping androgen deprivation. However, it is more likely to resolve when the duration of therapy is short (e.g. < 6 months).
5. Evaluation includes a breast and lymph node exam. Classify the breast size by Tanner stage or by measuring the breast. A mammogram and biopsy may be indicated in men with a family history of breast cancer, focal breast enlargement/pain, or a suspicious breast exam (lump, dimple, etc.).
6. Treatment of benign GM from androgen deprivation
   a. If possible, stop the causative agent.
   b. External beam radiation (XRT)—a single fraction of 12-15 Gy to the breasts *before* administering an antiandrogen or an estrogen has been shown to decrease the risk of GM. The long-term risks of breast XRT are unknown and some patients still develop GM.
   c. Tamoxifen—10 to 20 mg po per day can reduce breast size and pain. It is most effective when it is started before or soon after GM develops.
   d. Breast reduction surgery (liposuction or excision of tissue)—reduces breast size and can reduce breast pain. Surgery is often necessary when GM is severe (Tanner stage $\geq$ III) or long standing (> 1 year).

Osteoporosis from Androgen Deprivation

General Information

1. Osteoporosis is defined as low bone mineral density (BMD) and reduced bone mass that weakens the bones and increases the risk of bone fracture.
2. Medical and surgical castration can cause osteoporosis. Antiandrogen monotherapy and estrogens to do not cause osteoporosis.
3. *Most of the bone loss from androgen deprivation therapy (ADT) occurs within the first year of therapy.*
4. *A longer duration of ADT is associated with a greater decline in BMD and a higher risk of skeletal fractures.*
   a. Bone density may decline as much as 10% during the first year of therapy and by 1-3% per year thereafter.
   b. Men on long-term ADT have at least a 5 fold higher risk of osteoporosis related fractures than healthy, age-matched controls. Some fractures occur during the first year of ADT. *Pathologic fractures in men receiving ADT have been correlated with decreased overall survival.*
   c. *Most osteoporosis related fractures are caused by falling.* ADT causes fatigue and reduced muscle mass, which may increase the risk of falling.
5. Men about to undergo ADT have a lower BMD than healthy age matched controls. Thus, they are at risk for osteoporosis even before ADT is started.
6. Osteoclast inhibitors (such as bisphosphonates and denosumab) reduce the risk of osteoporosis and skeletal fractures in men on ADT.

Testing for Osteoporosis in Men on ADT

1. History and physical exam—including assessment for risk factors. *Since most osteoporosis related fractures are caused by falling, it is important to assess the patient's risk for falling and for osteoporosis.*
   a. Risk factors for osteoporosis—hypogonadism, current smoking, high caffeine intake, alcohol intake (> 3 drinks a day), steroid use, physical inactivity, thin body habitus, older age, vitamin D deficiency, low calcium intake, chronic metabolic acidosis.
   b. Risk factors for falling—*urinary urgency or frequency (causes more visits to the bathroom, and thus increases the circumstances when a fall can occur)*, impaired mobility, muscle weakness, poor balance, medications causing sedation or dizziness, orthostatic hypotension, impaired vision, impaired cognition, arrhythmias, previous falls.
2. Blood tests may be considered—blood tests may include serum calcium, creatinine, and vitamin D 25-OH.
3. Bone mineral density (BMD)—usually measured using dual energy x-ray absorptiometry (DEXA). *BMD correlates with bone strength and risk of future fracture.* Fracture risk increases exponentially as BMD decreases.
4. BMD from DEXA is reported using 3 measures
   a. Grams of mineral per area of bone scanned (g/cm^2).
   b. Z-score—the difference between the patient's actual BMD and the expected BMD for the patient's age and gender (expressed in standard deviations above or below the mean).
   c. T-score—the difference between the patient's actual BMD and the BMD of a young normal patient of the same gender (expressed in standard deviations above or below the mean).
5. The World Health Organization Fracture Risk Algorithm (FRAX®) provides the 10-year estimated risk of fracture for men based on BMD. FRAX® risk estimates can be determined using the online calculation tool or paper charts at the FRAX® website (www.shef.ac.uk/FRAX/).

Treatment of Osteoporosis in Men on ADT (Based on NOF Guideline)

1. Recommendations for all patients on long-term androgen deprivation
   a. DEXA at baseline and at least every two years thereafter to assess BMD.
   b. Adequate dietary intake of vitamin D and calcium—the recommended intake is vitamin D3 800-1000 IU po q day and at 1000-1200 mg calcium po q day (supplements may be necessary to achieve this).
   c. Reduce risk factors for osteoporosis—stop smoking, minimize alcohol and caffeine intake, avoid steroid use, and engage in weight bearing and muscle strengthening exercise.
   d. Minimize the risk of falling—in men with urinary urgency or frequency, consider using a portable handheld urinal, a condom catheter, diapers, or a bedside commode.
2. The National Osteoporosis Foundation (NOF) recommends treatment of osteoporosis when any of the following criteria are met.
   a. DEXA T-score ≤ -2.5 in the femoral neck, lumbar spine, or total hip.
   b. DEXA T-score between -1.0 and -2.5 in the femoral neck, lumbar spine, or total hip with either of the following criteria
      i. 10-year probability of hip fracture ≥ 3% (based on FRAX®).
      ii. 10-year probability of any major osteoporosis related fracture ≥ 20% (based on FRAX®).
   c. Vertebral or hip fracture
3. When treatment of men on ADT is indicated based on the NOF recommendations above, start denosumab or a bisphosphonate.
   a. Denosumab—FDA approved to increase BMD in men who are receiving ADT and who are at high risk for skeletal fracture.
   b. Bisphosphonates—zoledronic acid and alendronate have both been shown to increase bone mineral density specifically in men on ADT. Both drugs are FDA approved to treat men with osteoporosis regardless of the cause (thus, they are not specifically restricted to men on ADT).
4. After treatment for osteoporosis is started, the NOF recommends obtaining a DEXA in 1 to 2 years, and then every 2 years thereafter.

Denosumab 60 mg (Prolia®)

1. Denosumab 60 mg subcutaneous injection every 6 months is FDA approved to increase bone mass in men receiving androgen deprivation for *non-metastatic* prostate cancer and who are at high risk for skeletal fracture. At a higher dose and frequency (120 mg subcutaneous injection every 4 weeks), denosumab is FDA approved to prevent skeletal related events in patients with solid tumors that are *metastatic to bone* (see page 259).
2. Mechanism of action—*denosumab is a monoclonal antibody that binds to RANK ligand and prevents it from activating the RANK receptor; thus, denosumab prevents bone resorption by inhibiting osteoclast activity.*
3. Compared to placebo, Denosumab 60 mg significantly improves bone mineral density and reduces the incidence of new vertebral fractures (1.5% vs. 3.9%) over 3 years of treatment.
4. Prior to treatment
   a. Check calcium level and correct hypocalcemia.
   b. Perform routine oral examination. Dental examination and appropriate preventative dentistry should be considered in patients with poor oral hygiene, periodontal disease, dental implants, recent dental/oral surgery, or pocket risk factors that may increase osteonecrosis of the jaw.

5. Dose in men at high risk for fracture receiving androgen deprivation for *non-metastatic* prostate cancer—denosumab 60 mg subcutaneous injection (in upper thigh, upper arm, or abdomen) every 6 months, with oral administration of at least 1000 mg calcium daily and at least 400 IU vitamin D3 daily.

6. Side effects
   a. The most common side effects are arthralgia, back pain, and nasopharyngitis.
   b. Denosumab 60 mg causes severe hypocalcemia in < 2% of patients. Patients on dialysis or with creatinine clearance < 30 ml/min have a higher risk of hypocalcemia.
   c. Denosumab 60 mg may cause severe hypophosphatemia.
   d. Denosumab 60 mg rarely causes osteonecrosis of the jaw (< 1%).

7. During therapy
   a. In men with renal insufficiency, monitor calcium, phosphate, and magnesium.
   b. Monitor for symptoms of osteonecrosis of the jaw (pain, numbness, or swelling in the jaw or inside the mouth).
   c. Preventative dentistry is recommended during therapy. Stopping denosumab 60 mg for invasive dental procedures should be considered on an individual basis.

8. Patients should be transitioned to another antiresorptive agent if denosumab 60 mg is discontinued because vertebral fractures have been reported after stopping denosumab 60 mg. When denosumab is stopped, bone turnover increases above pretreatment level for about 24 months after the last dose of denosumab 60 mg.

REFERENCES

General

de Bono JS, et al: Abiraterone and increased survival in metastatic prostate cancer. N Engl J Med, 364: 1995, 2011.

Maatman TJ, Gupta MK, Montie JE: Effectiveness of castration versus intravenous estrogen therapy in producing rapid endocrine control of metastatic cancer of the prostate. J Urol, 133: 620, 1985.

NCCN—National Comprehensive Cancer Network clinical practice guidelines in oncology: Prostate cancer. V.1.2020, 2020 (www.nccn.org).

Smith Jr. JA, et al: Clinical effects of gonadotropin-releasing hormone analog in metastatic carcinoma of the prostate. Urology, 25(2): 106, 1985.

Yoon FH, et al: Testosterone recovery after prolonged androgen suppression in patients with prostate cancer. J Urol, 180(4): 1438, 2008.

5-α-reductase Inhibitors

Fleshner NE, et al: Dutasteride in localized prostate cancer management: the REDEEM randomized, double blind, placebo controlled trial. Lancet, 379: 1103, 2012.

Ashrafi AN, et al: Five alpha reductase inhibitors in men undergoing active surveillance for prostate cancer: impact on treatment and reclassification after 6 years of follow up. World J Urol, 2021 [e-published ahead of print] (https://doi.org/10.1007/s00345-021-03644-2)

Flare and Flare Prevention

Labrie F, Dupont A, Belanger A, et al: Flutamide eliminates the risk of disease flare in prostatic cancer patients treated with a luteinizing hormone-releasing hormone agonist. J Urol, 138: 804, 1987.

Noguchi K, et al: Inhibition of PSA flare in prostate cancer patients by administration of flutamide for 2 weeks before initiation of treatment with slow-releasing LH-RH agonist. Int J Clin Oncol, 6(1): 29, 2001.

Tsushima T, et al: Optimal starting time for flutamide to prevent disease flare in prostate cancer patients treated with a gonadotropin-releasing hormone agonist. Urol Int, 66(3): 135, 2001.

Castration Level of Testosterone and Microsurges

Morote J, et al: Refining clinically significant castration levels in patients with prostate cancer receiving continuous androgen deprivation therapy. J Urol, 178(4): 1290, 2007.

Oefelein MG, et al: Reassessment of the definition of castrate levels of testosterone: implications for clinical decision making. Urology, 56: 1021, 2000.

Tombal B: Appropriate castration with luteinizing hormone releasing hormone agonist: what is the optimal level of testosterone. Eur Urol, 4 (suppl): 14, 2005.

Side Effects: General

Famili P, et al: The effect of androgen deprivation therapy on periodontal disease in men with prostate cancer. J Urol, 177(3): 921, 2007.

Kumar RJ, et al: Adverse events associated with hormonal therapy for prostate cancer. Rev Urol, 7(suppl 5): S37, 2005.

Saylor P, Smith M: Metabolic complications of androgen deprivation therapy for prostate cancer. J Urol, 181: 1998, 2009.

Side Effects: Gynecomastia

Dobs A, Darkes MJM: Incidence and management of gynecomastia in men treated for prostate cancer. J Urol, 174(5): 1737, 2005.

McCleod DG, Iversen P: Gynecomastia in patients with prostate cancer: a review of treatment options. Urology, 56: 713, 2000.

Side Effects: Cardiovascular Disease and Diabetes

Alibhai SM, et al: Impact of androgen deprivation therapy on cardiovascular disease and diabetes. J Clin Oncol, 27(21): 3452, 2009.

D'Amico AV, et al: Influence of androgen suppression therapy for prostate cancer on the frequency and timing of fatal myocardial infarctions. J Clin Oncol, 25(17): 2007.

Efstathiou JA, et al: Cardiovascular mortality and duration of androgen deprivation for locally advanced prostate cancer: analysis of RTOG 92-02. Eur Urol, 54(4): 816, 2008.

Keating NL, et al: Diabetes and cardiovascular disease during androgen deprivation therapy for prostate cancer. J Clin Oncol, 24(27): 4448, 2006.

Levine GN, et al: Androgen deprivation therapy in prostate cancer and cardiovascular risk: a science advisory from the American Heart Association, American Cancer Society, and American Urologic Association. Circulation, 121(6): 833, 2010.

Nanda A, et al: Hormonal therapy use for prostate cancer and mortality in men with coronary artery disease induced congestive heart failure or myocardial infarction. JAMA, 302(8): 866, 2009.

Saigal CS, et al: Androgen deprivation therapy increases cardiovascular morbidity in men with prostate cancer. Cancer, 110: 1493, 2007.

Tsai HK, et al: Androgen deprivation therapy for localized prostate cancer and the risk of cardiovascular mortality. J Natl Cancer Inst, 99(20): 1516, 2007.

Side Effects: Osteoporosis

National Osteoporosis Foundation (NOF): Clinicians guide to prevention and treatment of osteoporosis, 2014 (www.bonesource.org/clinical-guidelines).

Daniell HW: Osteoporosis due to androgen deprivation therapy in men with prostate cancer. Urology, 58 (suppl 2A): 101, 2001.

Kiratli BJ, et al: Progressive decrease in bone density over 10 years or androgen deprivation therapy in patients with prostate cancer. Urology, 57:127, 2001.

Neto, AS, et al: Bisphosphonate therapy in patients under androgen deprivation therapy for prostate cancer: a systematic review and meta-analysis. Prostate Cancer and Prostatic Diseases, 15: 36, 2012.

Oefelein MG, et al: Skeletal fracture associated with androgen suppression induced osteoporosis: the clinical incidence and risk factors for patients with prostate cancer. J Urol, 166: 1724, 2001.

Shahinian VB, et al: Risk of fracture after androgen deprivation for prostate cancer. N Engl J Med, 352: 154, 2005.

Smith MR, et al: Bicalutamide monotherapy versus leuprolide monotherapy for prostate cancer: effects on bone mineral density and body composition. J Clin Oncol, 22(13): 2546, 2004.

Smith MR, et al: Gonadotropin releasing hormone agonists and fracture risk: a claims based cohort study of men with non-metastatic prostate cancer. J Clin Oncol, 23(31): 7897, 2005.

Smith MR, et al: Randomized controlled trial of zoledronic acid to prevent bone loss in men receiving androgen deprivation therapy for non-metastatic prostate cancer. J Urol, 169(6): 2008, 2003.

Smith MR, et al: Denosumab in men receiving androgen deprivation therapy for prostate cancer. N Engl J Med, 361: 745 2009.

Stoch SA, et al: Bone loss in men with prostate cancer treated with gonadotropin-releasing hormone agonists. J Clin Endocrinol Metab 86: 2787, 2001.

Side Effects: Cognitive Dysfunction

Green HJ, et al: Quality of life compared during pharmacological treatments and clinical monitoring for non-localized prostate cancer: a randomized controlled trial. BJU Int, 93: 975, 2004 [update of BJU Int 90: 427,2002].

Jenkins VA, et al: Does neoadjuvant hormone therapy for early prostate cancer affect cognition? Results of a pilot study. BJU Int, 96(1): 48, 2005.

Joly F, et al: Impact of androgen deprivation therapy on physical and cognitive function, as well as quality of life of patients with non-metastatic prostate cancer. J Urol, 166(6, part 1): 2443, 2006.

Shahinian VB, et al: Risk of the "androgen deprivation syndrome" in men receiving androgen deprivation for prostate cancer. Arch Intern Med, 166(4): 465, 2006.

Side Effects: Hot Flashes

Barton DL, Loprinzi CL, Quella SK, et al: Prospective evaluation of vitamin E for hot flashes in breast cancer survivors. J Clin Oncol, 16(2): 495, 1998.

Gerber GS, Zagaja GP, Ray PS, et al: Transdermal estrogen in the treatment of hot flushes in men with prostate cancer. Urology, 55: 97, 2000.

Hammar M, Frisk J, et al: Acupuncture treatment of vasomotor symptoms in men with prostatic carcinoma: a pilot study. J Urol, 161(3): 853, 1999.

Irani J, et al: Efficacy of venlafaxine, medroxyprogesterone acetate, and cyproterone acetate for the treatment of vasomotor hot flushes in men taking gonadotropin releasing hormone analogues for prostate cancer. Lancet Oncol, 11(2): 147, 2010.

Loprinzi CL, Michalak JC, Quella SK, et al: Megestrol acetate for the prevention of hot flashes. N Engl J Med, 331(6): 347, 1994.

Loprinzi CL, et al: A phase III randomized, double blind, placebo controlled trial of gabapentin in the management of hot flashes in men. Ann Oncol, 20(3): 542, 2009.

Quella SK, Loprinzi CL, Sloan J, et al: Pilot evaluation of venlafaxine for the treatment of hot flashes in men undergoing androgen ablation therapy for prostate cancer. J Urol, 162(1): 98, 1999.

Quella SK, Loprinzi CL, Sloan JA, et al: Long term use of megestrol acetate by cancer survivors for the treatment of hot flashes. Cancer, 82(9): 1784, 1998.

Smith Jr. JA: Management of hot flushes due to endocrine therapy for prostate carcinoma. Oncology, 10(9): 1319, 1996.

PROSTATE SPECIFIC ANTIGEN (PSA)

General Information

1. PSA, a glycoprotein in the kallikrein family, is produced by the prostate epithelial cells and deposited in the seminal fluid.
2. PSA acts as a serine protease and cleaves semenogelin, a protein in seminal fluid. Cleavage of semenogelin reduces semen viscosity (i.e. it causes semen liquefaction) and leads to greater sperm motility.
3. The mechanism by which PSA enters the systemic circulation in unknown. The PSA blood test measures the concentration of PSA in the circulation.
4. In the circulation, total PSA = free PSA + complexed PSA. Complexed PSA is bound to other proteins (mostly to $\alpha 1$-antichymotrypsin, with a smaller amount bound to $\alpha 2$-macroglobulin), whereas free PSA is not bound to other proteins.
5. PSA half life is approximately 2.2 to 3.2 days.
6. PSA does *not* vary during the day (no variance with circadian rhythms).
7. PSA is androgen dependent (its production is stimulated by androgens).

Conditions That Can Alter The PSA Level

1. Conditions that can elevate total PSA
   a. Prostate cancer
   b. Benign prostatic enlargement (BPH)
   c. Infections (prostatitis, bacterial cystitis)—antibiotic treatment will cause the PSA to decline in nearly 30% of men with chronic prostatitis.
   d. Prostate manipulation or trauma within the past several days (e.g. cystoscopy, urethral catheterization, prostate massage, prostate biopsy, bicycling). Prostate exam (without excessive prostate pressure) does not alter PSA appreciably.
   e. Ejaculation within a few days before the test may increase PSA levels.
   f. PSA increases with age.
2. Conditions that can reduce total PSA
   a. 5α-reductase inhibitors (finasteride, dutasteride) typically reduce total PSA by approximately 50% after 6-12 months of treatment, although the maximum PSA reduction and the time to reach it are highly variable. These medications usually do not alter the percent free PSA. Using a 5α-reductase inhibitor appears to improve the ability of PSA to predict the presence of prostate cancer, particularly high grade cancers. Men whose PSA does not decline by 50% within 12 months after starting a 5α-reductase inhibitor or whose PSA rises while on a 5α-reductase inhibitor have a higher risk for prostate cancer; therefore, prostate biopsy is often recommended in these men.
   b. Low serum testosterone—e.g. hypogonadism, testosterone lowering medications (e.g. ketoconazole, LHRH agonists, antiandrogens).
   c. Prostatic surgery—for surgery that removes or destroys part of the prostate, PSA may rise immediately after surgery because of prostate manipulation, but with longer follow up, PSA usually declines.
   d. Prostate radiation often elevates PSA during and immediately after radiation; however, with longer follow up, PSA usually declines.

3. Hemodialysis and peritoneal dialysis do not alter total PSA, but they do alter free PSA. Therefore, *free PSA should not be used in dialysis patients.*
4. There are several different PSA assays. *The PSA can vary by up to 25% between different assays; thus, PSA values from different assays are not interchangeable.* There is no reliable conversion factor between assays.

BPH and PSA
1. In men with BPH, a high PSA increases the risk of prostate growth, deterioration of urinary symptoms, low urine flow rate, acute urinary retention, surgery for BPH, and BPH progression.
2. In men with BPH, serum PSA is proportional to prostate volume. Thus, men with larger prostates tend to have a higher PSA.

Prostate Cancer and PSA

Using PSA to Screen for Prostate Cancer—see page 172.

Risk of Prostate Cancer Based on PSA—see page 184.

Prostate Cancer and Pre-treatment PSA—see page 198 and page 201.

Prostate Cancer and Post-treatment PSA—see page 231.

PSA Kinetics
1. PSA doubling time (PSADT) versus PSA velocity (PSAV)
   a. PSAV is based on the assumption that PSA increases in a linear fashion, and it can be calculated using a simple formula.

$$PSAV = 0.5 \times \left(\frac{PSA_2 - PSA_1}{Time_1} + \frac{PSA_3 - PSA_2}{Time_2} \right)$$	PSA_1 = 1st PSA (ng/ml) PSA_2 = 2nd PSA (ng/ml) PSA_3 = 3rd PSA (ng/ml) $Time_1$ = years from PSA_1 to PSA_2 $Time_2$ = years from PSA_2 to PSA_3

   b. PSADT is the number of months it takes for the PSA to double. PSADT is based on the assumption that PSA increases in an exponential fashion. The calculation of PSADT is complex and usually requires a sophisticated computer algorithm.
   c. At least 3 PSA values are required to calculate PSA kinetics. The PSA values must be far enough apart in time to reflect meaningful changes (e.g. at least 3 months apart when PSA kinetics are used for prostate cancer screening, and at least 1 month apart when used for advanced prostate cancer). PSA kinetic calculations may be more reliable when using a greater number of PSA values.
   d. A short PSADT and a high PSAV are indicators of poor prognosis.
2. PSA doubling time (PSADT)
   a. In men with biochemical relapse after curative therapy, local recurrence is more likely when the PSADT is long (e.g. > 1 year), whereas systemic recurrence is more likely when PSADT is short (e.g. < 6 months).
   b. In men with biochemical recurrence after curative therapy (M0 with rising PSA) or with metastatic disease (M1), *PSADT < 3 months (at any time before or after castration) is associated with a higher risk of death from prostate cancer.* Prognosis improves as the PSADT increases.
3. PSA velocity (PSAV)
   a. PSAV can be used for prostate cancer screening (see page 182).
   b. *Men with a pretreatment PSAV > 2 ng/ml/yr before curative therapy are more like to have high grade tumors, high T stage, and lymph node metastasis. They are also more likely to recur and more likely to die from prostate cancer.*

REFERENCES

General

Catalona WJ, Partin A, Slawin KM, et al: Use of the percentage of free prostate-specific antigen to enhance differentiation of prostate cancer from benign prostatic disease. JAMA, 279 (19): 1542, 1998.

D'Amico AV, et al: Preoperative PSA velocity and the risk of death from prostate cancer after radical prostatectomy. N Engl J Med, 351: 125, 2004.

Draisma G, et al: Lead times and over detection due to prostate specific antigen screening: estimated from the European Randomized Study of Screening for Prostate Cancer. J Natl Cancer Inst, 95(12): 868, 2003.

Partin AW, et al: Complexed prostate specific antigen improves specificity for prostate cancer detection: results of a prospective multicenter clinical trial. J Urol, 170, 1787, 2003.

Thompson IM, Pauler DK, et al: Prevalence of prostate cancer among men with a prostate specific antigen level ≤ 4.0 ng/ml. N Engl J Med, 350: 2239, 2004.

PSA Kinetics

Arlen PM, et al: Prostate Specific Antigen Workshop Group guidelines on prostate specific antigen doubling time. J Urol, 179: 2181, 2008.

D'Amico AV, et al: Preoperative PSA velocity and the risk of death from prostate cancer after radical prostatectomy. N Engl J Med, 351: 125, 2004.

D'Amico AV, et al: Pretreatment PSA velocity and risk of death from prostate cancer following external beam radiation therapy. JAMA, 294: 440, 2005.

Eggener SE, et al: Prediagnosis prostate specific antigen velocity is associated with risk of prostate cancer progression following brachytherapy and external beam radiation therapy. J Urol, 74(4: Part 1), 1399, 2006.

Freedland SJ, et al: Death in patients with recurrent prostate cancer after radical prostatectomy: PSA doubling time subgroups and their associated contributions to all cause mortality. J Clin Oncol, 25(13): 1765, 2007.

Hussain M, et al: Absolute prostate specific antigen value after androgen deprivation is a strong independent predictor of survival in new metastatic prostate cancer: data from Southwest Oncology Group Trial 9346 (INT-0162). J. Clin Oncol, 24(24):3984, 2006.

Kwak C, et al: Prognostic significance of the nadir prostate specific antigen level after hormone therapy for prostate cancer. J Urol, 168(3): 995, 2002.

Loeb S, et al: PSA velocity is associated with Gleason score in radical prostatectomy specimen: marker for prostate cancer aggressiveness. Urology, 72(5): 1116, 2008.

Patel DA, et al: Preoperative PSA velocity is an independent prognostic factor for relapse after radical prostatectomy. J Clin Oncol, 23(25): 6157, 2005.

Sengupta S, et al: Prostate specific antigen kinetics in the management of prostate cancer. J Urol, 179: 821, 2008.

Stewart AJ, et al: Prostate specific antigen nadir and cancer specific mortality following hormonal therapy for prostate specific antigen failure. J Clin Oncol, 23(27): 6556, 2005.

Tomioka S, et al: Significance of prostate specific antigen doubling time on survival of patients with hormone refractory prostate cancer and bone metastasis. Int J Urol, 14(2): 123, 2007.

Wieder JA, Belldegrun A: The utility of PSA doubling time for prostate cancer recurrence. Mayo Clin Proc, 76(6): 571, 2001.

Zhou P, et al: Predictors of prostate cancer specific mortality after radical prostatectomy or radiation therapy. J Clin Oncol, 23(28): 6992, 2005.

Index

A

B